COMMUNICATIVE DISORDERS
IN CHILDREN

C. Weiss

COMMUNICATIVE DISORDERS IN CHILDREN

fifth edition

Jon Eisenson

SAN FRANCISCO STATE UNIVERSITY

Mardel Ogilvie

PROFESSOR EMERITA
HERBERT H. LEHMAN COLLEGE OF THE CITY UNIVERSITY OF NEW YORK

MACMILLAN PUBLISHING CO., INC.
NEW YORK
COLLIER MACMILLAN PUBLISHERS
London

Macmillan Publishing Co., Inc.
866 Third Avenue, New York, New York 10022

Collier Macmillan Canada, Inc.

Library of Congress Cataloging in Publication Data

Eisenson, Jon, 1907–
   Communicative disorders in children.

   Includes bibliography and index.
   1. Communicative disorders in children.
I. Ogilvie, Mardel, 1909–   II. Title.
RJ496.C67E47   1983   618.92′855   82-15331
ISBN 0-02-332100-8   AACR2

Printing: 1 2 3 4 5 6 7 8   Year: 3 4 5 6 7 8 9

PREFACE

Communicative Disorders in Children, 5/e was initially intended to be a fifth edition of *Speech Correction in the Schools*. However, as we the co-authors revised materials and shared viewpoints with one another, we appreciated that we were involved with a book, sufficiently different in scope and content, to deserve a new title. The present effort is intended for professionals who will have the responsibility of identifying and improving the language and speech—the communicative abilities—of children with impairments of sufficient degree to interfere with normal communication. The professional persons include speech/language clinicians, psychologists, teachers of children with learning disabilities, and the classroom teacher. The impact of Public Law 94-142 and the recent emphasis on "mainstreaming" rather than segregating and separately teaching exceptional children who are handicapped increase the incidence of contacts that the classroom teacher has with children with communicative disabilities. Now, more than ever before, the professional person working in an educational setting, must share much of the knowledge and to some degree the responsibilities of co-professionals in the team effort to identify and provide remedial services to the handicapped child. These children who have communicative handicaps add to this challenge.

Although the contents and the organization of *Communicative Disorders in Children*, 5/e are the responsibility of the authors, we have been helped by the suggestions of critic-readers. These, for the most part, are colleagues who, at our request, advised us as to the weaknesses as well as the strengths of the predecessor to this book and indicated what modifications and additions they would like to see in a revision of our textbook. We feel that we were graciously and well advised.

We decided on the title *Communicative Disorders in Children* 5/e, as most appropriate for the contents and emphasis of this book. Other titles that we considered included *Language and Speech Disorders of Children, Remediation for Children with Language and Speech Disorders,* and *Disorders of Communication in Children.* We note that each of the titles includes the word *children* as an indication of the limitation of the scope of the book. Problems of adults—the acquired aphasias, dysarthrias, and apraxias—are well covered in several recently published textbooks. We continue to devote our efforts in this volume to as full an exposition of the communicative problems of children as the size of the book allows.

We are using the term language/speech clinician rather than speech pathologist because we believe that the former term has more positive implications than the latter. Admittedly this is a personal preference. Other terms, appropriate for professional persons who work with children with communicative disorders related to impairments of language and speech, include speech clinician, teacher of speech and hearing handicapped, speech and hearing therapist, and logopedist— the last a term used in much of the Western world outside of the United States. Whatever the designation, we are identifying persons whose professional education and clinical training have prepared them to diagnose and provide remedial services to children whose linguistic, motor, vocal, or hearing handicaps impair their potential for effective communication.

The first half of the book deals with general considerations and background knowledge basic for an understanding of the child with a communicative impairment. We begin with a chapter which defines language, shows its relationship to communication, and explains how a speech and/or language handicap can impede effective communication. The ensuing chapters are based on the assumption that fundamentals of information about normal speech and language precede a discussion of speech and language disorders. Accordingly, we include material about inter- and intra-cultural language usage, the clinician's and the child's role in the communicative act, the mechanism for speech, the production of speech sounds, the development of language in children, and the stimulation of language development.

The second half of the book includes a discussion of the specific speech, language, and hearing disorders found in children. We explain the nature and cause of the speech/language disorder and the remediation involved. Because so many children are "mainstreamed" today, we indicate how teachers can supplement and reinforce the work of the speech/language clinician.

CONTENTS

1

Language and Communication

In this book we are concerned with proficiencies in the oral communication act which involves: 1) the speaking of words and sentences intended to have an impact on the listener or listeners, 2) thinking about
the ideas and concepts represented by these words and sentences,
and 3) responding to the ideas expressed. This communicative act, no
matter at what level of maturity, involves not only linguistic skills but
also perceptive, cognitive and social skills. Furthermore, these communicative acts occur in particular settings with different participants
who take on varying roles which result in many kinds of interplay
among the participants.

In such situations, language is the tool which makes the communicative act work. Like all tools, it varies in degree of sophistication. The
language used by participants in "Meet the Press" is much more complex than the language used by a child asking his Mother for his teddy
bear. But this tool that helps the speaker get his message across to his
listeners consists of components which again vary in sophistication according to the situation and the maturity of the speaker. These components, to be considered in more detail later in the chapter, are:

- Phonological—articulated sounds of American English, their com-
  binations, and rules governing them.
- Morphological—pattern of word construction.
- Syntactical—conventions of ordering words and producing sen-
  tences.
- Suprasegmentals or prosody—audible features accompanying one

1

or more speech sounds—features of pitch, stress and juncture, more or less conventional to the language.
? • Pragmatic—meaning of language—taking into account its intent and the social environment in which it occurs.
  • Semantic—meanings of utterances in the light of all of the above.

Obviously this tool, language, does not operate in a vacuum, but rather within a context. Even the physical surroundings affect its use; a classroom, a formal reception hall, a ball field, an elevator, a clinic session have a bearing on the speaker's choice of all the components of language. How the listeners receive the message, how they react to the speaker's ideas and personality, influence the success or lack of success of the message. And the listeners are influenced by the partic-

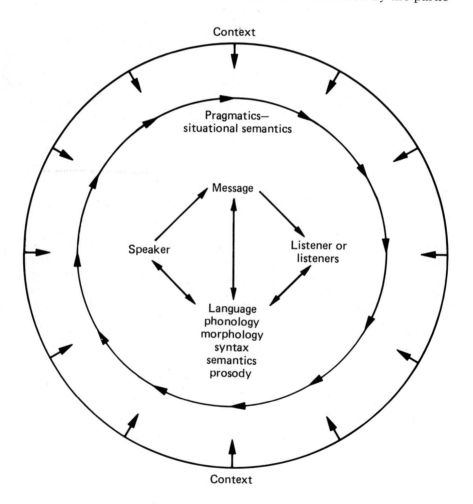

ular components of the language of the message, and in turn influence the use and choice of these components. All of these factors are intertwined as is evident in the diagram.

FUNCTIONS OF LANGUAGE

Since we look at language as a tool of communication, we believe the comprehension of language on any occasion is clearly related to the listener's understanding of the intended use of language by the speaker. We are, therefore, reviewing Halliday's (1977b) categories of the functions of language.

Halliday (1977, pp. 16–18) reports the results of a study of the language of one particular child from nine to eighteen months. He emphasizes that language evolves in the service of certain particular human needs. He constructed the various strands that make up a pattern of thinking about language in functional terms. In the light of his observations of the child, theoretical considerations about linguistic functions—both those essentially linguistic and those extra-linguistic in nature—and lastly sociological theories embodying some concepts of cultural transmission and processes of socialization, he evolved the following set of functions:

1. Instrumental (I want)—language used to satisfy the child's needs or desires, e.g. *I want to go with Daddy.*
2. Regulatory (do as I tell you)—language used to control another person's behavior, feelings, or attitudes, e.g. *Find my doll. Don't be mad at me. Let's go.*
3. Interactional (me and you)—language used in the give and take of social dialogue, particularly with the child's mother and other important individuals. Includes such items as teasing, conversational greetings, and invitations, e.g. *Hi! How are you?*
4. Personal (here I come)—language used to express the child's own individuality, pride in himself/herself, feelings, e.g. *I did the best drawing.* Includes expressions of interest, pleasure, disgust, etc.
5. Heuristic (tell me why)—language used for finding knowledge, e.g. *Tell me what makes the light go on.*
6. Imaginative (let's pretend)—language used in make-believe play, e.g. *I'm a princess* or *I'm the big, bad wolf.* Here, the child creates an environment of his own.
7. Representative or informative (I've got something to tell you)—language used to give information, to describe a deed or object; in other words, to represent experience to others, e.g. *Let me tell you about my trip to the Fair.* This function is more sophisticated than the others in that it depends on the internalization of a whole complex set

of linguistic concepts that the young child does not possess. (Halliday
[1977, pp. 18–32 and 37])

We have added examples to clarify the use of the functions. The examples we have given are not those of the very young child. However,
since these functions are often cited in literature about language in
school age children, this particular use of example seemed wise. Halliday believes that these functions develop in approximately the order
listed; but, in any case, the "informative" is significantly last.

Halliday (1977, pp. 54–58) explains that the origins of language development can be interpreted as the learning of a set of functions,
each with its associated "meaning potential." The system is one in
which function is identical with use—with each function having one
predominant purpose. But he makes clear that at a certain age, the
child begins to use language in a *mathetic* function—to learn—arising from a generalization from the personal and heuristic. About the
same time, a generalization of the remaining functions occur under a
pragmatic rubric—including the use of language to satisfy one's own
needs and to control and interact with others. Consequently, as the
child matures, he/she needs to employ increasingly sophisticated language to make sure that his utterance achieves at least its predominant
purpose.

Smith (1977) adds three categories to Halliday's seven. They are:

Divertive—language used for enjoyment as puns, jokes and riddles.
Authoritative, contractual—language used to indicate how life must be
   (stated laws, agreements, contracts).
Perpetuating—language used to indicate how life was in the past (records, histories, diaries, notes).

In looking at language as a tool, Smith (1977) also includes alternatives, other than spoken language, for the various functions. They are:

1. Instrumental—pantomime, facial expression, screaming, pointing,
   grabbing.
2. Regulatory—pushing and pulling people around; modelling behavior for others to copy.
3. Interactional—waving, smiling, linking arms, holding hands, shaking fist, sport.
4. Personal—art, music, dress, cosmetics, ornamentation.
5. Heuristic—exploration, investigation, experimentation.
6. Imaginative—art, mime.
7. Representational—pointing, rituals, diagrams, maps, mathematics.
8. Divertive—games, puzzles, magic.
9. Authoritative or contractual—roles, regalias, uniforms, architecture.
10. Perpetuating—photographs, sculpture, documents, memorials.

As children develop language (see Chapter 7), many make themselves understood through some of these alternatives. The first three of these uses are important for the speech/language clinician to examine.

THE COMPONENTS OF LANGUAGE

As just noted, the components of language are intertwined with the function and with the context. These components are phonology, morphology, syntax, suprasegmentals from all of which, in the light of pragmatics, semantics emerges.

Phonology

Phonology refers to the sound system of a natural language. In English this system comprises consonants, vowels, and diphthongs. The differences in the initial consonants of the words *tab, dab*, and *nab* which distinguish the words, one from the other, are phonemic differences. When you listen carefully to the variety of /t/ in *tab, stab*, and *cat,* you find that they do not sound exactly alike, for they are produced somewhat differently; but you do not perceive them as significantly different from one another nor do they alter the meanings of the words because of their incidental feature differences. /t/ is, therefore, a phoneme. The *phoneme* is a linguistic unit significantly different from all other sounds within a language system. This material is covered in more detail in Chapter 6.

As noted in Chapter 7, children begin their phonological development during the first nine months. They discriminate among phonemes according to broad categories, i.e. stops, fricatives, nasals, vowels. Early in the development often one member of the category seems to "stand" for the entire category. They produce sounds starting usually with /p/ and /m/ and then go on to /t/ and /k/. Even as late as the second and third year, children reduce clusters such as /sp/ and /str/ and "simplify" words by omitting phonemes or substituting one phoneme for another. Eventually almost all children produce the sounds accurately both alone and in contextual utterance.

Morphology

Normally children by the end of their first year combine phonemes to make morphemes. A *morpheme* is a minimal unit that carries meaning. *Fast* consists of four phonemes: /f/, /æ/, /s/, and /t/. Since all four phonemes are needed to make a unit that carries meaning, *fast* is a morpheme which can stand alone and is accordingly a *free morpheme.* But when *er* is added, producing *faster,* two morphemes are present; *er* is a *bound morpheme* which cannot stand alone but does carry meaning. There are also two morphemes when *s* is added to *cat* and when *ed* is added to *melt.* Morphology involves the pattern of making words which in larger contexts become phrases and sentences.

Suprasegmentals—Prosody

Bolinger (1975, p. 46) notes that "prosody or suprasegmentals are a kind of musical accompaniment of speech, just as gesture is a kind of histrionic accompaniment," He goes on to explain that intonation is the broad undulation of the pitch curve that carries the ripples of accent on its back.

MacKay (1978, pages 213–216) divides suprasegmentals into: stress—emphasis given to a syllable or word, manifested as increased distinctiveness or loudness and reduced assimilation; timing involving rate of speech and pauses; and intonation—patterns of changes in the fundamental frequency of the voice, related to the grammatical structure of the sentence or discourse that convey meaning. He makes clear that not every syllable is stressed in an English sentence but that strongly stressed syllables occur because of syntactic, semantic, and emphatic considerations.

Try the example, given by MacKay (1978, page 213) which illustrates differences in stress and intonation. The sentence is, "He didn't stay because I was there." Speak it with two different meanings: 1) He stayed—and my being there was the reason for his staying and 2) He left because I was there. What are the differences in stress and intonation between the two sentences as you speak them with the two different meanings?

Junctures are used to set apart syllables or words within phrases, to set off phrases and sentences or to terminate them. Bolinger (1975, page 59) notes that special phonic events are tied to the separation of words—which events are identified as junctures. He goes on to emphasize that they are "slippery entities." He cites one interesting example of juncture:

> Is it a real rock? No, it's a sham rock.
> Is it a red rose? No, it's a shamrock.

Juncture then sets boundaries which boundaries rely on context.

Prosodic or suprasegmentals are relative in a way that phonemes are not. For example, a stressed vowel in a word cannot be established without comparing the vowel with another segment or in the sequence. If we are talking about pitch, the pitch is high or low in relation to other syllables within the phrase or sentence. We can usually agree on which syllables to stress. For example, if we ask the question, "What is Jane doing?" the answer may well be "Jáne's báking a cáke." But when we ask, "Who's going to bake the cake?, we say "Jáne's báking the cáke." (Sommerstein, 1977, pages 35–40)

Recording segmentals takes a variety of forms. We are indicating but one of them. We are using numbers for pitch, various signs for stress, and short lines and arrows for juncture. Stress is sometimes expressed through various sized black dots; intonation patterns by a wavering line which indicates where pitch rises and where it falls.

Most native speakers of English use one level below and two above their habitual pitch. When the speaker is surprised, the pitch level rises, often two levels above the habitual pitch level. Using 1, 2, 3, and 4 levels of pitch with 4 as the highest, the following sentence states a
fact. $\overset{2}{He}$'s $\overset{3}{been}$ $\overset{1}{killed}$. But $\overset{2}{He}$'s $\overset{1}{been}$ $\overset{4}{killed}$ asks a horrified question.

Dictionaries provide stress marks to help you determine the pronunciation of a word. Frequently you find two stress marks—one indicating major stress and the other indicating a minor stress. When, however, you speak in phrases, you are likely to use four distinct stress marks. One system of recording these is: /ˊ/—heavy stress, /ˆ/—medium stress, /ˋ/—light stress, and /ˇ/—weak stress. *A rolling stone gathers no moss* is likely to be spoken thus. *Ă rôlliñg stóne gàthěrs nô móss.* As in pitch, the degrees of stress are relative.

Lastly, juncture may be expressed thus: /+/ which sets apart syllables or words within phrases. This juncture would, for example, distinguish between *cupful* and *cup full*. The other three are used to set off phrases and sentences or to terminate them. They are: /↑/—the rising juncture, /↓/—the falling juncture, and /→/—the level juncture. The following are examples:

> When he plays football ↑ , he eats at the training table ↓ ,
> By eight o'clock→ I'll be through ↓ Are you coming ↑

Again we should like to emphasize that the suprasegmentals help to express the meaning dictated by the intent of the speaker and the context. We should also like to point out that the suprasegmentals (musical accompaniments) will vary from individual to individual.

Syntax

As children grow older, they become more sophisticated in arranging in an orderly (rule observing) way the practices we observe in contextual speech. These practices are syntactic rules (the grammar of an utterance). One word productions become fewer and are expanded into two words, then three words, then four words, then whatever the number adults usually use in keeping with the needs and purposes of their linguistic productions. For example, in early syntactic development, one child may say "light out;" another, "me find dog." Both of these utterances involve an agent, action and object. Still another child's "Me go home" involves agent, action, and location. As children mature, further syntactic development includes such items as declaratives, negative, *wh* questions, and passive voice. Syntax, then, involves the constructing of sentences. The development of this area and its relationship to the other areas are explained in detail in Chapter 7.

Semantics

Semantics has to do with the meaning of a word or words in relationship to different and specific situations. Referents are important in attaching meaning to words. For example, when adults are asked whether they grew up *rich* or *poor*, the referents differ greatly. On the one hand, the referents may include quality of life—the amount of affection, attention, and feelings existing in the family, the community relationships, and the kind of childhood friendships. These referents depend upon feelings created by the childhood environment. On the other hand, the referents may depend on the money available for growing up in a family. They may consist of a home with bathroom fixtures of real gold, a reception hall large enough for a dance furnished with oriental rugs and priceless antique furniture, educational opportunities for attending a prestigious preparatory school and an Ivy League college, to see Broadway shows, to travel abroad. Or they may consist of living in a housing project, being on relief, wearing hand-me-down clothes, being inured to a ghetto neighborhood, and never having quite enough to eat. Rich in relationship to what? Poor in relationship to what? The words carry quite different meanings dependent on their referents. In extreme instances, because of different referents, *poor* may seem to equal *rich*.

Children's language usually reveals kinds and types of referents. They begin with words like *ball* and *milk*, then proceed to specific people and pets as *Mommy, Daddy,* and *Fido,* and then to action words like *up* and *down.* For one child *fufu* meant not only his play dog but all kinds of four legged animals. Eventually he differentiated among animals and acquired individual names for those he knew. In semantics, as in other aspects of language, children become more sophisticated as they grow older. Sophistication is usually indicated by differential responses and productions.

Semantic relationships are linked with syntax. The syntactic construction helps the listener to understand the semantic relationships not always easy to discern. A child may use a word or phrase which for him has a meaningful intent. The receiver of the message may, however, get a message different from the one intended. When a child says, "She's a dog," he has most likely named an animate object. But obviously the same words uttered by an adolescent or adult have quite a different meaning. When Joey says, "Bob, the ball," one child may understand that Joey meant that Bob threw the ball whereas another child may understand him to mean to go get the ball that Joey threw.

Speech and language clinicians, teachers, and parents have traditionally helped children acquire the sounds of language—correcting the *th* sound in *the, then,* and *them* when another sound is substituted for the *th*. Similarly they have encouraged children to become more sophisticated in their syntactical usage—using phrases like *a good dog, a better dog, the best dog* or by suggesting they combine sentences. For instance, *Tom is my cousin* and *Tom is learning to drive* are combined into *My cousin Tom is learning to drive*. And they encourage the development of vocabulary.

Pragmatics

There exists another factor, the study of language in context. The sound, the word, the sentence are not the basic units of communication. Rather the basic unit is the speech act which involves the intended impact, the spoken form, and structure, and the perceived influence and/or effect on the listener. For speech and language clinicians to be effective, they must understand the child in communicative situations. Such analysis may be called *pragmatic*. This approach focuses not only on the phonological, morphological, syntactic, and semantic competencies of language structure but also on the child's abilities to understand their intended import. It also includes the child's ability to impart the intent of his/her message. Bates (1976) defines pragmatics as the study of rules governing the use of language in context. He further notes (p. 412) that context does not just cause language, but is an integral part of the structure of language. Meanings are conveyed through a creative combination of utterances and social settings.

The study of pragmatics emphasizes that a message is more than the particular words selected or the way they are strung together. Rather a word, sentence, or string of sentences may communicate quite different messages according to their different contexts. In the following speech act, in one context the word *doll* indicates to one listener appreciation and pleasure but to another disgust while in another context the same word indicates to still another listener hurt and dismay. In the first context, a father is about to take his ten-year-old daughter to dinner to celebrate her tenth birthday. As she comes down the stairs, dressed in her best, he exclaims, "Doll!" She is delighted with his use of the word. But her mother, not at all amused, is aghast at her husband's use of the word, for to her it signifies an unacceptable stereotype. In the second context, an eleven-year-old on her birthday receives from her aunt an expensive doll with an array of beautiful clothes. As she opens the box, she reveals her utter disbelief and some amusement in her, "A doll . . . ." Her aunt, noting the child's disaffection and amusement with her carefully selected gift, says to herself, "She is growing up faster than I realized but she could have been more appreciative of my intention." Thus, the word *doll* had quite different impacts on these three individuals.

When the message is not clear, the listener in some way indicates that he/she does not understand, Whereupon the speaker attempts to clarify the meaning. For instance, Joan said to her friend that she went to the movies with Bill. When her friend looked puzzled, Joan cleared up the mystery with "Bill Johnson." Children clarify their meaning when adults or other children do not respond appropriately to their messages. Gallagher (1977) found that normal children around the age of two, regardless of language stage, primarily revise the linguistic form of the message when they perceive that the listener does not understand. In this study, the experimenter, pretending that she did not understand what the child had said, would ask, "What?" The revisions followed this pattern:

1. No response.
2. Repetition. The child repeats what was said before the "What?"
3. Revision. The response differed structurally from the first response. These revisions fall into four categories:
   a. Phonetic change. For example, *he kit the ball* became *he kick the ball*.
   b. Constituent elaboration. A morpheme not in the original contribution was added as *It ball* became *It big ball*.
   c. Constituent reduction. The first response *It big ball* became *It ball*.
   d. Constituent substitution. Another word replaced the word in the first attempt as *He kick it* for *He kick ball*.

An overwhelming majority of the responses were revisions.

Gallagher and Darnton (1978) did a similar study but with language-disordered children. They found that these children are also sensitive to the conversational demands inherent in a communicative failure and respond to these demands as do the normal children, by revising the structure of the original utterance. But unlike the normal children, the language-disordered children's selection of revision strategies and their execution of these strategies appear unsystematic —undifferentiated relative to the level of language-structure knowledge they have achieved. Such children are using their knowledge of language structure to meet the demands of conversation in a qualitatively different way from the normal children. This research suggests that language strategies used by speech/language clinicians and teachers should take pragmatics into account, for children do not communicate in drill words and phrases but rather use language rules in conversation—in the classroom, at home, and in the playground.

We emphasize the area of pragmatics because we believe that an understanding of the speech act and its import are essential both in the diagnosis of difficulties in language and speech and in their remediation. Prutting (1978) has summarized the major behaviors of the communicative system (pragmatic, semantic, syntactic, phonological) in five stages from the pre-linguistic through adult. Her summary provides guidelines for the content and sequencing of communicative behaviors.

SETTINGS FOR COMMUNICATION

Communication changes complexion because of variation in settings and factors within the settings: the physical environment, the ideas and concepts, the emotional overtones of the situation, and the participants and the interplay among them. A conversation between two friends in a quiet coffee shop involves helping a mutual friend plan her first European trip; the young woman is apprehensive about going by herself. The two speakers have warm, sympathetic feelings for their mutual friend; they themselves are sensitive, perceptive individuals. On the other hand, a professor lectures to an audience of two hundred in a large lecture hall. The listeners, mathematics majors, are intent, for they find his message about differential equations interesting and stimulating. Besides, they may need this information for a forthcoming quiz. But behind the message is the man whom students, on the basis of several office visits and one to his home, see as a worthy, respected mentor and a good friend. In both instances certain social attributes such as friendly, warm, interested participants with positive interplay among them are conducive to effective, useful communication. But the ideas and concepts expressed in the two situations are quite different. Those in the coffee shop are relatively simple and clear although emotionally charged. Those in the lecture hall may be complicated and abstract but with little or no emotional charge. The one setting is intimate, comfortable; the other—because of the size of the room, the rigid seating, the large number of persons involved—may well project a certain feeling of anonymity.

Consider the players on a football field getting ready for an important contest. What are the likely functions of their communicative endeavors? What is the setting like? What is the relationship of the participants to each other and to their coach? How complex are the ideas being generated? What is the physical environment like? How do these factors affect the communication act? Or consider the actors and actresses at a dress rehearsal. How do the social aspects, the setting, the role of the participants and their interplay, the concepts involved affect the communication act? In both of these situations language is the medium being used for learning.

In Chapter 4 we will consider communication in the school in more detail. But we note here that generally adults in most situations participate more equally in the give-and-take of a communicative situation than do children in a classroom. In many classrooms the functions of language most frequently used are heuristic and informational. Some of the functions are rarely utilized. Hopefully the classroom is a place where there are many opportunities for such activities as sharing information, discussion, problem-solving, debate, and dramatic play— activities where the participants are comfortable, where they accept each other and each other's ideas, where they are motivated to use a wide variety of the functions of language, and where they are learning to learn. This idea of learning leads us to the role of cognition in language.

COGNITION

Cognitive processes include thought, perception, memory, learning, and activities involving problem solving. Children codify the product of these processes through language. They further develop strategies to keep what they know so that they can continue in their pursuit of knowledge about their culture and environment. Cognitive processing in children involves both their learning to learn and their becoming increasingly proficient in attaining and using knowledge. Through this process, they code their sensory perceptions, store them, and call on them for use as they need them. As they analyze the sensory data that they have received on the basis of past experiences, they may well react to only a portion of the data. The relationship of this processing to language development is explored in Chapter 7 on "The Development of Language."

The theory of cognition, illustrated in Chapter 8 on "Stimulating Language Development," is based on Piaget's hypothesis that cognitive development is a coherent process of successive qualitative changes of cognitive structures with each structure and its concomitant changes deriving logically and inevitably from the preceding one. (Wadsworth, 1973, p. 25) Piaget believes that the child controls the producing and organizing of experiences in his own environment. In other words, the child feeds relevant data into his/her machine and rejects the irrelevant data.

Obviously, the cognitive attainment of the child is closely related to semantic development and, it would seem, to environmental influences. Bruner (1972) notes

> As to how language becomes internalized as a program for ordering experience, I join those who despair for an answer. My speculation, for what it is worth, is that the process of internalization depends upon interaction with others, upon the need to develop corresponding categories and transformations for communal action. It is the need for cognitive coin that can be exchanged with those on whom we depend. (Bruner 1972, page 166)

Bruner goes on to say that what is significant about the growth of mind in the child is to what degree it depends not upon capacity but upon the unlocking of capacity by techniques that come from exposure to the specialized environment of a culture. For all of those involved in language development, Bruner's concept that the course of human development cannot be viewed independently of cultural priorities and the educational process and that we arrange to make that development possible is especially important.

To summarize, children develop language as they use it in a meaningful way. Using their own bank of experiences, they develop a potential to convey meaning, to communicate with others, and to create a view of what the world is like. Along the way they become more sophisticated in their use of the components of language. Children achieve this sophistication partly through hearing adults and other children using language in a variety of situations, through their responding with their own language, and through the feedback they receive from their listeners as to the appropriateness of their language.

Language, a symbolic code used to serve the functions of communication, may be verbal or non-verbal. When verbal, the physical output of the code is speech. Speech, then, is the manner of communication with its many functions, as distinguished from the means—language.

But the manner, the means, and the functions of communication cannot be separated; they are inextricably interwoven.

Rees (1974) examines the relationships among language, communication, and speech.

> *Language* is a code with structural properties characterized by sets of rules for producing and comprehending sentences. *Communication* is the process of sharing or giving information, feelings, and attitudes. Language may serve as a tool in the process of communication, and also as an instrument for learning. *Speech* occurs when the rules of the language are applied in oral production; more specifically, speech is the articulatory-acoustic output of the linguistic code.

THE DEFINITION OF A
SPEECH/LANGUAGE DISORDER

With this information as background, what then is a speech/language or communication disorder? A speech/language disorder is a serious interference or obstruction of the communicative act that reduces or prevents its intended impact on the listener. For example, when the listener cannot perceive the intent because so many consonants are deviant or omitted, he/she cannot react to the meaning of the message. Or "wrong" words may have been selected. Or the voice may be so unpleasant and so far from an acceptable norm that it interferes with the import of the message. Or the meaning may be distorted because of the speaker's or the listener's lack of understanding of the significance of particular words. Or the speaker may be hesitating unduly, repeating sounds, words, and phrases more frequently than normal. Or the speaker may make glaring errors in word order. Or, for their age, speakers may use many tenses and pronouns inaccurately. Or the speaker may use syntax too complex for the listener to appreciate if not understand. In such situations a degree of failure exists for both the speaker and the listener in the communicative situation.

Specialists in the field classify these obstacles to communication differently: Van Riper (1978) uses the categories articulation, time, voice, and symbolization; Curtis (1978) disorders of language, speech, and hearing; Nation and Aram (1977) phonology, syntax, semantics, pragmatics. Van Hattum (1980) is more inclusive; he divides disorders into (1) receptive, which includes hearing loss and impairment and disorders of auditory processing, and (2) expressive, which includes speech (articulation, voice, and rhythm) and language (phonology, morphology, syntax, and semantics).

Teachers, parents, and others may perceive some less serious interferences in communication as speech/language disorders. In these instances, however, the interferences are often applicable only to a particular class of listeners or to a particular setting. Such interferences include:

1. *Nonstandard pronunciations and language usage.* In this instance many or most of the child's classmates understand him/her with little or no difficulty.
2. *Regional dialects.* Again children from the child's home region undoubtedly understand the communicative effort.
3. *Poor oral reading.* This difficulty occurs only in one setting.
4. *Articulation and fluency patterns*—not adult, but normal for the developmental stage of the child. Once again, the other children usually can interpret the message—often better than the teacher.
5. A *psychological disturbance* that manifests itself as a speech/language symptom. Cooperating specialists help teachers plan programs of speech/language improvement in such instances.

An eight-year-old girl says, "I din't recognize dat neighbor wid de fedders in her hair—de one who's awiz pretendin'. She's actin' in de Cender play." This girl is not in need of help from the speech/language clinician. Half of her classmates and even her parents say *dat* for *that* and *de* for *the.* Her observation gives evidence of a fairly sophisticated use of language for her age. Her classroom teacher, however, plans a program to improve the level of speech and language of all the students in the class. Undoubtedly, this child communicates effectively at home and with most if not all of her classmates. But time and occasion will arrive when such non-Standard pronunciations may handicap her. We discuss this problem in Chapter 3.

Children may transfer from sections of the country where people speak differently from most people in the area where the children now live. The teacher and classmates of these children may be very conscious of the differences in pronunciations and melody patterns in the speech of these children. In fact, at times the teachers and classmates may be unable to understand what these transferred children are saying. But as the children live in their new community for some time, the differences in their speech patterns will tend to disappear, and they will acquire the speech patterns of their playmates. The teacher can help the adjustment of the transferred children by accepting their speech and by explaining the differences in their speech to the other members of the class. Regional differences in speech are also discussed in Chapter 3.

Oral reading presents problems for some children because of their difficulty in understanding the meaning of the words printed on the page. As a result, their oral reading is uncommunicative; it is hesitant and hard to understand. The conversation of the same children, however, may be quite adequate. Their main problem in communication is one of oral reading although, as mentioned in Chapter 10 on articulatory defects, reading, speech and language problems are often related. It has been our experience that as children improve in one ability, they frequently improve in another.

Kindergarten and first-grade teachers find that many of their children articulate some sounds inaccurately. Fourth- and fifth-grade teachers find decidedly fewer children with "inaccurate" articulation. Some of the more accurate articulation has resulted from speech remediation but most of it has resulted from the children's own phonological development. In many instances, a child's "inaccurate" articulation is the result of the stage in development rather than of a deficit in development. Speech/language clinicians, therefore, prognosticate which children must have clinical help. Ways of successful prognostication for correcting deficient articulation are discussed in Chapter 10.

Similarly, children in kindergarten sometimes exhibit disfluencies that are part of the normal development of children. The aspects of language development are discussed in Chapter 7.

In some instances, the major problem is not one of speech but of social adjustment. One little girl whose voice is consistently thin and weak and who speaks with little or no inflection surely exhibits a problem of voice. This problem, however, may be closely related to the child's concept of herself—she feels she cannot do anything very well. She says, "I feel like a big stupid lump most of the time." Her stooped posture, her halting walk, her untidy dress, her sloppy compositions, her lack of enthusiasm, and her dull, thin, weak voice are all part of a syndrome. In such an instance, the voice is merely the symptom of a personality difficulty. The speech/language clinician can help only in cooperation with other members of the school personnel.

INCIDENCE AND TYPES OF SPEECH/LANGUAGE DISORDERS

Leske (1981) reviews the major sources of prevalence data on communicative disorders in the United States. Her first paper is on speech disorders; and her second, on language, hearing and vestibular disorders. She quotes a study mady by Hull and Timmons (1971) that examined a nationwide sample of 38,802 public school students in Grades 1–12. Trained examiners evaluated the presence of articulation errors, voice problems, and stuttering. According to this survey, speech problems were present in 5.7 per cent of children 6–18 years of age. The table follows:

Per Cent Prevalence of Speech Disorders, by Sex[1]

Type of Disorder	Males	Females	Total
Articulation	2.4	1.5	1.9
Voice	3.7	2.1	3.0
Stuttering	1.2	0.4	0.8
Total	7.3	4.0	5.7

[1] National Speech & Hearing Survey, 1971, from Leske, 1981, p. 219.

However, it should be noted that Hull and Timmons (1971) found that the category of moderate and severe articulation deviation declined from 9.7 per cent in the first grade to .5 per cent in the twelfth grade. Voice deviations varied from 5.6 per cent in the first grade to 1 per cent in the twelfth grade. Leske (1981, p. 223) further notes that available evidence suggests that less than 1 per cent of children entering school have a marked language delay. She also indicates that the number of persons who lost hearing ability for speech before 19 years of age is estimated at .2 per cent and that many of these persons have severe language impairment.

THE TEACHER'S ROLE IN LOCATING SPEECH DEFECTS

Classroom teachers frequently refer the speech/language-defective child to the speech/language clinician—often carrying the major responsibility for identifying the speech-defective child. When the speech/language clinician does not screen the school population, the teacher should be trained to hear and locate symptoms of the various speech/language defects. The training may be accomplished by college courses, in-service courses, or a series of lectures by the speech/language clinician.

The need for training teachers to recognize speech/language handicaps is emphasized in a survey of teachers conducted by Clauson and Kopatic (1975). They report that teachers are uncertain about the particular speech/language handicaps that the school speech and language clinician handles; in fact, only one teacher out of 50 answered the question pertaining to this subject correctly. Only 58 per cent of the teachers felt certain they could recognize a speech/language-defective child in their class. A majority of the teachers believes that children will outgrow their speech/language problems even when the children are past the third grade.

Damico and Oller (1980) found that teachers who were taught to use pragmatic criteria to identify language-disordered children identified significantly more children and were more correct in their identification than teachers taught to use syntactic criteria. They assigned 54 regular teachers (K–5) to one of two matched groups. One group received training in the traditional approaches of assessing language disability: morphological and syntactic criteria including such areas as noun-verb agreement, tense marking, pluralization, pronoun case or gender, and syntactic transpositions. This group received training material from current language tests. The second group received similar training except that the criteria of interest were pragmatic in nature. Referral criteria included:

1. Linguistic nonfluency. The child's speech production is disrupted due to a disproportionately high number of repetitions, unusual pauses and excessive use of hesitation forms.
2. Revisions. Speech production is broken up by numerous false starts or self interruptions. The child revises what he has already said as if he keeps coming to dead ends in a maze.
3. Delays before responding. Attempts at communication initiated by others are followed by pauses of inordinate lengths.
4. Nonspecific vocabulary. In this instance we are concerned with the use of deictic[1] expressions such as *this* or *that, the, he, over there,* and the like when no antecedents have been provided by the speaker and when the listener has no way of knowing what is being referenced. Also, children displaying this chracteristic will tend to use generic terms such as *thing, stuff, these* and *those* when more specific referring expressions would seem to be required.
5. Inappropriate responses. These are easy to spot but difficult to explain. It is as though the child were operating on an independent discourse agenda, rather than attending to the prompts or probes of the adult or others.
6. Poor topic maintenance. The child makes rapid and inappropiate changes in the topic without providing transitional clues to the listener.
7. Need for repetition. Multiple repetitions are requested without any indication of improvement in comprehension. [Damico and Oller (1980, p. 88)]

[1] Without stable meaning.

The last criterion may indicate a hearing problem; but the class-room teacher does not ordinarily do audiological testing. Rather, audiological testing is accomplished by a variety of specialists in the public school system, including speech and hearing clinicians, nurses, physicians, school audiologists, and health department personnel. Almost all schools, however, provide for regular audiological screening. In Chapter 14, we indicate how up to 40 children can be audiologically screen-tested in about 15 minutes.

THE CLASSROOM TEACHER AND SPEECH AND LANGUAGE PROBLEMS

It is very important for classroom teachers to have training in recognizing speech and language difficulties, in planning strategies for the reinforcement of clinical work, and in differentiating between what language and speech work falls into the realm of speech and language *therapy* and what falls into the realm of speech and language *improvement* and *stimulation*. The evidence for teachers' need for training in the identification of speech defects has already been given. As stressed earlier, the need for this training is particularly important because the teacher frequently carries the responsibility for referral of speech- and language-handicapped children to the school speech/language clinician.

Teachers should also know what is going on in the speech/language clinic, for when this work is reinforced in the classroom, the improvement in communication is more rapid. If the child uses one set of rules for speech and language in the clinical setting and another set in the classroom, the improvement in the child's speech can be hindered. Furthermore, the teacher and clinician should approach the problem from the same basic philosophy; otherwise the reinforcement may be negative rather than positive. For example, while the clinician may be helping children to accept their stuttering, the teacher may be asking them to stop, to think before they speak. The combination of these two behaviors is counterproductive. We suggest close cooperation between the teacher and the specialist. The members and the roles of the speech and language team are discussed in the next chapter.

Teachers must also be able to recognize which language and speech problems are in their province and which are in the province of the speech/language clinicians. For instance, teachers show good judgment in refusing to accept primary responsibility for the rehabilitation of the speech of the stutterer, of the speech and voice of the child with a cleft palate or with a hearing defect, or of the voice of the child with a serious vocal handicap. However, teachers often have had the training and have the competence to handle the child with a minor functional articulatory difficulty, such as the child who says *tree* for *three*. And teachers should be able to distinguish whether this substitution is a dialectal difference or a functional articulatory error. In some instances, most of the children in the class may say *tree* for *three*, for this substitution is a product of their environment. The classroom teacher, however, is almost always responsible for the program that stimulates speech and language development of the entire class. Frequently, the speech/language clinician or another educational specialist, such as the learning disabilities resource teacher, aids in planning this work.

Fortunately today much of classroom study is experientially based and is designed to further communication between the teacher and the students and among the students. For example, kindergartners visit the supermarket and upon returning to the classroom talk about the manager, the customers, the checkout clerk, and the arrangements of the products. Or in their housekeeping corner, they play "Mother," "Daddy," "Doctor," and "Sister." After the second graders have planted corn seeds, pumpkin seeds, avocado seeds, and cuttings from such plants as coleus or wandering jew, they read about and talk about various ways of propagation and the need for light and water for growth; that is, they set up criteria for growing living plants.

If a teacher had a child such as six-year-old Eloise in class and heard her explain that Sabine, a rag doll, "has absolutely no face at all partially because she came from Jamaica by Air Express" and that her very large doll Saylor is armless because "she was in the most terriblest accident and she bleeded so hard she almost choked in the night and this ambulance came and took her to this hospital and it was an emergency,"[2] she would describe the language as imaginative and giving evidence of considerable vocabulary and syntactic development. She would be pleased that Eloise had provided a reason for the armless state of Saylor and for her choking in the night. She would not be concerned with *bleeded* or *most terriblest*, for these show some understanding of the rules.

Today an increasing number of language-handicapped children are enrolled in regular classrooms. This situation is partly the result of national and state movements to provide education for all handicapped children in the "least restrictive environment." An environment con-

---

[2] From the child's book *Eloise* by K. Thompson New York: (Simon & Schuster, Inc., 1955).

ducive to the kind of communication that activates the development of language and meaning should meet this criterion. This environment, then, involves the physical surroundings, the participants, their roles, and their opportunities to interact; it also involves providing opportunities for a variety of functions of language.

Pinnell (1975b) found that the functions of language that children use are closely tied to the activities and the environments of their classrooms. For instance, situations that call for problem-solving encourage heuristic language whereas playing house invites imaginative language. Teachers can help develop competence in using language for different purposes by creating situations that require such differentiation. In such situations children learn to ask questions, to interact with others, to persuade others to their way of thinking, to seek out new information, to impart it to others, to make believe . . . and perhaps to pun and make up riddles. At the same time they will be enlarging their vocabularies, making longer and more complex sentences, and learning to pronounce difficult words. Throughout these communicative acts, they will also be adding to their knowledge of the world.

Problems

1. Visit a lower-grade classroom and try to screen the children into the following categories: (a) those who have speech and language that will probably meet their social and educational needs; (b) those whose speech and language may be faulty but likely to improve with maturation; (c) those who need language stimulation; (d) those who have more serious difficulties that will require the attention of a speech clinician.
2. Visit one of the sessions held by a speech clinician. Indicate the problem of one of the children and the kind of help he/she received.
3. Visit a kindergarten and a fifth-grade class. Indicate whether the number of articulatory errors decreases or increases and whether the disfluencies decrease or increase in the two grades. Lastly, indicate some differences in vocabulary and syntactical development between the groups. Be as specific as you can.
4. Visit a session held by a speech clinician. Indicate in two specific ways how you as a classroom teacher could reinforce the teaching done in this session in your classroom.

    or

    Visit a first- or second-grade class. Indicate suggestions you might make as a clinician to the teacher to help a particular child with a specific language disability.
5. Visit a primary-grade classroom. Using Halliday's classification of functions, note the various functions used in the classroom and give samples.

6. Watch children playing—in a yard, at a pool, at home—anywhere. Note the functions of language used. Give examples.
7. Watch some young children playing. Note their use of nonverbal language. Describe one of them.
8. How many morphemes do the following words have?
   singers   best   cats
   thinking   heated   bright
9. Indicate some possible referents for *beautiful*, for *clever.*

References and Suggested Readings

Bates, E., "Pragmatics and Sociolinguistics in Child Language." In D. Morehead and A. Morehead, Eds., *Normal and Deficient Child Language.* Baltimore: University Park Press, 1976, pp. 411–463.

Bolinger, D., *Aspects of Language,* 2nd Edition, New York: Harcourt, Brace, Jovanovich, 1975.

Bruner, J. S., "The Course of Cognitive Growth," in *Language of Education,* prepared by the Language and Learning Course Team for the Open University, A. Cashdan, Chairman, London and Boston: Routledge and Kegan Paul, 1972, pp. 161–168.

Clausen, G. M., and N. J. Kopatic, "Teacher Attitudes and Knowledge of Remedial Speech Programs." *Language, Speech, and Hearing Services in Schools,* 6 (October 1975), 206–210.

Curtis, J. F., Ed., *Processes and Disorders of Human Communications.* New York: Harper & Row, Publishers, 1978.

Damico, J. and J. W. Oller, Jr., "Pragmatic Versus Morphological-Syntactic Criteria for Language Referral. *Language, Speech, and Hearing Services in Schools,* 11 (April 1980), 85–94. Reprinted by permission.

Des Roches, C. P., "Speech Therapy Services in a Large School System: A Six-year Overview," *Language, Speech, and Hearing Services in Schools,* 17 (1976), 207–219.

Gallagher, T. M., "Revision Behaviors in the Speech of Normal Children Developing Language." *Journal of Speech and Hearing Research,* 20 (1977), 303–313.

——— and B. A. Darnton, "Conversational Aspects of the Speech of Language-Disordered Children: Revision Behavior." *Journal of Speech and Hearing Research,* 21 (March 1978), 118–135.

Gillespie, S. K., and E. B. Cooper, "Prevalence of Speech Problems in Junior and Senior High Schools." *Journal of Speech and Hearing Research,* 16 (December 1973), 739–743. (Indicates that in Tuscaloosa, Alabama, 5.5 per cent of junior and senior high school students have speech problems.)

Halliday, M. A. K., *Explorations in the Functions of Language.* London, Edward Arnold & Co., 1973.

Halliday, M. A. K., "The Functional Bases of Language." In B. Bernstein, Ed., *Applied Studies Toward a Sociology of Language.* Boston: Routledge and Kegan Paul, 1973.

Halliday, M. A. K., *Learning How to Mean: Explorations in the Development of Language:* New York, American Elsevier, Inc., 1977.

Hull, F. M., and R. J. Timmons, "The National Speech and Hearing Survey: Preliminary Results, *ASHA,* 13 (1971), 501–509.

James, H. P., and E. B. Cooper, "Accuracy of Teacher Referral of Speech-Handicapped Children," *Exceptional Child,* 30 (September 1966), 29–33.

Leske, M. C., "Prevalence Estimates of Communicative Disorders in the United States; Speech Disorders." *ASHA,* 23 (March 1981), 217–228. (Reviews the sources for national estimates of prevalence of speech disorders and lists prevalence estimates for different types of speech disorders.)

——, "Prevalence Estimates of Communicative Disorders in the United States: Language, Hearing and Vestibular Disorders." *ASHA,* 23 (March 1981), 229–236. Reviews studies on prevalence of hearing impairments, language disorders and vestibular disorders.

Lieberman, P. *Intonation, Perception and Language.* Research Monograph 35 Massachusetts Institute of Technology Press, Cambridge, Mass., 1967

MacKay, I. R. A. *Introducing Practical Phonetics.* Boston: Little, Brown and Company, 1978.

Moerk, E. L., *Pragmatic and Semantic Aspects of Early Language Developments.* Baltimore: University Park Press, 1977.

Nation, J. E. and D. M. Aram, *Diagnosis of Speech and Language Disorders.* St. Louis, Missouri: C. V. Mosley Co., 1977.

Neal, W. R., "Speech Pathology Services in the Secondary Schools." *Language, Speech, and Hearing Services in Schools,* 7 (January 1976), 6–16.

O'Connor, J. D. and G. F. Arnold, *Intonation of Colloquial English,* London: Longman, 1973

Pinnell, G. S., *Language Functions of First Grade Students Observed in Informal Classroom Environments.* Ph.D. Dissertation, Ohio State University, 1975a.

——. "Language in Primary Classrooms." *Theory Into Practice,* 14 (1975b), 318–327.

Prahl, H. M., and E. B. Cooper, "Accuracy of Teacher Referrals of Speech-Handicapped School Children." *ASHA,* 6 (October 1964), 392.

Prutting, C., "Process \präǀᵢses\n: The Action of Moving Forward Progressively from One Point to Another on the Way to Completion." *Journal of Speech and Hearing Disorders,* 44 (February 1979), 3–30.

Rees, N. S., "The Speech Clinician cum Language Clinician." *Language, Speech, and Hearing Services in Schools,* 4 (October 1974), 185–186. (Gives knowledge and therapeutic strategies that the speech clinician needs. Contains definitions of *language, communication,* and *speech.*)

Schiste, I. *Suprasegmentals,* Cambridge, Mass., Massachusetts Institute of Technology Press, 1970.

Searle, J. R., *Speech Acts: An Essay in the Philosophy of Language.* London: Cambridge University Press, 1969.

Smith, F., "The Uses of Language." *Language Arts,* 54 (Sept. 1977), 638–644.

Sommerstein, A., *Modern Phonology*, Baltimore: University Park Press, 1978.

Van Hattum, R. J., *Communication Disorders: An Introduction.* New York, Macmillan Publishing Co., Inc. 1980.

Van Riper, C., *Speech Correction: Principles and Methods*, 6th ed. Englewood Cliffs, N.J.: Prentice-Hall, Inc., 1978, Chap. 2. (Describes the types of disorders of speech.)

Wadsworth, B. J., *Piaget's Theory of Cognitive Development.* New York: David McKay Co., Inc., 1973.

Wertz, R. T., and M. D. Mead, "Classroom Teacher and Speech Clinician Severity Ratings of Different Speech Disorders." *Language, Speech, and Hearing Services in Schools,* **6** (July 1975), 119–124.

2

Speech and Language Services in the Schools

On one day a speech/language clinician may work with a group of stutterers, with a client who has cerebral palsy, with another who has had vocal nodules removed, with still another who is language-disordered, and, in addition, may serve as a member of a team to assess the degree of language disability of a language-disordered child. This clinician ideally has at least a Master's degree and holds the American Speech-Language-Hearing Association Certificate of Competency in speech and language pathology; consequently this individual presumably is competent in diagnosing speech and language disorders and in planning, carrying through, and evaluating remediation for clients with communicative handicaps. The profession of this pathologist involves

> the application of principles, methods, and procedures for measurement, testing, identification, prediction, counseling, and instruction related to the development and disorders of speech, voice or language for the purpose of identifying, preventing, managing, habilitating, ameliorating, or modifying such disorders and conditions in individuals or groups of individuals." (Van Hattum, 1980, p. 34).

COMPETENCIES OF SPEECH/LANGUAGE CLINICIANS

The duties mentioned above point to the need for certain competencies on the part of the speech/language clinician. We assume that all clinicians will have solid academic backgrounds in human development, including knowledge about language acquisition and its relationship to the normal development of children, in the area of language and language behavior, in understanding the anatomical, physiological, acoustic, psychological, and linguistic parameters underlying linguistic competence and performance, in the theory of the causes, diagnosis, and treatment of the various types of speech, hearing, and language disorders, and in the current philosophies, curricula, and organization of the public schools. Having assumed this academic background, we present the following list[1] of competencies for the speech/language clinician:

1. To organize screening procedures which will help identify the speech, language and hearing disordered.
2. To identify accurately and efficiently those individuals who give evidence of disorders of speech, language and/or hearing.
3. To plan appropriate programs of remediation for each individual with such a handicap.
4. To evaluate in an organized fashion the effectiveness of each intervention program.
5. To organize an effective overall program for the speech, language, and hearing handicapped.
6. To plan and supervise the activities of the aide or aides whom the school assigns to the program.
7. To identify and use the resource programs, personnel, and facilities within the school district, town, city, state, and United States that can provide assistance to the speech, language, and/or hearing handicapped.
9. To interpret a child's speech and language problems to his/her parents.
10. To function effectively as a member of the learning disabilities team and to determine the nature, etiology, and severity of the specific handicaps of those children with language disabilities.
11. To program one's own continual professional growth through activities of speech, hearing, and language associations, attendance at summer schools, and professional reading.
12. To prepare reports on the number of speech and language disabled children, the results of hearing, speech and language testing, schedules of schools and classes, therapy progress reports and final reports.

[1] For a detailed discussion of competencies, see "A Competency Based Teacher Education Program for Education of Teachers of the Speech and Hearing Handicapped," *ASHA* **20** (February 1978), 84–91.

Blanchard and Nober (1978) completed a survey which rates the following competencies for the school speech/language clinician in the order of their importance: *1. getting along with others*

1. Preschool screening.
2. Kindergarten screening.
3. Preparing educational plans.
4. Interpreting data of other specialists.
5. Administering and interpreting speech tests.
6. Participating in case conferences with parents.
7. Team decision making.
8. Preparing progress reports.
9. Preparing final reports.
10. Treatment—elementary age students.
11. Treatment—articulation disorders.
12. Treatment—language disorders.
13. Treatment—auditory discrimination.
14. Consultation with parents, teachers, and specialists. (Blanchard and Nober, 1978, pp. 79–80.)

Some clinicians have all of these competencies; others most of them. The American Speech-Language-Hearing Association requirements for the certificate of clinical competence in speech and language assumes the possession of such competencies. Some public school clinicians, however, do not possess this certificate; instead they possess a state certificate or license for following their profession. Undoubtedly, meeting the requirements of the American Speech-Language-Hearing Association and the State Association certifications, the M.A. and/or Ph.D. degree in the area, attendance at national and state conventions, reading in the field, and supervision from a qualified supervisor do further the acquisition of these competencies.

Taylor (1980), reporting that only 14 states require the M.A. degree, notes that basic requirements in state certification for speech/language clinicians vary widely. For example, the requirements in semester hours for speech pathology and audiology vary from 12 to 78 semester hours and the clinical practicum in schools from 50 clock hours to 100. Requirements also differ in such related areas as psychology, where about half of the respondent states require 16 semester hours in psychology. Obviously, widely different preparations and widely different types of personalities of speech/language clinicians affect the degree of achievement of the competencies just mentioned.

Clearly, the acquisition of competencies will vary in degree because of differences in training and in job requirements.

THE INFLUENCE OF STATE AND FEDERAL
LEGISLATION ON THE HANDICAPPED

In 1974, the Education Amendment of 1974—Public Law 93–380—helped to promote the right to an education for all handicapped children. The law required states receiving financial assistance under title VI-B of the Education for All Handicapped Children Act to: (1) Develop due process procedures. (2) Initiate procedures to identify and evaluate all handicapped children. (3) Establish a goal of providing full educational opportunities for all handicapped children and to submit a plan indicating how the state would meet the goals.

Public Law 94–142 was the result of the 1970s concern for the handicapped. As reported in Section 602 (b) of Public Law 94–142 in 1975, a congressional hearing that included parents and special educators found that one-half of the nation's eight million handicapped children were not receiving an appropriate education and about one million received no education at all. In some instances, schools did not admit handicapped children at all; other schools placed them on long waiting lists; and still others diagnosed them inaccurately; often, as a result, the children were not taught according to their potential. At the time of this writing, the fate of federally mandated speech and language services has not been determined. In all likelihood, however, many states will fill the void and mandate help for the speech, language, and hearing handicapped. The relationships of the provisions of P.L. 94–142 to the speech/language-handicapped are included in Appendix II.

We continue to believe that federal and state laws will provide for most of the speech/language-handicapped children a free appropriate education including special education and supportive services that meet the needs of these children. These laws apply to the *speech impaired, deaf,* and *hard of hearing.* Definitions of these terms may vary but we are including those given in Public Law 94–142 (121 a.5). *Speech impaired* means a communication disorder such as stuttering, impaired articulation, language impairment or a voice impairment which adversely affects a child's educational performance. *Deaf* means a hearing impairment so severe that the child is impaired in processing linguistic information through hearing with or without amplification, which impairment severely affects educational performance. *Hard of hearing* means a hearing impairment, whether permanent or fluctuating, that adversely affects a child's educational performance, but is not included under the designation *deaf.* (See Chapter 14 for more exact definitions of *deaf* and *hard-of-hearing.*)

The passing of legislation dealing with handicapped children and the growth of research and knowledge in language acquisition, diagnosis of language disorders, and language intervention have promoted change and expansion in the field of communicative disorders. Titles of speech/language clinicians have changed. Originally they included terms such as *speech clinician, speech correctionist, speech and hearing therapist, teacher of the speech handicapped.* Now, you more frequently hear *speech/language pathologist, speech/language clinician, speech/language/hearing specialist* and *language clinician.* Similarly course titles have changed from such titles as *Speech Disorders* or *Speech Defects* to *Speech and Language Pathology* or *Communication Disorders.*

Previously speech/language clinicians programmed children for a certain period weekly or biweekly, usually taking them out of regular classes. The clinicians travelled from school to school as they treated children who in the main could function adequately in the classroom. Their case load involved predominantly articulation cases (about 80 percent). Whereas the teacher, parents, school nurse, learning disabilities teacher, psychologist and/or guidance director provided insight into the needs of each child, the clinician usually planned the speech/language program and had the ultimate responsibility for it.

Today the role of the speech/language clinician has changed. Speech/language clinicians are primarily concerned with developing children's communicative abilities, with all aspects of language— phonology, morphology, syntax, semantics, and pragmatics—as noted in Chapter 1. Children are more often placed, if possible, in a regular classroom even when they are seriously handicapped in language. The speech/language clinician serves as a member of a team the members of which diagnose and train children who are language handicapped, sometimes playing a major role and at other times a supportive one. Speech/language clinicians enhance their own standing and background by working cooperatively with other professionals in the field of psychology, reading, mental retardation and learning disabilities. All such personnel are aware that a delay in the development of speech and language is usually a predictor of potential academic problems.[2]

The supporting role of the speech/language clinician in the area of language disabilities is particularly important. According to Public Law 91–230, children with *specific learning disabilities* exhibit a disorder in one or more of the basic psychological processes involved in understanding or in using language spoken or written that may mani-

[2] For a clarification of the role of speech/language clinician in learning disabilities, see ASHA Task Force on Learning Disabilities, "Position Statement of the American Speech and Hearing Association on Learning Disabilities," *ASHA*, **18** (1976), 282–290.

fest itself in an imperfect ability to listen, think, speak, read, write, spell, or do mathematic calculations. The term includes conditions such as perceptual handicaps, brain injury, minimal brain dysfunction, dyslexia, and developmental aphasia. The term does not include learning problems that are the result of visual, hearing, or motor handicaps or that are primarily caused by mental retardation, emotional disturbance, environment, cultural or economic disadvantage.

Blanchard and Nober (1978) found that after 14 months a Massachusetts law requiring mainstreaming for all handicapped children had a significant impact on speech, language and hearing programs. Their data revealed that since the implementation of the law, there was a 38 per cent reduction in case load numbers and a 22 per cent increase in the number of clinicians hired.

Blanchard and Nober (1978) also note that clinicians today are working as a more integral part of the total service delivery process, which is now mandated by law. Consequently, the specialized services of the speech, language, and hearing clinicians are much more visible than formerly to teachers, parents, and the school administrators. The case loads have changed and now reflect significantly greater numbers of children with language disorders and more severely handicapping conditions. The need to place children with special handicaps in the least restrictive educational environment has led to an increase of supportive services of the speech, language, and hearing clinician.

Federal Public Law 94-142 has had notable effects on speech/language services. Consequently, we have given details concerning some of the law's requirements and their effects on speech/language clinicians' responsibilities in Apendix II. We have placed this information in an appendix because some readers will not be immediately interested in the details of the law.

THE SERVICES OF THE
SPEECH/LANGUAGE CLINICIAN

In allotting time for clinical services, the area that formerly received the largest share, was, as noted earlier, that of articulatory problems. Whereas children with serious articulatory disorders are still seen by the speech/language clinician, children with less serious articulatory problems are now helped through other services. In some instances, maturity alone takes care of the difficulty. But where the difficulty is of concern to the parents, to the child because of the reactions of his friends and classmates, to the teacher who may believe that the defect is retarding either his social or intellectual growth, the speech/language clinician uses his/her best judgment about servicing the child. In other instances, the speech/language clinician trains volunteers, paraprofessionals or high school or college students to help in the remediation program.

The time thus saved can be spent with children more seriously in need of speech/language services. Those seriously in need include children with noticeable voice problems, with hearing problems, with speech/language problems such as those related to organic difficulties or to neurological disturbances, those who stutter, and those who have serious phonological difficulties. In these instances, the defect does seriously interfere with communication. We believe, however, that each state should be held responsible for the funding of speech/language services even though the speech/language problems are not noticeably handicapping.

The need for speech/language clinicians to be able to diagnose and offer intervention to the language-disordered has already been noted. But the need for the supportive services of the speech/language clinician is apparent. Special Education Directors frequently ask for assistance from the speech/language clinician for help for handicapped individuals with language problems; this need for help includes both the learning-disabled and the mentally retarded. In addition, the speech/language clinician often serves as a resource person for the classroom teacher. The clinician serves as a consultant in planning a language arts program that will facilitate the language development of those children who are language-disabled at the same time that it services normal children. Whereas the teacher has the responsibility for programs to facilitate language development, the speech/language clinician provides remediation; but necessarily the clinician and teacher must help each other in their viewing of the child as a whole person in need of language development.

That speech/language clinicians base their selection of children to be helped on a logical and appropriate rationale is important, and that they use this rationale in defending the inclusion or omission of a child from their caseload is imperative. When teachers, administrators, and concerned specialists have been involved in working out this rationale, parents and other concerned individuals are more likely to accept the omission of a particular child from the case load gracefully.

THE TEAM APPROACH

The need for effective teamwork in helping the speech- and language-disordered child has already been demonstrated in the preceding pages. Both the assessment and the development of programs of remediation for language-deficient children are the result of team-work. The members of the team may vary but they inevitably include the speech/language clinician and the teacher; in addition, the school health personnel, the learning disabilities teacher, the reading specialist, and the school psychologist are often part of the team. At times, other specialists such as an orthodontist, otologist, neurologist, or psychiatrist are invited to join the group. Very important members of the team are, of course, the parents of the children involved. The team assesses the children's difficulties, works out programs for them, sees that the programs are carried through, and helps evaluate progress.

The Classroom Teacher

Surely classroom teachers know the children better than other members of the team, for they are with the children all day. Because they are interested in all of the child's development, they see the child's speech and language as part of a total development. Of the members of the team, teachers in all likelihood have the most opportunity to observe and understand the child. They know how the child acts in the playground and in class. They recognize the child's ability to lead, to be a good student, to build birdhouses, or to throw a baseball. Furthermore, they usually have more contact with the parents than any of the other members of the team. Consequently, they are the ones most intimately acquainted with the child.

Ideal classroom teachers for the language- and speech-handicapped children are good teachers for both the children with normal speech and language and those wth defective speech and language.

First, and most important, they accept children with handicaps, whether the handicaps be speech, physical, or emotional, and help the classmates of these children to be accepting. When teachers control their feelings of sympathy and accept handicapped children with their difficulties in a matter-of-fact way, the handicapped children and their classmates are likely to adopt a similar attitude.

Second, teachers make sure that their classrooms invite oral communication. When the children plan their work together, when they like to play with each other, they talk and listen. As they go on purposeful trips, as they act in a play, or as they build a bookcase, they have worthwhile discussions. Their classroom, with its interesting bulletin board, with its work corner, invites conversation.

Third, the teacher fosters good human relationships among the children. When a warm friendly feeling exists in the classroom, when youngsters like each other and their teacher, when the teacher helps to build a positive concept of self in the child, when activity is stimu-

lating, speaking is both necessary and enjoyable. As children participate in decisions, as they realize that they are the most important part
of the school program, they have a feeling of belonging to their school
group.

Last, the good teacher is a cooperative person who reinforces the
learning taught by other teachers and who contributes factual information about the child to other colleagues when it will prove useful.

The Speech/Language Clinician

Speech/language clinicians must appreciate that they are working
members of an educational team. As such, they must have a professional awareness and attitude and must cooperate with school personnel and with parents. Since so many of their clients will be mainstreamed, it is particularly important to cooperate with classroom
teachers.

Cooperation with the Classroom Teacher

The teacher and the clinician must be cognizant of the roles and
functions of communication and, furthermore, they must work together to provide motivation for the child to develop language in various contexts. When the child feels the need to communicate—to ask
for more paper, to make clear how his calculator works, to persuade
the teacher to read a favorite story, to applaud verbally a classmate's
rendition of a song, to respond to the student chairman's invitation to
join a committee—he is motivated to develop language. This type of
cooperation implies that the speech/language clinician may well be
involved in language arts curriculum development, textbook selection
in relation to children's language skills, planning and implementing
language activities in the classroom, and generally serving as a consultant to the classroom teachers in matters involving language.

Since the speech/language handicapped children are usually enrolled in regular classrooms (mainstreamed), the teacher of these children asks for advice and counselling from the speech/language clinician on the handling of these children and their difficulties. This
advice and counselling is particularly applicable to the child who is
hard of hearing and to the child who is learning-disabled. Learning-
delayed children display discrepancies between their suspected intellectual potential and their academic achievement, which discrepancy is due to a disturbance in the components and processes of language. Many of these children succeed in the regular classroom with
the help of the speech/language clinician, who often works with them
daily in a language resource room. Those children who do achieve ac-

ademically in the regular classroom tend to be those who are not more than two years behind their peers in reading, mathematics, and visual-motor areas. In such situations, the speech/language clinician and classroom teacher cooperate closely to find and use strategies for the good of the child.[3]

Speech/language clinicians work closely with reading specialists, who emphasize the importance of language abilities in learning to read. We believe that reading involves the ability to think in the language of the text, including the mastery of requisite syntax, a vocabulary adequate to the task at hand, and a feeling for and understanding of the intent of the printed message. We believe that reading based on language experience furthers the development of language generally. This matter is discussed further in Chapter 8.

Two articles provide examples for the kind of cooperation of school personnel that we believe in. In the first article Pickering and Kaelber (1978) describe a project undertaken cooperatively by the speech/language pathologist and teachers designed to help kindergarten and first-grade teachers integrate three principles of language development into regular classroom curriculum.

To begin with, the speech/language clinician noted these needs for teachers' interactions with children.

1. Teachers could modify their own listening habits and skills to present a model of someone who attends to a speaker, thereby making talking more rewarding for the speaker.
2. Teachers could expand, reformulate, and combine the children's utterances.
3. Teachers could simplify, shorten, reformulate or restate their own questions and directions when a child apparently does not comprehend or respond.
4. Teachers could ask more questions to develop logical or abstract thinking. (Pickering and Kaelber, 1978, p. 45)

Next, the speech/language pathologist identified and defined with the teachers the objectives involved in the children's understanding and expression of spoken language within the class curriculum. Thirdly, the speech/language clinician aided in the implementation of the teachers' instruction objectives by providing techniques, activities and materials. The teachers moved from the concrete to the abstract,

---

[3] From the Superintendent of Documents, U.S. Government Printing Office, Washington, D.C. 20402 at a cost of approximately $3.75, you may obtain *Guides to Mainstreaming Pre-Schoolers*. These guides, prepared to help teachers and parents, include *Children with Speech and Language Impairments, Children with Hearing Impairments, Children with Mental Retardation,* and *Children with Learning Disabilities.* These guides have been prepared to help teachers and parents.

from pantomime to verbal expression, and from simple to complex areas of comprehension and expression. For this purpose, the children were grouped according to need and were provided with activities directed toward their known cultural and social experiences. Lastly, an individualized program for children with language needs was devised wherein children with language needs received additional instruction from the classroom teachers. The fundamental goal of this program was for the speech/language clinician and the teachers to develop their own resources to provide a language development program for all the children in their classes.

The second such article is a report by Neuman (1979) on a beginning reading program planned and implemented by an interdisciplinary team. This program, designed to coordinate developmental language patterns, had five aims: (1) To increase receptive language ability. (2) To increase sight vocabulary. (3) To increase expressive vocabulary. (4) To increase expressive use of sentences. (5) To create an awareness of language as being patterned, predictable and meaningful. The project made use of puppets, flannel board, pictures, and games. The program included suggestions for the words to be used, the activities involved, the rules for sentence structure when applicable, and an evaluation.

Professional Status and Attitudes

Now that the study of speech/language disorders has reached maturity, clinicians should be aware of the need for maintaining professional status and attitudes. The first factor in awareness is gaining the necessary training. The American Speech-Language-Hearing Association lists the requirements for the certificate of clinical competence. Speech/language clinicians who work in the schools should preferably meet these requirements upon beginning their employment. If they do not, they should take whatever additional course work they need. Neal (1976) notes that of the clinicians in public schools that he surveyed, 81 per cent held the American Speech-Language-Hearing Association's Certificate of Clinical Competence in Speech Pathology, 89 per cent held a Master's degree, and 2 per cent held a doctoral degree. A second factor is the clinicians' relationships with other professions. They must recognize the delimitations of their field from those of the doctor, psychologist, psychiatrist, dentist, and physical therapist. Clinicians should neither criticize these workers nor make even a hint of a diagnosis in a field other than their own. The third factor is the knowledge of their own limitations. When clinicians do not understand a voice case or when they have difficulty with parents, they must seek help from someone who knows more than they do. Professors in universities, experienced workers in the field, and administrative officials of a school are all available to help young clinicians.

Because the clinicians are working with individuals and with small groups, they must be particularly careful to maintain a professional and workmanlike attitude and to allow no undue familiarity between themselves and their students. They should be friendly but at the same time keep the necessary professional distance. They should not respond emotionally to a child's problem, for their attitude must remain objective. Although they undoubtedly desire a permissive atmosphere for their speech/language intervention, clinicians should set their limits and hold strictly to them. A permissive attitude should not mean a laissez-faire attitude. Some behavior should be discouraged.

Human Relationships

Another part of being an effective clinician is getting along well with others—having good personal relationships with the members of the community, with the school personnel, and with the parents of their children. Clinicians must be able to work and interact with people effectively. The success of their programs depends to some extent on how well the members of the community receive the programs. Clinicians must be able to explain their programs to service clubs such as the Rotary Club or the Lions Club, and to others who are already sympathetic to the handicapped child. Clinicians must, however, be able to make them understand that the language-, speech-, or hearing-handicapped child can receive help and that their community is responsible for offering this help. One clinician, talking to a club in the town about the kind of help being given to three children with quite different difficulties, persuaded its members of the advantages of the program; in turn, these men and women were supportive of the program when the need arose.

Clinicians, as noted earlier, need the cooperation and help of the classroom teachers. In turn, they must appreciate the teachers' work. One clinician made it his duty to visit a classroom when he had some free time because of the absence of a child in his case load. His few warm words of appreciation to the teacher at the end of the visit aided in building a good relationship between the two.

The support of the parents of the handicapped children is as important as that of the classroom teacher. One father remarked recently, "I'll only live in this town three years, but I'll always be thankful for Davy's speech help. Suppose I'd happened to be in a place where there was no help." Sincere appreciation by parents is an asset in firmly establishing and maintaining a speech/language therapy program. The conferences with parents and the home visits are most important. The clinician must be able to gain the confidence of the parents so that they will cooperate for the good of the child and the success of the program.

Parent Counseling

Many speech/language clinicians meet regularly with the parents of the children they service. In one area of an inner city, the clinician meets frequently with the parents of her children in groups of about 25. Their discussions have ranged from helping the child to build a strong self-image to the verbalizing of feelings of guilt and anger by the parents. Members of this group talked frankly about their relationships with their youngsters and about their own needs and feelings, which were often reflected in their children's attitudes and behavior. As they discussed these problems with each other and with the clinician, they were better able to understand their own feelings and the feelings their children had about themselves and about their parents.

One parent lived in fear that his son, a stutterer, would become a dope addict. He kept repeating, "I try to set him straight." When questioned, he acknowledged that the reason for his fear was the boy's anger, which was often expressed in "beating up" his younger brother and other kids on the block. He began to understand why the boy felt angry and to be able to communicate this understanding to him. Even though the boy's behavior was unacceptable, the father *did* accept the fact of his anger, even when it was unprovoked. As the boy perceived his father's understanding and acceptance of his feelings, he began to communicate. The father, who had communicated mostly nonverbally, to reprimand, began to communicate verbally, and particularly at times such as when the boy was elated at his success in writing poetry. The father previously had looked on this activity as a foolish waste of time. Admittedly, the severity of the boy's stuttering did not diminish, but he became a happier and much more communicative member of his family and of his school community. The other parents in the group, mostly mothers, were instrumental in helping the father to look at himself and his son realistically and honestly.

That speech/language clinicians frequently become involved with parents is supported by Cartwright and Ruscello (1979) who surveyed speech and hearing clinics in United States and Canada to determine the amount of parent involvement in such clinics. They found that over half of the clinics hold parental conferences as clinical policy; the other half indicated that scheduling conferences is at the discretion of the clinic. In almost 80 per cent of the clinical cases, parental observation is clinical policy. Over half of the clinics hold parent discussion groups. With training, over a third of the parents carry out home practice. Parent involvement is obviously an important facet of speech, language, and hearing intervention, as is evidenced by this study.

In-Service Courses

In some schools, clinicians not only treat the children but also lead discussions and give lectures or in-service courses so that teachers can reinforce the clinician's work given in therapy sessions. Clinicians give the teachers the necessary training to locate the children with speech/language difficulties and send out mimeographed bulletins to help the teachers understand the various speech and language handicaps of the children. Clinicians explain to teachers the relationship of speech and language difficulties to academic achievement, such as reading, and to behavior problems. They report to teachers on research that relates the study of language and speech disorders to classroom teaching.

Preparing Schedules

The clinician must serve as a team member in preparing a schedule of intervention sessions and in making reports. Many variables make the preparation of a therapy schedule difficult. The clinician may want to place students homogeneously in terms of defect and age, to work with certain cases in the morning, or to cut across several classes and age levels for stuttering groups. In addition, the clinician usually has to work around the schedules of the classroom teachers and other specialists; for example, the classroom teacher may not wish a child to lose certain fundamental work that is usually given at a particular time. Because so many of the school personnel are involved, their cooperation and that of the administration is essential in working out a schedule. Consultation with the teachers and the administration helps to ensure the prompt and regular attendance of the speech-handicapped children. Lastly, the IEP with its suggested times of meeting with the handicapped child must be considered. (See Appendix)

The resulting schedule should be placed in the hands of the administrator and the teachers involved. All the members of the team should adhere to the schedule except for necessary absences.

When contemplating assigning students to the speech/language intervention sessions, the clinician should notify the parents. The need for this notification is explained in the appendix.

Before enrolling a child in speech/language intervention sessions, the clinician should make sure that the child is not receiving help from a speech and hearing center or from a private individual. Speech/language instruction from both a school and another source usually are not advantageous to the child, although overanxious parents often believe that the more help their child receives the better, and consequently enroll the child for private help without informing the school. Local centers and school personnel should cooperate to do what is best for the youngster. In some instances, the child is better treated at a center; in other instances, at school. A school administrator may coordinate the work by approving the child's taking therapy from an outside source and by excusing the child from school therapy. A signed slip is then sent to the outside source. The superintendent or another official should also request information on the amount and kind of therapy being given the child by outsiders. The work of the agency and the school should be related.

Records and Reports

Records tend to be of three types in the speech-language-hearing school center: (1) A general report available to local school agencies, (2) A report with records that provides for a study of the accountability and cost-effectiveness of the program, and (3) Case studies for individual children.

The general report tends to be made up of:

- The number of speech/language screenings.
- The number of hearing screenings.
- The number of children seen.
- The number of speech, language, and hearing disorders identified.
- The number of speech, language, and hearing disorders treated.
- The number of referrals by category of referral.
- The number of hours spent in screening, diagnosis, and therapy.
- The number of hours counselling parents, teachers, and others.

These in turn may be subdivided on the basis of the primary disorder, such as articulation, aphasia, cleft palate, cerebral palsy, hearing, language, rhythm-fluency, speech and language, and voice. They can be further subdivided into the amount of time spent on each disorder, on individual versus group therapy, on screening, diagnosis, and consultation with other personnel. The referrals can be subdivided as to who referred the child—neurologist, physician, psychologist, dentist, home care, and others. In some instances any absences of either the children or the clinician are recorded with the reasons for the absences.

The second type of report is for studying the accountability and cost effectiveness of the speech-language-hearing program. This information includes material having to do with *case selection*—the testing instruments used, the rationale for using these instruments, the use of the scores of these tests in determining admittance to the program, and other criteria such as teacher evaluations, use of language samples, or consultation with other school personnel. How is the screening program developed, organized and administered? Who is to receive the information which the screening program divulges? Information concerning accountability also includes material having to do with *diagnosis*. What instruments are available? What are used? How is this information recorded? What is the role of parents in the program? What other school personnel are involved? How is the information reported?

In addition, records for this purpose usually include material on *treatment* — scheduling and means of speech/language intervention. The scheduling section indicates how the children are scheduled, a rationale for the grouping of children, the role of the teacher of the child in the scheduling plan, the dissemination of information to the administrators and teachers about scheduling. The therapy program records should identify the groups of children according to type of disorder, age, and severity, the goals devised for each type of disorder, any provision for special programs for particular children, the dissemination of therapeutic goals to teachers and to parents (including what kind of cooperation is to be offered), and lastly an evaluation of the speech/language intervention in each case. Records are kept as to attendance, the progress of each student at each session, and the ability of each child to meet the designed goals.

Lastly, a case history is kept on each child. Recently because of innovation in the medical field, many speech/language clinicians are adopting problem-oriented records for their clients. Since this system is being widely used in medicine, occupational therapy, physical therapy, and social work, the communication among these specialists is more effective when they start from the same base. According to Kent and Chabon (1980, p. 151), this process includes four basic operations:

1. Collection of comprehensive data base for each client.
2. Identification and specification of the client's problems from the data base.
3. The formulation of objectives and plans to affect favorably or resolve the problems.
4. Maintenance of documentation of the therapeutic process including the progress or lack of it made toward the satisfactory solution of the problem.

The base includes such items as the history, the results of the diagnosis, and reports. The problem is revealed by the client but is substantiated through testing procedures. The base also includes the duration, frequency, severity, and current and past management of the problem, and objectives and plans for its management. The plans note the behavioral objectives for each problem and how they are to be achieved. The progress notes evolve from the documentation of the service plan, service delivery, therapeutic process and results of the program. The IEP form usually includes this data. Forms to guide the supplying of this data for IEP are often planned and printed for school usage. (See appendix for clarification of IEP).

The Psychologist

The psychologist helps the teacher, speech/language clinician, and the parents to understand the child. The results of the testing program may help all three in handling the child. For example, in one case a psychometric test showed a child to be far brighter than the teacher, clinician, or parents had thought. In another case, the administration of the Children's Thematic Apperception Test revealed a definite adjustment difficulty for the child. Because of the information and advice given by the psychologist, both the teacher and the clinician were able to treat these children more wisely.

In still aother case, the counseling services of the psychologist were of inestimable value. A stutterer was determined to become a lawyer. The choice definitely appeared to be his own. But the psychologist discovered in talking with him that the choice was really his grandfather's. The boy was deeply interested in science and mathematics. As a result of conferences with the psychologist and the boy's parents, the boy changed his high school major from social science to science and mathematics. The pressure to major and to do well in social studies, about which he was not enthusiastic, was removed.

A mother and father, both college graduates, set high academic standards for their boy who was struggling through an academic high school course. The psychologist helped the parents to understand their son and his academic problems—and in the process to better understand themselves. The boy is now doing very well in a general course. He spent some of his free time selling Christmas cards, which until recently was a forbidden activity. The suggestions and advice of the psychologist are particularly helpful in the adjustment of children such as these.

The psychologist's services may be of a more general nature. The problem may be one of social adjustment. Some children with speech difficulties need help in becoming a vital part of a group.

Medical Personnel

When a speech/language defect is the result of an organic or psychological difficulty, the health authorities contribute to solving the speech problem by arranging for appropriate medical treatment. They talk the health problem over with the parents and frequently refer the child to medical specialists. For instance, the nurse's home visits may be the beginning of a sound health program for the child. At times the need for the help of other specialists is obvious. For example, when the results of the audiometric examination reveal a hearing loss, the child is referred to an otologist. The child with a cleft palate will be under the care of an oral or a plastic surgeon and an orthodontist. A stutterer with a serious adjustment difficulty may require psychiatric help. The situation where many specialists work together for the benefit of the child is ideal.

As the specialists work together, an appreciation for and an understanding of the work of the others comes about. Inevitably, some overlapping takes place. The speech/language clinician, for example, surmises that certain problems of the speech-handicapped child need investigation by the psychiatrist, psychologist, or doctor. The pediatrician, on the other hand, is concerned that a child has developed a stutter and recognizes that the child's speech difficulty needs treatment. The psychologist, in examining the speech/language-handicapped child, may uncover a deep-seated personality problem that the psychiatrist must handle. Each specialist is learning from those in other fields, and each is primarily interested in helping the child to develop into an effective, well-functioning and communicative human being.

Aides

Aides, paraprofessionals, or other supportive personnel contribute to the educational programs of most school systems. Speech/language clinicians usually find that aides have added support to speech-language-hearing programs in that the aides have done routine work that frees the clinicians for language, speech, and hearing problems that require their special expertise.

In almost every instance, aides begin with a training program that is normally around two to three weeks long and which the speech/language clinician plans and administers. That the aides be selected carefully is very important. They need to be able to communicate with children effectively, to emphathize with the communicatively handicapped, to understand the cultural and linguistic heritage of certain pupils, and to establish ground rules for children's behavior. More specific qualifications of the aides involve their own ability to perform as a communication aide. These qualifications include the acceptable articulation of the sounds of English, and the ability to discriminate between phonemes and among the obvious variations within a phoneme, to follow specific instructions in the remediation (as in a programmed remediation kit), and to learn to operate tape recorders, duplicating machines, and other equipment used in the speech/language program.

Scalero and Eskenazi (1976) note that the training program for supportive personnel should include among other things these items:

- General information in the field of communicative disorders.
- Orientation to the speech and hearing unit.
- Knowledge of the role of supportive personnel in the unit.
- General knowledge of articulation disorders and the roles of the aides in this program.
- General knowledge of language disorders and the roles of aides in this program.
- Operation of programmed instruction.
- Instruction on how to keep up with the daily paper work. Preparation of materials for therapy under the direction of the speech/language clinician.

The presence of supportive personnel reduces the amount of time that speech/language clinicians spend with largely routine work and augments the time spent with the more severe, complicated cases. Aides perform well when the program is carefully planned with articulated progressive steps, and when correct and incorrect responses are based on criteria carefully worked out by the speech/language clinician and clearly understood by the aide. Costello and Schoen (1978) report on the effective articulation intervention by aides with elementary-school children with functional [th] for /s/ substitutions. These aides, all mothers, were trained as paraprofessionals in speech/language pathology. Their educational background ranged from two to four years of college.

Two successful programs where university and high school students participated in public school speech/language remediation are described in the journal *Language Speech and Hearing Services in Schools*. The first, reported by Hall and Knutson (1978) describes a cooperative program between a university and a public school wherein preprofessional undergraduate students were trained as communicative aides. They worked only with children who could correctly produce their error sound with verbal or visual stimulation. The speech/language clinician ran two orientation meetings to explain the respective roles of the clinician and the preprofessional worker in the program. The program benefited the students, the school, and the university.

The second program (Groher, 1976) involved the use of high school students to administer speech remediation for public school elementary children with articulatory difficulties. This program, too, was successful.

Paraprofessionals can also assist in screening children for speech and language problems. In rural Maine, Pickering and Dopheide (1976) report on a practical way to meet the need for immediate speech and language screening. In this instance, existing school personnel were trained for this task. Two workshops, led by two instructors holding Certification in Clinical Competence in Speech Pathology from the American Speech-Language-Hearing Association, trained 37 aides who had no previous background in speech and language training. They were first trained, through demonstrations by videotapes, to score and record imitative responses on the Templin-Darley Screening Test of Articulation. They were then prepared to assess language, voice, and fluency. Throughout, their abilities in these areas were evaluated. Finally they were given practicum experience. Their results encourage the use of existing school personnel to conduct this aspect of speech and hearing programs. The speech/language clinician must, however, continuously and carefully examine and evaluate such a program.

Problems

1. Outline the help your state provides for programs for language-, speech-, and hearing-handicapped children. How does this help compare with that of one of your neighboring states?
2. Indicate the general organization of the services for the language-, speech- and hearing-handicapped children in your town. What do you think can be done to improve them?
3. What are the certification requirements for a school language-, speech-, and hearing-clinician in your state? How do they compare with the requirements in one of your neighboring states?
4. Compare the competencies needed by the language and speech clinician with those you believe the classroom teacher requires.
5. Attend a section of an educational meeting having to do with children needing services from a speech, language, or reading specialist. Indicate how the concepts discussed in this meeting could further your education in the area.
6. Using as a base an article in *Language Arts, Reading Teacher,* or a language arts test, describe one strategy for reinforcing language remediation by a classroom teacher.

References and Suggested Readings

American Speech-Language-Hearing Association, "Association Advisory Comments Report." *ASHA*, **22** (January 1980), 33–35. (Defines speech and language pathologist and audiologist.)

——, "Code of Ethics of the American Speech-Language-Hearing Association." *ASHA*, **22** (January 1980), 41–43.

——, "Guidelines for the Employment and Utilization of Supportive Personnel in Audiology and Speech-Language Pathology." *ASHA*, **21** (November 1979), 980–984.

——. "Recommendations for Housing of Speech Services in the Schools." *ASHA*, **11** (April 1969), 181–182. (Describes room, equipment, furniture and storage space for the speech therapy room.)

——, "Requirements for the Certificates of Clinical Competence." *ASHA*, **20** (April 1978), 334–342.

——, "Guidelines for the Employment and Utilization of Supportive Personnel in Audiology and Speech-Language Pathology." *ASHA*, **21** (November 1979), 980–984

Andrews, J. R., "Applying Principles of Instructional Technology in Evaluating Speech and Language Services," *Language, Speech, and Hearing Services in Schools*, **4** (April 1973), 66–71. (Includes five questions that apply to the evaluation of speech and language therapy.)

Blanchard, M. M. and E. H. Nober, "The Impact of State and Federal Legislation on Public School Speech/Language and Hearing Clinicians." *Language, Speech, and Hearing Services in Schools*, **9** (April 1978), 77–84. Reprinted by permission.

Bouchard, M. M. and H. C. Shane, "Use of the Problem Oriented Medical Record in the Speech and Hearing Profession." *ASHA*, **19** (March 1977), 157–159.

Bountress, N. G., "The Ann Arbor Decision: Implications for the Speech/Language Pathologist." *ASHA*, **22** (August 1980), 543–545. (Discusses a court ruling requiring a school to develop a plan for teaching standard English to students who use dialectal variations.)

Bown, J. C., "The Communication Disorders Specialist as a Support Team Member of a Resource Program." *Language, Speech, and Hearing Services in Schools*, **4** (April 1973), 77–85.

Caracciolo, G. L., E. B. Morrison, and S. Rigrodsky, "Supervisory Relationships and the Growth in Clinical Effectiveness and Professional Self Esteem of Undergraduate Student Clinicians During School-Based Practicum." *Language, Speech, and Hearing Services in Schools*, **11** (April 1980), 118–126.

Cartwright, L. R. and D. M. Ruscello, "A Survey on Parent Involvement Practices in the Speech Clinic." *ASHA*, **21** (April 1979), 275–279.

Chapey, R. and G. Chapey, "Supervision: A Case Study." *Language, Speech, and Hearing Services in Schools*, **8** (1977), 256–263.

Chapey, R. *et al.*, "The Availability of Language, Speech and Hearing Centers in Day Care Centers." *ASHA*, **20** (December 1978), 1030–1034.

Cooper, E. B., "Case-Selection Procedures for School-Aged Disfluent Children." *Language, Speech, and Hearing Services in Schools*, 8 (1977), 264–269.

Costello, J. and J. Schoen, "The Effectiveness of Paraprofessionals and a Speech Clinician as Agents of Articulation Intervention Using Programmed Instruction." *Language, Speech, and Hearing Services in Schools*, 9 (April 1978), 118–128.

———, S. Rigrodsky and E. R. Morrison, "A Rogerian Orientation to the Speech-Language Pathology Supervisory Relationship." *ASHA* 20 (April 1978), 286–290.

Culatta, R., "A Competency-Based System for the Initial Training of Speech Pathologists." *ASHA*, 18 (October 1976), 733–739.

———, "Competency Based Teacher Certification." *ASHA*, 20 (March 1978), 206–210.

——— and H. Seltzer, "Content and Sequence Analysis of the Supervisory Session: A Report of Clinical Use." *ASHA*, 19 (August 1977), 523–526.

Dopheide, W. R., and J. R. Dallinger, "Improving Remedial Speech and Language Service Through Clinician-Teacher In-Service Interaction," *Language, Speech, and Hearing Services in Schools*, 6 (October 1975), 196–205.

Emerick, L. L., *Diagnosis and Evaluation in Speech Pathology;* 2nd Ed. Englewood Cliffs, N.J.: Prentice-Hall Inc., 1979. (Includes material on diagnosis, assessment, parent counselling, and report writing.)

Feldman, R. L., "Special Report: A Competence Based Teacher Education Program for Education of Teachers of the Speech and Hearing Handicapped." *ASHA*, 20 (February 1978), 84–91.

Flocken, J. M., "Personality Characteristics of Communication Disorders Graduate Students." *ASHA*, 22 (January 1980), 7–16.

Galloway, H. F., and C. M. Blue, "Paraprofessional Personnel in Articulation Therapy," *Language, Speech, and Hearing Services in Schools*, 6 (July 1975), 125–130. (Describes a three-year project in which paraprofessionals were trained to administer programmed materials to first- through fifth-grade students with articulatory errors.)

Gearheart, B. T., and M. W. Weishahn, *The Handicapped Child in the Regular Classroom*. St. Louis: Missouri; The C. V. Mosby Company, 1976. (Contains chapters on strategies and alternative for educating the hearing impaired, speech problems, and the importance of good personal interaction. Gives a clear indication of the role of the teacher in helping the handicapped child.)

Groher, M., "The Experimental Use of Cross-Age Relationships in Public School Speech Remediation." *Language, Speech, and Hearing Services in Schools*, 7 (1976), 250–258.

Hall, P. K., and C. L. Knutson, "The Use of Preprofessional Students as Communication Aides in the Schools." *Language, Speech, and Hearing Services in Schools*, 9 (July 1978), 162–175.

Healey, W. C., Coordinator, "Position Statement of the American Speech and Hearing Association on Learning Disabilities." *ASHA*, 18 (May 1976), 282–

290. (Includes material on definition of a learning disability, the preparation of speech pathologists for servicing learning disabled children, the roles and responsibilities of speech pathologists engaged in the treatment of learning disabled children, and designs for services for learning disabled children.)

Helmick, J. H., *et al.*, "Guidelines for the Employment and Utilization of Supportive Personnel." *ASHA*, **23** (March 1981), 165–169. (Includes material on the qualifications of the speech-language assistant and the audiology assistant, on the training of both of these individuals, on their roles as assistants, the competencies needed to fulfill these roles, and the supervision involved.)

Hester, E. J., "Health-Planning Agencies and Speech-Language Pathology." *ASHA*, **23** (February 1981), 85–92. (Explains role of health-planning agencies and lists them by state.)

Kamara, C., "Special Report—Computer Billing Service Analysis and Financial Reporting in a Hearing and Speech Agency." *ASHA*, **20** (April 1978), 229–231.

Kent, L. R. and S. S. Chabon, "Problem Oriented Research in a University Speech and Hearing Clinic." *ASHA*, **22** (March 1980), 151–158.

Madrid, J. H., "A Method for Determining Speech, Hearing and Language Staff Assignments to Schools in Cooperative Agreements." *Language, Speech, and Hearing Services in Schools*, **8** (1977), 209–216.

Muma, J. R., "Language Training in Speech-Language Pathology and Audiology: A Survey." *ASHA*, **21** (July 1979), 473.

Neal, W. R., "Speech Pathology Services in the Secondary Schools," *Language, Speech, and Hearing Services in Schools*, **7** (January 1976), 6–16.

Neidecker, E., *School Programs in Speech-Language: Organization and Management Supervision*, Englewood Cliffs, New Jersey: Prentice-Hall, Inc., 1980. (Provides information in organizing, developing, managing and evaluating school programs in speech-language.)

Neuman, K. H., "A Team Approach to a Language-Based Beginning Reading Program." *Language, Speech, and Hearing Services in Schools*, **10** (July 1979), 152–157.

Oratio, A. R., "Computer Assisted Interaction Analysis in Speech-Language Pathology and Audiology." *ASHA*, **21** (March 1979), 179–184.

Pannbacker, M., "Diagnostic Report Writing." *Journal of Speech and Hearing Disorders*, **40** (August 1975), 367–379. (Reviews purposes and types of diagnostic reports and provides guidelines for report writing.)

Phillips, P. P. "Variables Affecting Classroom Teachers' Understanding of Speech Disorders." *Language, Speech, and Hearing Services in Schools*, **7** (1976), 142–149. (Lists the significant variables that affect classroom teachers' attitudes toward an understanding of children with speech disorders.)

Pickering, M., "An Examination of Concepts Operative in the Supervisory Process and Relationship." *ASHA*, **19** (September 1977), 607–610.

—— and W. R. Dopheide, "Training Aides to Screen Children for Speech and Language Problems." *Language, Speech, and Hearing Services in Schools*, **7** (1976), 236–241.

———— and P. Kaelber, "The Speech-Language Pathologist and the Classroom Teachers: A Team Approach to Language Development." *Language, Speech and Hearing Services in Schools*, 9 (January 1978), 43–49. Reprinted by permission.

Sarnecky, E., S. Dublinske and M. Laney, "Notes from the School Service Program." *Language, Speech, and Hearing Services in Schools*, 11 (April 1980), 129–136. (Delineates five major problems of the speech/language clinician in the public school.)

Scalero, A. M. and C. Eskenazi, "The Use of Supportive Personnel in Public School Speech and Language Programs." *Language, Speech, and Hearing Services in Schools*, 7 (1976), 150–188.

Shafer, R. E. "The Work of Joan Tough: A Case Study in Applied Linguistics." *Language Arts*, 55 (March 78), 308–314. (Talks about resources for language arts work, language, and literature.)

Shriberg, L. D., *et al.*, "Personality Characteristics, Academic Performance and Clinical Competence in Communicative Disorders Majors." *ASHA*, 19 (May 1977), 311–321.

Task Force Report, "Task Force Report on Data Collection and Information Systems" *Language, Speech, and Hearing Services in Schools*, 4 (April 1973), 57–65.

Taylor, J. S., *Speech-Language Pathology: Services in the Schools*. New York: Grune and Stratton, 1981. (Contains material on federal legislation affecting the speech-language-and hearing handicapped, on the identification and assessment of children with communicative disorders, on case selection and management, on scheduling, and on the speech-language clinician's role with other school personnel and with parents.)

————, "Public School Speech-Language Certification Standards: Are they Standard?" *ASHA*, 22 (March 1980), 159–166.

Traywick, H., "A Rural County Speech and Language Program." *Language, Speech, and Hearing Services in Schools*, 8 (1977), 250–255. (Describes in some detail a program for providing help for the teachers and services for the speech, language, and hearing handicapped. Includes a flow chart that shows how the plan was implemented.)

Van Hattum, R. J., Chairman, "Report from the Association Advisory Committee." *ASHA*, 22 (January 1980), 33–35. (Defines the scope of the profession. Includes definitions and descriptions of practice of the speech and language pathologist and of the audiologist.)

————, "Services of the Speech Clinician in Schools: Progress and Prospects." *ASHA*, 18 (February 1976), 59–63. (Discusses the changing role of the speech clinician in the schools with less emphasis on articulatory difficulties and more on language and the clinician's contributions to the learning disabled professional team.)

Van Riper, C., *A Career in Speech Pathology*. Englewood Cliffs, N.J.: Prentice-Hall, Inc., 1979. (Presents a sample of the wide variety of speech-language clients, and solutions to their problems.)

Work, R. S. *et al.*, "Accountability in a School Speech and Language Program. Part II, Instructional Materials Analysis." *Language, Speech, and Hearing Services in the Schools*, (1976), 259–270.

3

Intercultural and Intracultural Speech and Language Usage

The following scenes represent a variety of reactions to particular speech patterns:

Scene 1. Front porch of a large, white house.
YOUNG MAN, A PH.D., SON OF A COLLEGE PROFESSOR (*to a black cat*):
Youz a beautiful kitty-cat.
FRIEND OF HIS FATHER'S: *Youz!* Ugh!

Scene 2. A reception room in a college dormitory.
HANDSOME SENIOR (*to his friend*): I say you're wrong again. (*again rhyming with rain.*)
FRESHMAN (*not so handsome*): Dumb guy—clothes, hair, walk, and *again!*

Scene 3. A train.
CONDUCTOR (*calling loudly*): Silver Creek. (Rhyming with *brick.*)
PASSENGER: Someone should tell him it's *Creek.* (Rhyming with *meek.*)

Scene 4. At the side of a large, comfortable house.
EIGHT-YEAR-OLD BLACK GIRL (*to her black friend*): I'll axs Mom for fifty cent.
MOTHER: Don't axs me for fifty cent; ask me for fifty cents!

In all four instances, the emotion of the tone and the inflection with which the comments are uttered are easy to identify but difficult to understand. If the young man feels good about saying *Youz* to the cat and if, in turn, the cat feels good about this salutation, why not? Surely this young man would not say *Youz* to his research assistant. If the second young man has somewhere picked up his particular pronuncia-

49

tion of *again,* why not? If the conductor calls *Silver Crick,* fine. In the United States as a whole, his *crick* is used as commonly as the passenger's *creek.* The small black girl, communicating to a peer, could just as easily have said, "I'll ask Mom for fifty cents" but she uses one of two dialects depending upon the circumstances. Sometimes she combines the two dialects as she did here.

The amount of interest and even of emotion generated by the pronunciation and syntactic differences in such instances as these far outweigh their importance in communication. If we were teaching actors to read the lines in these four scenes, what motivations would they ascribe to the four speakers who did the commenting? Perhaps the first commentator would add these words to the script: *with some condescension;* the second, *with derision;* the third, *with ill-concealed superiority;* and the mother, *with annoyance.* This mother may not want her child ever to use any aspect of Black English dialect, regardless of the circumstances.

In the first place, such interest in pronunciation and in syntax arises partly because these aspects of spoken language are perceived as social skills. Educated, cultured speakers tend to sound alike, to communicate with many of the same speech patterns. Admittedly, their patterns do vary somewhat as they come from different regions, but the similarity of their speech patterns outweighs the differences. Dictionaries reflect this concept. For instance, *The Random House Dictionary of the English Language* (the Unabridged Edition, 1966) contains these two definitions:

> **Standard English.** The English language as written and spoken by literate people in both formal and informal usage, and that is universally current while incorporating regional differences (p. 1385).

> **Nonstandard English.** Differing in usage from the speech or writing of those whose language is generally considered to be correct or preferred (p. 981).

In the second place, the emotional attitudes represented in the comments reflect one of the characteristics of language—that it is closely related to self. Our language is part of us and part of our family heritage. When a teacher criticizes children's language, they may feel rejected both for themselves and for their families. Many teachers believe that children who apply sets of "incorrect" pronunciation or grammatical rules must be brought into line. Their way of bringing the children into line may be humane and compassionate but negative feelings may still persist.

When teachers put the emphasis on clear communication of meaning and feeling to a particular audience, the situation is conducive to good feelings, to clear expression and reception of ideas, and frequently to the acquisition of Standard English. The understanding and feelings that are expressed and received must represent accurately the intentions of the speaker. They can represent the intent powerfully even when the pronunciation and grammar are far from standard. Edwin Newman in *Strictly Speaking* (1974, page 6) exemplifies this notion:

> Harry Truman used to say *irrevelant* and stress the third syllable in *comparable*. But Mr. Truman never had any trouble getting his points across.

Newman again represents this thesis:

> As a veteran, I was in an army hospital in 1947, and a fellow patient asked me what another patient did for a living. I said he was a teacher. "Oh," was the reply, "Them is my chief dread." A lifetime was summed up in those six syllables. There is no way to improve on that.

WHAT STANDARDS OF SPEECH FOR THE CLASSROOM?

Every young child develops language to express ideas and feelings, using whatever language feels most comfortable. In a few instances, the young child's language necessarily may be almost entirely pantomimic. But it is better to communicate through gesture than not to communicate at all. Eventually the child can be weaned from pantomimic language to spoken language. In other instances, the child's language may possess many nonstandard features. In still others, it may represent the prestigious dialect of the community. Regardless of dialect, young children must first speak in sentences to develop their particular linguistic potential; furthermore, in their early years, they do better with their native tongue than with a superimposed one.

We believe, however, that at some point children must be able to read, speak, and write Standard English if they are eventually to succeed in school, in most jobs, and in almost all professions. They may, of course, later wish to pursue a life-style outside of the middle- and upper-class milieu. But the school should provide boys and girls with the tools to cope with the demands of education in elementary school, high school, and college, in certain vocations, and in most, if not all, professions. Thus, this concept conflicts with the one that children should communicate each as an individual in a dialect of choice that may well have a code and structure all its own and that fundamentally has as much right to attention as any other dialect.

Admittedly, some educators and some linguists, believing that teachers should not confuse the middle-class social stigma of a particular dialect with its linguistic capacities as a linguistic tool, are not concerned with presenting children with the option of learning the "prestigious" dialect. They consider the sum total of dialectal variations as self-contained, systematic, ordered systems that are different from but neither communicatively more or less effective than Standard English. They believe that a nonstandard dialectal system with its logical and consistent rules is an effective code for expressing ideas and concepts. Most educators today recognize that a Black English dialect is a viable tool for communication, that a speaker can use it to communicate abstractions on any level, and also that it is based on a variant of the linguistic system that is recognized as Standard American English. As communication is needed, language develops.

Whenever speakers of different languages are thrown together through business, war—or in earlier days at slave stations—they devise a language for the necessary communication, a contact language or pidgin. African pidgin was one language of this type. The Portuguese in their travels and conquests established pidgins around the world. A pidgin is a nonnative shared language resulting from intersocietal rather than intrasocietal contacts. Occasionally, when the need for communication disappears so does the need for the pidgin. In such cases, the pidgin may be learned as a native language and the process of creolization begins; consequently Creole then evolves like any other language (Bolinger 1975, p. 356).

Bailey advocates that teachers understand the creolization processes:

> Specialists in Creole linguistics believe that the verb system of the Negro speakers of non-Standard English is much more like that of the English-based Creoles than of Standard English, and that unless teachers understand that this is a valid system with its own grammatical rules, they cannot intelligently guide the children into an acquisition of the new system that is so much like their own that the possibility of linguistic interferences increases at every turn. The Creole languages express the possessive relationship, the number distinction in nouns and verbs, the past tense in verbs, and the cases of pronouns by different means from the Indo-European languages, in which such relationships are indicated by suffixation of some kind. Grammatical relations in the Creoles are largely expressed by juxtaposition of words, by the aid of special function words, or by the stress and pitch patterns (Bailey 1968, p. 573).

We believe that language and culture are entwined. If in Hawaii pidgin is part of an individual's culture and of his image of himself, it should not be ridiculed but accepted. However, it should be possible to learn Standard English as part of another culture. We believe that the child must learn first to communicate in his native-born dialect. The kindergartner who omits the final *t* and *d* for the past tense in *I like her* for *I liked her* and *I lug the box* for *I lugged the box* is using a morphological system that is different from those of children speaking Standard American English. It is important for the teacher to accept this as one mode of communication but, at some point, the child must build a second mode of communication, for a nonprestigious social dialect in a local community can be a handicap. A candidate for district attorney who says "tooim" and "dis" and "dat" detracts from the appeal of his message to some of his audience even though what he says may have real and significant import to the community. Blacks, too, at some point in their school career need to learn to speak, read, and write Standard English. Dr. Bernard Gifford,[1] a research scholar at the Russell Sage Foundation and former Deputy Chancellor of the New York City School System, says, "English is the language that blacks have to learn how to read and write and speak if they want to achieve anything in America."

WHEN DO WE TEACH CLASSROOM STANDARD SPEECH?

Having stated our position that at some point the teacher should teach Standard English or the "prestigious dialect" as a second mode of communication, the question arises: When? Baratz (1970) advises that standard English be taught in the junior and senior high school years. Loban (1968) suggests that children start learning standard English during the third grade:

> The strategy is merely that the pre-school stage and kindergarten are much too early to press him to be concerned about using Standard dialect continuously. Such teaching only confuses small children, causing them to speak much less frequently in school. Usually from grade three and after, the children's daily recitation should adhere to standard English, but in the early years the teacher would accept "him a good dog." At this stage the teacher would be more interested in eliciting from the child, "him a good dog but with three fleas"; indeed, the teacher would be very much interested in such qualification and amplification (Loban 1968, p. 595).

Loban further talks about when to begin the discussion of social language discrimination:

[1] As reported in *The New York Times*, November 27, 1979, p. C4.

Eventually the time comes when the teacher must talk over with these pupils the facts of social language discrimination, and that time, to my way of thinking, usually is grade five, six, or seven. Teachers differ on the ideal age for introducing the concept, but I see no point in telling children this earlier. Before they can really see the value of learning standard English, pupils need to understand the social consequences the world will exact of them if they cannot handle the established dialect. Grade five, six, or seven, therefore, would be the point at which the concept would be discussed, although parts of the total concept might be sketched in earlier as answers to questions children ask. At this grade level I would select most carefully teachers who do not have snobbish attitudes about language, the scholar-linguist-humanists whom the school could most safely entrust with the important task of explaining sociological truth to these children, aged 11 and 12 (Loban 1968, p. 519).

Bountress (1977) indicates that while a gradual decrease in the use of Black English characteristics occur as a function of age, the tendency for the most pronounced dialectal decline in the language occurs between six and seven years of age for most of the linguistic functions. As a result of this study, Bountress believes that a readiness period exists in the linguistic development of school-age children who speak Black English; he suggests that this period begins at approximately seven years of age.

Geiger and Greenberg (1976), as a result of their study of the black child's ability to discriminate dialectal differences, similarly believe that the process of recognizing dialectal distinctions is a developmental one. The development proceeds from the use of paralinguistic features (including topic, message content, age, and sex of speaker) to reliance on logical differences and, finally discrimination of syntactic features. They indicate that children may be ready for training in the paralinguistic and lexical features of social dialects during the primary school years. They further note that these distinctions should be made before the syntactic ones.

HOW DO WE TEACH STANDARD CLASSROOM SPEECH?

Having indicated *when* we would begin teaching Standard English, we now need to be concerned with *how*. The base of literacy is the child's existing language and the ability to use it proficiently and effectively. The first important principle in establishing the base combines two concepts: (1) Teachers speak in manners that are natural to them; they do not need to speak in the local dialect even when most of the children use it, and (2) Teachers understand and accept the children's particular dialects. The class may contain children with a variety of dialects: those coming from foreign countries and having a definite "foreign accent," those speaking Black English; those speaking little or no English; those speaking non-Standard English; those speaking Standard English. The second important principle is that the child be permitted, even encouraged, to respond to what he/she has read or experienced in his/her own language. The third principle is that as much of the curriculum as possible be experientally based. Our own preference would be that reading be taught through language experience. This strategy utilizes the child's own language patterns, naturally reflecting the phonology, morphology, syntax, semantics, and pragmatics of native speech. The experiences in the class should be those that will expose the children to vocabularies they do not already possess, to more complicated sentence structure, to Standard English, and to experiences that will encourage talk.

Attitudes Toward Standard and Non-standard Speech

Both children and adults seem to attribute more positive qualities to speakers of Standard English than to speakers of non-Standard English. Light (1970) studied how eight- and nine-year-old children from different socio-economic backgrounds react to Standard and non-Standard English and the extent to which they conceptualize their attitudes. Fifty-two children listened to a speech sample recorded by a well-educated black woman who spoke Standard English and to one recorded by another black woman who, less educated, spoke non-Standard English. The children responded to each of the two recordings by completing a semantic differential scale, which scale included the categories of intelligence (smart—dumb), appearance (pretty—ugly), personality (nice—mean), economic background (rich—poor), and race (black—white). In general, the children's responses attributed the positive qualities (smart, pretty, and nice) more often to the Standard-English-speaking voice and the negative qualities (dumb, ugly, poor) more often to the non-Standard-English recording. Light notes that these children had learned to stigmatize others on the basis of non-Standard speech—to judge others harshly on a basis that has no actual worth. The study does indicate, however, that their judgments about the speakers functioned independently of perceived race to a degree not previously suspected. These children, nevertheless, are "well on their way to developing linguistic attitudes held by society at large," (Ibid., p. 137). Similarly Giles and Farrar (1979) report that studies show that the more prestigious the accent speakers adopt, the more intelligent, competent, educated, self confident, and industrious they are perceived. Likewise, Cazden (1972, p. 174) reports research that demonstrates that teachers evaluate children more negatively when the children's speech has the features of non-Standard English.

Color alone may have an effect on the perception of speech and language by some teachers. Williams (1971) asked teachers to evaluate speech patterns of a black child and a white child whom they saw and heard on videotape. In spite of the fact that Standard speech patterns were superimposed on the tape of the black child, teachers perceived the black child as speaking less standard American English than the white child.

Recent evidence indicates that school personnel are developing more flexible and positive attitudes toward non-Standard English and in their teaching reveal that different varieties of English have a place in our society. As noted later, most of us have a repertoire of speech styles that we adjust to the particular occasion and audience. We hope, too, that teachers are motivating their children to learn to speak Standard English.

Receptive Language Abilities of Inner-city Children

Current research seems to indicate that upon entrance to school, inner-city children are able to comprehend the Standard English of the teacher even though this dialect is different from their own. We have selected some recent reports of research that support this thesis: Quay (1971) tested 100 black four-year-olds with the Stanford-Binet Test using (1) Standard English and (2) Negro dialect and found no reliable difference in the two modes of expression. Levy and Cook (1973) studied the relationship between dialect proficiency in Standard and in Black non-Standard English and auditory comprehension of stories presented in Black non-Standard and Standard English. The subjects, 32 black second-grade boys and girls, did consistently better on performance based on stories that were told in Standard English. Similarly, Ramsey (1972) found no significant difference in the ability of first-grade Negro dialect speakers to answer literal comprehension questions about stories presented orally in Standard English and in Black non-Standard English. Again, Frentz (1971) found no relationship between the dialect of third-grade users and the comprehension of sentences presented orally in the two dialects.

A similar finding is reported by Marwit and Neumann (1974) who used a black and a white examiner to administer Standard English and non-Standard English forms of the Reading Comprehension section of the California Reading Test to 60 black and 53 white second-graders.

The investigators found that black children did not comprehend non-standard English materials better than those in Standard English and that white children did not comprehend Standard English better than non-Standard English. This research has to do with the receptive aspects of language that precedes production aspects.

In other words, young children understand many facets of the language before they are able to produce them. Teachers and clinicians need to understand the differences between the receptive and productive language processes and, in addition, be aware of what young children are listening to and understanding, to be supportive of the children's communicative efforts in their own dialects, and to avoid over-emphasizing the production of Standard English. They need to recognize that children may have more language proficiency than they exhibit in talking.

FACTORS INVOLVED IN ADOPTING THE LANGUAGE OF THE SCHOOL

In helping students to adopt the language of the school, teachers recognize a variety of factors: (1) that words are rarely spoken singly, but are almost always a part of a phrase or sentence and that in this process pronunciations of words change because of the influence of sounds in context; (2) that language is constantly changing; (3) that there are regional differences in speech; (4) that speech styles vary from one communicative situation to another and that the social group of the speaker influences the speaker's patterns; (5) that spelling is frequently not helpful in learning to pronounce words; and (6) that dictionaries, while useful guides, are not wholly dependable when a particular word is to be used in a conversational phrase. These factors are considered in more detail in the following pages.

Contextual Utterance

Words, almost never spoken singly, are usually part of a phrase or a sentence. As your friend asks, "Are you going to buy a red or blue dress?" you may respond, "Red." Even here, however, you are likely to respond with, "A red dress" or "I need a red one to match my shoes and purse." Speech moves or flows onward from word to word within a phrase. In onflowing speech contextual influence is always at work and the sounds of syllables of different words may be linked as "Aredress," [ərɛd:rɛs] for *a red dress. What is* usually becomes "Whats" or "Wats" [hwɑts] or [wɑts].

Children eat *a napple* [ənæpl] long before they become aware of *an apple*. Part of the change in pronunciation is the result of the influence of adjacent sounds. *Assimilation,* the modification of pronunciation, has usually occurred over the decades in the direction of simplicity and economy of effort. For instance, *Captain* sometimes becomes *Capm* [kæpm̩]. [p] is made with both lips and this position influences [n] to become [m]. But the nasal characteristic of the [n] is maintained. [t] is dropped entirely, however. In *horseshoe* [s], too, is completely lost; [ʃ] takes over [s].

Some assimilations are widely used; others are not. *Nature* and *picture* are commonly pronounced *nacher* [netʃɚ] and *pikcher* [pɪktʃɚ]. Almost all of us take these pronunciations with their assimilations for granted. Almost none of us attempt to say *natyer* [netjɚ] or *pictyer* [pɪktjɚ]. The same kind of change occurs when we say *wonchu* [wontʃə] for *won't you* [wontju]. Some persons are loath to accept the assimilation in *wonchu* although they themselves use the same kind of assimilation in *nature*. Types of assimilation will be discussed in Chapter 6.

Another example of change in onflowing speech is the use of *weak* rather than *strong* forms. The following are examples: When we read the word *to* in a list of words, we pronounce it as *two* or *too*. But when we read *to* in the sentence, "I want to do it," the vowel in *to* is no longer a long o͞o but a short o̅o̅ or even the schwa /ə/, the sound in the last syllable of *sofa*. The *to* pronounced like *two* is the strong form, whereas the *to* pronounced like [tə] is the weak form. When we say, "We live in Apartment 2A," we pronounce the *a* to rhyme with *day*. But when we say, "We live in a house," the *a* is the same sound as we use in the last syllable of *sofa*, the schwa. The *a* that rhymes with *day* is the strong form; the one that is the schwa is the weak form. The *a* in *and* in a list of words is pronounced with a short *a*, but the *a* of *and* in the phrase *Mary* and *John* is likely to be the schwa. The first *a* is the strong form; the second *a*, the weak form. Ordinarily we use the weak forms of pronouns, prepositions, articles, auxiliaries, and conjunctions in conversation, except where we stress a particular word. For example, when we want to stress that *both* Mary and John are going, we may use the strong form of *and*. In strong forms, the vowel is stressed; in weak forms it is unstressed.

Changes in Language

Styles of pronunciation change. Many of these changes are obvious. We do not pronounce the *k* in *know, knight,* and *knee*. These words began to lose their *k* sound in the seventeenth century and completed the loss in the eighteenth century. *K* does remain the Germanized pronunciation of such proper names as *Knag* or *Knode*. The seventeenth-century poet Alexander Pope rhymed *join* with *thine*. We know that *join* was then pronounced *jine* [dʒaɪn]. Furthermore, he rhymed *obey* and *tea*. *Tea* was then pronounced *tay* [teɪ]. Changes may occur in the pronunciations within families from one generation to the next. A father and mother may say *erster* [ɜrstɚ] for *oyster* and *boin* [bɒɪn] for *burn*. Their daughter, however, pronounces *oyster* and *burn* the way most of the rest of us do. Here some outside influence, perhaps that of the child's playmates or her teachers, brings about the change.

Not only pronunciations change but so do meanings of words. Slang varies from decade to decade. Once an exciting person was *hot stuff,* then *cool,* and more recently just plain *hot. Super* or *super-duper* has now become *"awesome."* Such language creeps even into reporting in *The New York Times.* In a recent review of a television documentary,[2] "Only the Ball Was White," the performance of a black, quiet, modest Bob Gibson, who had hit at least fifty home runs a season, was described as "awesome." Shortly *awesome* will be supplanted by another word or phrase.

Regional Differences

We have spoken about "prestigious" pronunciations and have indicated that pronunciations, voice, and vocabulary differ in varying speech situations. We have talked about the influence of particular social cultures and subcultures. Another difference exists—that of region. Kenneth Goodman points out that socially acceptable speech varies from region to region and that no dialect of American English has ever achieved the status of some imaginary standard that is correct everywhere and always. He writes:

> It is obvious that a teacher in Atlanta, Georgia, is foolish to try to get her children to speak like cultured people in Detroit or Chicago . . . cultured speech, socially preferred, is not the same in Boston, New York, Philadelphia, Miami, Baltimore, Atlanta, or Chicago. The problem, if any, comes when the Bostonian moves to Chicago, the New Yorker to Los Angeles, the Atlantan to Detroit. Americans are ethnocentric in regard to most cultural traits, but they are doubly so with regard to language. Anybody who doesn't speak the way I do is wrong. A green onion is not a scallion. I live in Detróit not Détroit. (Goodman 1967, p. 41).

The educated person from Boston has little difficulty understand-

---

[2] *New York Times,* February 16, 1981, page C-18.

ing the educated person from Atlanta. The backwoodsman from Minnesota with little education may, however, have difficulty understanding the mountaineer from Tennessee with little education. Differences in speech among the educated are not as wide as those among the uneducated, even though admittedly there are discernible differences in the speech patterns of educated persons of different areas.

The differences among the areas are, however, not too numerous. A New Englander and a Southerner may say *bahn* for *barn*, whereas an Ohioan is likely to pronounce the *r* in the same word. A New Englander approaches *pahth* for *path*. The Ohioan is likely to use the same vowel in *path* that he uses in *cat*. In the South the *o* in *glory* is usually the same *o* as in *tote;* whereas in some other regions, it may be the *aw* sound in *law*. The vowel in the word *scarce* in the North Central and Eastern areas may be either the vowel found in *hate* or the one in *let* or in *there* in the South, for the word *scarce* the vowel in *hat* is heard frequently. In *greasy* and the verb *grease*, the New Englander uses the *s* sound whereas the Southerner uses the *z* sound.

A dialect miscue may result from these different pronunciations, although most children make instant translations. Rigg (1978) defines dialect miscues as "differences between the author's dialect and the readers." She points out that if children use the same vowel /ɪ/ in *pen* and *pin*, the teacher should not attempt to teach the aural and oral discrimination of these two words. She further notes that since all of us translate an author's sound system into our own, differences between the author's and the reader's sound systems have little effect on comprehension. She notes that most readers change, "'You might right,' said Mrs. Slater with a sigh" in Lois Lenski's *Strawberry Girl* to "You're mighty right." She suggests that teachers provide students with material of literary worth in a variety of dialects and then show them how to read dialects different from their own without losing meaning. This type of teaching is also applicable to oral communication.

When teachers consider regional differences as pronunciation errors and try to correct the pronunciations, they find themselves in trouble. In the first place, the children will have difficulty in differentiating the two sounds themselves and, in the second place, they will not be hearing the differentiation in the community in which they live. The teachers themselves may not make the distinctions except in the classroom and even there, they may be inconsistent. Teachers must accept such regional differences, for no single standard of pronunciation exists in North America.

The Influence of Spelling on Pronunciation

Until the fifteenth or sixteenth century spelling, changing frequently, kept pace with changes in pronunciation. As we look at the following extract from the Prologue to *The Canterbury Tales*, we realize how different our spelling is today. This excerpt is representative of Middle English.

THE PRIORESSE:

Ther was also a nonne, a Prioresse,
That of hir smylyng was ful symple and coy;
Hir gretteste ooth was but by Seint Loy;
And she was cleped Madame Eglentyne.
Ful wel she soong the servyce dyvyne,
Entuned in hir nose ful semely, ...

For the last 400 or 500 years spelling has remained relatively constant while pronunciations have changed. Spelling today, therefore, does not always approximate the pronunciation of words. For example, the *t* sound in *castle* and *whistle*, the *b* sound in *limb* and *comb*, the *w* sound in *write*, the *s* sound in *island*, and the *l* sound in *calm* are not pronounced. The *i* /ɪ/ sound is variously spelled as *o* in *women*, *y* in *myth*, and *i* in *linen*.

The discrepancy between sound and spelling has caused some persons to ask that the writing conform to the sounds. Thus, over the years, many attempts have been made to change spelling to reflect the spoken word. Before George Bernard Shaw died, he specified in his will that a considerable sum of money be used for spelling reform. Such systems are frequently proposed, then abandoned. The same discrepancy has caused others to try to make the sound conform to the spelling. Some people today try to pronounce both *p* and *b* in *cupboard* and all the sounds in *indict*. Although the *t* in *often* was dropped, it is creeping back. The same is true of the *l* in *almond*. Some of our American pronunciations as distinguished from British pronunciations show that we have placed some value on spelling. For example, the name *Anthony* in Britain is pronounced with a *t* for the *th* and *secretary* in British English usually has three syllables as compared to our four syllables.[3]

---

[3] For information on influence of writing on spoken language, see F. W. Householder, *Linguistic Speculation*, Cambridge, England; Cambridge University Press, 1971, ch. 13.

The Influence of Dictionaires on Pronunciation

Long before dictionaries existed, people understood the words that others pronounced. Today, however, lexicographers record pronunciations. One function of the dictionary is to describe the pronunciation of a word, not to dictate or prescribe it. The early lexicographers based their recording of pronunciations not only on the pronunciations of the cultured people of the time, such as statesmen and actors, but also on their own idiosyncracies. Daniel Webster, however, realized that pronunciations must be based on the pronunciations of the people. Mencken says of Webster:

> He was always at great pains to ascertain actual usages and in the course of his journeys from State to State to perfect his copyright on his first spelling book he accumulated a large amount of interesting and valuable material, especially in the field of pronunciation. . . . He proposed therefore that an American standard be set up, independent of the English standard, and that it be inculcated in the schools throughout the country. He argued that it should be determined not by "the practice of any particular class of people," but by "the general practice of the nation . . ." (Mencken 1946, p. 9).

Today, lexicographers try to record accurately the pronunciations of the educated, cultured citizens of our country and to keep the recordings current. They try to inform on the basis of the facts of usage. When a substantial proportion of the population pronounces a word in a certain way, they record it.

A pronunciation given in a dictionary is a generalization of the way many persons say a word. The recording of this generalization differs from dictionary to dictionary. Dictionaries frequently record more than one pronunciation. In some instances, the first pronunciation is the one held to be more widely used; in others, the editor makes no attempt to show which pronunciation is the more prevalent. At least one dictionary indicates pronunciations current in regional areas. Most do not. Some dictionaries record the pronunciations using diacritic markings; others record them with phonetic symbols. Some adopt for representation the style of formal platform speech; others include informal pronunciations. Teachers should read the introduction to a dictionary to learn what its levels and procedures are. They should also note its date to determine whether the pronunciations recorded are current.

Dictionaires are useful in assisting us to pronounce unfamiliar words. When students come across a word such as *esophageal,* the dictionary is an excellent source of information for pronunciation. But for the usual, everyday words, students do better to train their ears to listen rather than to find the pronunciations in the dictionary, for we learn pronunciation largely through imitation. Those desiring to improve their pronunciations must listen to the speech of the educated, cultivated members of their communities who have had certain social advantages. In addition, they must listen to themselves (often with a recorder) so that they know how their speech differs. If we look up *duty* in the dictionary, we may find the *y* sound before the *u*; however, careful reading of the introduction of the dictionary usually indicates that the word is pronounced both with and without the *y* sound. Surely to listen and to perceive the differences is more helpful than to use the dictionary. Furthermore, dictionaries give pronunciations of a word as it is used individually. When we speak, however, we rarely speak in single words, but rather in phrases or sentences. The same words used in different phrases with different rhythm, tempo, intonation, and meaning intended by the speaker do not sound alike. For instance, dictionaries usually include the strong forms (stressed ones), not the weak forms (unstressed). The student, whether in elementary or in secondary school, should learn to use the weak forms both in speaking and in reading aloud.

Whereas almost all children learn pronunciations of words from hearing them, they need to be introduced to dictionaries as early as the second or third grade. They should look up unfamiliar words to find their meanings and their pronunciations. Throughout our lives, most of us have used dictionaries as reference books. Now that dictionaries have been written and edited just for children, they can become accustomed to using them for reference in the primary grades. In addition, dictionaries, especially those that are attractive to children, can arouse an interest in language through their appeal. *Beginning Dictionary*[4] is an example of a dictionary that children not only learn from but enjoy. The definitions are clear and normally within the ability of third to sixth graders to understand. This dictionary includes, in addition to a phrase defining the word, sentences with the word used in context. For example *heavy* is defined as: *Large in size and amount*. But this definition is followed by: *We were late because we got stuck in heavy traffic* and *We had a heavy snowfall last night*. Sometimes there is no specific definition but the word is used in a variety of contexts. For example, *this* is defined thus: *This house is ten years old. This dress is cheaper than that one. Is this your coat? This*

---

[4] Wm. D. Halsey, Editorial Director and C. G. Morris, Editor, *Beginning Dictionary*. New York: Macmillan Publishing Co., Inc., 1977.

is mine; that is hers. Is it this hot here every day? At the end of the
entry, the pronunciation, part of speech and inflection are included.
The key for pronunciation is based on diacritical markings, with the
exception of the schwa /ə/, which is explained clearly. One of the advantages of this dictionary is that the pronunciation key appears on
every page; another is that many words are illustrated with pictures.

Another dictionary useful for approximately the same age group is
Webster's New Elementary Dictionary.[5] The entries have been selected largely on the basis of their occurrence in textbooks and in assigned reading in the elementary curriculum. Again the pronunciation
key is easy to use. This dictionary, also, is illustrated. Further, it includes at the end lists of Presidents and Vice-Presidents, states of the
union, Canadian provinces, the world's nations and their largest
cities.

A more sophisticated dictionary is *School Dictionary,*[6] which is designed for junior high school students. This dictionary is written on a
higher level than the others and meets the needs of children in grades
6–9. It includes clear, useful definitions and many pictorial illustrations of the meanings of words.[7]

Speech and Language Styles in Context

The particular speaking situation influences the speaker's speech patterns. Joos (1962) notes that people use a wide variety of speech and
language styles—varying from the most intimate to the most formal
and that they automatically shift to whatever is appropriate to the social situation. When children play ball in an open field, they speak
more loudly than usual, more quickly, often in shorter phrases, and
with a quite different choice of language from when they are playing a
word game in which they are concentrating to recall unusual words.
As they speak together in the classroom, they are likely to speak more
formally, in longer phrases, and be more careful of their pronunciations than they are when they call to each other on the playground. In
a school assembly, the child who introduces the speaker speaks still
more formally—more slowly, with more stresses, with more careful

---

[5] *Webster's New Elementary Dictionary.* Springfield, Mass: G. and C. Merriam
Company, 1975.

[6] *School Dictionary,* New York: Macmillan Publishing Co., Inc., 1974.

[7] Dictionaries for still younger children are available. These include L. Hayward,
Ed., *The Sesame Street Dictionary,* New York: Random House; T. J. Baehr and S.
Krensky, Eds., *My First Dictionary,* Boston: Houghton Mifflin Company; *Webster's Beginning Dictionary,* Springfield, Mass.: G and C. Merriam Company. Since we believe
that dictionaries generally have little academic value until the second or third grade, we
have not reviewed them here.

choice of language. Thus, the continuum goes from very informal speech and language often with many nonstandard pronunciations, to formal speech and language with few nonstandard pronunciations. We believe that the particular communicative situation determines the kind of language used: the vocabulary, the pronunciations, the syntax, the morphology, the voice, the rate of speaking. All of us tend to modify our styles of speaking in different situations according to the styles of the persons to whom we are talking. Within the limits of their speech repertoires, two persons meeting for the first time tend to become alike in their speech styles, including rate, pauses, pronunciations, and syntax. The language of the speakers reflects the need of both speakers to be socially integrated (Giles and Thakerer, 1980).

In today's world, to attempt to modify children's speech and language styles without their seeing the need for change and wanting to make the change is foolish. Parents often see the need for change. For example, one parent vehemently said to her child's teacher, "Jamie's gotta speak good—not like me." Obviously this mother encourages (perhaps too strongly) her child to adopt a speech and language style different from hers. Children should recognize early that they have a repertoire of speech and language styles and that a particular person, group, or situation demands a particular style from this repertoire.

CULTURAL DIFFERENCES IN SPEECH AND LANGUAGE AND THE TEACHER'S ROLE

Teachers are aware that voice and pronunciation characteristics exist on all kinds of local, cultural, and subcultural levels and that the influence of the social group on the speaker's voice and pronunciation is important. Teachers usually are sensitive to the needs of the child who speaks other than Standard English. But to some teachers, the child who speaks Black English may seemingly not do as well as a child of the same intellectual ability who speaks Standard English. In such instances, the speech/language clinician helps these teachers become sensitive to the notion that the most important aspect of communication is getting meanings and feelings across to others successfully. The clinician also helps the teachers to recognize that language either adds or detracts from communicative intent. Henry Higgins convinced Eliza Doolittle in Shaw's play *Pygmalion* to change her speech patterns. Teachers, like Henry Higgins, must, as noted earlier, recognize the importance of language as a measure of social success in adult life. If their students want to achieve in America, it is important that they graduate from high school with an ability to speak Standard English.

Improving Pronunciation

Having established (1) the need for the teacher to recognize the variety of speech and language styles and the use of them in different communicative situations, (2) the prime importance of successful communication—the achievement of the speaker's communicative intent, and (3) the need for most high school graduates to speak Standard English, the question arises *what* to improve. Teachers are not concerned with regional differences, or with pronunciations that are widely accepted. They are concerned with those characteristics that tend to generate the impression that speech is not prestigious, that it contains many nonstandard pronunciations. These nonstandard deviations, unlike articulatory defects, which are definitely speech difficulties, are not the responsibility of the speech/language clinician but of the classroom teacher. The ten-year-old boy who substitutes *f* and *v* for the two *th*'s and says *acrost* for *across* is in need of help from the teacher to understand and sometimes to eliminate the nonstandard speech.

Obviously, as noted earlier, there is a time for teachers to motivate their students to achieve Standard English and a time for them to help students reach this goal. Just as obviously not all substandard speech characteristics can be eliminated during two or three grades; rather such elimination usually is a process that occurs directly or indirectly in all language arts activities in the course of the school years.

Nonstandard Speech Characteristics

Teachers frequently need make but few formal attempts to change nonstandard speech patterns—particularly when the students are participating in communicative situations where there is a kind of standardization of language based on the prestigious dialect of the community. As children and their teachers are thrown together in the classroom, the children's own pronunciations tend to move toward a class standard. Consequently, many of them discard their nonstandard variants. As they share each others' thoughts and feelings in a variety of classroom experiences, their language and speech differences tend to be ironed out.

The guidance of the teacher, however, may be needed in eliminating

1. substitution of one sound for another,

2. omission of sounds,
3. addition of sounds,
4. transposition of sounds, and
5. addition of features that are not usually part of a sound.

SUBSTITUTION OF SOUNDS. Nonstandard pronunciation frequently involves the substitution of one sound for another; for example, one consonant may be substituted for another. A common substitution is that of /d/ for ð, as *dem* and *dose* for *them* and *those*. The teacher must remember, however, that many substitutions are made by educated people. For example, many educated speakers pronounce *when, where,* and *what* with an initial *w*, though others do use the *wh* sound. Other assimilations frequently used by the educated are *ingcome tax* for *income tax, grampa* for *grandpa,* and *pangcake* for *pancake.*

Many vowel substitutions are so widely employed that they have become acceptable. *Git* for *get* is heard so frequently that many speakers would not even notice the substitution. Other vowel substitutions are regional. Many Midwesterners use the same vowel in *merry, Mary,* and *marry.* Almost no one notices this variation in vowel usage. On the other hand, as *milkman* becomes *mulkman,* as *been* becomes *ben,* the substitution may distract from the message.

OMISSION OF SOUNDS. In informal speech most of us omit many sounds even though they are included in the orthographic representation of the word. For example, the word *clothes* is frequently pronounced *cloz,* omitting the *th* sound. Both the *American College Dictionary* and Webster's *New Collegiate Dictionary* accept these variants. Before a teacher insists on the inclusion of a sound, we recommend consultation of a good, recent dictionary. The following are some of the omissions that probably do not occur in formal speech; *bout* for *about; Bufflo* for *Buffalo; kunt* for *couldn't; ask* for *asked; mosly* for *mostly; simily* for *similarly; reconize* for *recognize.*

ADDITION OF SOUNDS. Sounds are frequently added or inserted. Historically we have added sounds; for instance, *against* was once *agens.* Although dictionaries for years did not recognize the *t* in *often* or the *h* in *forehead,* some dictionaries now include both of these pronunciations. Many speakers pronounce *mince* as if it were *mints* or *dance* as if it were *dants.* The insertion of excrescent [t] makes for easier, more economical pronunciation by all, including the educated. But some additions and insertions are less common in the speech of the educated. Examples of these are *athaletic* for *athletic; anywheres* for *anywhere; oncet* for *once; drownded* for *drowned; wisht* for *wish; pursh* for *push; filum* for *film;* and *theayter* for *theatre.*

TRANSPOSITION OF SOUNDS. Children frequently and adults sometimes transpose sounds. Most of us have heard a child ask for *pisghetti* (spaghetti). Here again, dictionaries record that educated persons use some of these transpositions. Kenyon and Knott list both *children* and *childern* and *hundred* and *hunderd.* Transpositions rarely used by educated persons include *prespire* for *perspire; plubicity* for *publicity; modren* for *modern; revelant* for *relevant; I akst him* for *I asked him; pernounce* for *pronounce; tradegy* for *tragedy; patrin* for *pattern;* and *osifer* for *officer.*

DISTORTION OF SOUNDS. Sometimes a child approximates a given sound but changes some of the features somewhat. The child may make an *s* so that it cannot be readily distinguished from an *sh.* The problem arises as to how liberal to be in accepting these changes. The first part of the diphthong of *now* is normally a back sound. Many Americans, however, raise the tongue on the first part of this diphthong so that it is in the same position as the vowel in *cat.* Many Americans raise the tongue on the vowel sound in *hat* nearly to the position of the vowel sound in *met.* The teacher must make a value judgment on whether to motivate the child to change the pronunciation of the diphthong in *now* and the vowel in *cat.*

Establishing Prestigious Dialects

As noted earlier, some children need to learn to speak Standard English as a second language. The work of Shuy (1964) suggests methods for accomplishing this. Other children need to be made aware that to speak well is an economic and social advantage. For this second group, the teacher leads a discussion by asking such questions as: What do we mean by "speaking well?" Who speaks well? Are there various degrees of speaking well? Should we always speak equally well? When do we need to speak particularly well? Where do we need to speak particularly well? How can we help each other to speak well?

As children talk about effective speech, they will not only list "correct" pronunciation, pleasant voices, and saying the sounds "correctly" but they will also include other factors such as sounding friendly, making oneself clear to others, and having others respond favorably. One child said that speaking well was really a way of getting along well with others. This idea, at first rejected by the children, provided the basic impetus for the children's speech work. A teacher can help children to realize that our speech today is a living, changing medium of communication. Children are interested in the idea that pronunciations have changed, that meanings of words have changed, and even that grammar has changed over the centuries.

As children talk about who speaks well, they are really setting up standards against which to compare their own speech. They usually include some of the educated members of the community, some of the well-known broadcasters. Analyzing what makes the speech of a particular broadcaster effective is helpful. Such talk encourages children to listen to the pronunciations of broadcasters and, as a result, often to be critical of their own pronunciations. Many times they imitate some of the pronunciations of broadcasters. One teacher employs a very interesting device to teach the influence of varying speech situations on those involved in them. She uses puppets dressed in various ways— as a king, a queen, a bedraggled beggar. As the children manipulate the puppets, they speak as they think the characters would. This device serves as a basis for a discussion of how people in various walks of life speak differently.

The question "Why do we need to speak well?" is provocative. Some students frankly feel little need to speak well; they say that nobody seems to have trouble in understanding them and that the quality of their speech makes no difference in their relationships with people. Other youngsters, however, consider good speech a valuable asset. One boy said that when he collected for his newspapers he talked carefully. He said he thought his customers might not consider him a good salesman if he spoke carelessly. He also made the point that his attempts at good speech and good manners paid dividends in terms of tips. He ended by admitting that he enjoyed speaking well and being courteous to his customers.

This topic leads naturally into a discussion of the places where acceptable speech is important. Children usually agree that whatever their jobs are going to be, they will have to speak well. This objective is not immediate. Therefore, children must think of present situations where they need good speech. One child said that while he works in his father's shoe repair shop, he must wait on customers with good manners and with good speech so that they will feel right toward him and understand him easily.

In this discussion the teacher's own voice and pronunciations are important. Unconsciously, the child thinks of how the teacher sounds. As children feel warm and friendly toward their teachers, they imitate them, wearing similar clothes, walking like them, and talking like them.

Defining Unacceptable Vocal Qualities

The teacher is concerned that students' voices serve their communicative purposes as well as they can. The student's voice problems may be serious. The more serious difficulties of voice production are discussed in Chapter 12. When a child has a consistently hoarse voice, the teacher may assume that the difficulty calls for specialized help. Many times, however, children's voices are adequate for communicative purposes but they would be more effective if improved. In such instances, the teacher works for improvement, taking into consideration four aspects of voice: volume, pitch, quality, and rate of speaking. (See Chapter 12 for a discussion of correcting significant vocal difficulties.)

LOUDNESS. Childrens' voices should not be too loud or too soft. They should be able to adjust the loudness of their voices to the demands of the room in which they are speaking. Florence always spoke rather quietly. In the classroom, children heard her fairly well although sometimes they had to listen carefully. But when she was to act as mistress of ceremonies in the auditorium, she discovered that the children in the back of the room could not hear her. She had to learn to adjust the volume of her voice to the size of the larger room. She further learned that speaking more slowly and articulating more clearly helped her to be heard. Harry, a ten-year-old, seemed to be yelling. He rarely spoke quietly. He appeared afraid that his classmates would not heed him and felt that when he spoke loudly they listened more attentively. He came from a family where the person who spoke loudest received the most attention. With the teacher's direction Harry came to realize that he was more effective as a personality and easier to listen to when he spoke more softly.

PITCH. Children's voices should be appropriate to their age, sex, and physical maturity. They should express the meaning and emotion of what they desire to communicate. The material on pitch, in Chapter 12, is important in consideration of children's pitch. No child's habitual pitch should be changed without careful diagnosis. Many changes in pitch can safely be made, however. Mark's voice tended to be monotonous, for he spoke on one pitch level. Although he was a lively youngster, he had acquired the habit of speaking with little inflection. The school psychologist believed that Mark's monotonous speech was a carry-over from a time when he had had many adjustment problems. These problems were no longer evident, but the monotonous voice was. The teacher helped Mark to make his voice more lively.

QUALITY OF VOICE. Quality of voice refers to the tone that distinguishes one voice from another. The tone differs because of the way the resonating system acts to modify it and because of the particular way in which vocal cords vibrate. The quality may be clear, pleasant, resonant; or it may be breathy, muffled, or nasal. The changing of a consistent quality of voice is discussed in Chapter 12. Quality, however, is also used to help express a person's feelings and emotions. The teacher can help the child to use a quality of voice that does express feeling. One child, partly because of personality difficulties, always spoke as if he were angry. With the teacher's help, the child began to realize that his attitude toward life tended to be negative rather than positive. With the guidance of the school psychologist and with such classroom work as creative dramatics, the boy changed his tone from one of almost consistent anger to one of friendliness.

RATE OF SPEAKING. Few children speak too slowly. A large number of them speak at too fast a rate. Some are in a hurry to get their words into the conversation. Others tend to run fast, to work fast, and to talk fast. They need to realize that their listeners may miss part of what they are saying because of their speed. One 14-year-old boy sang very well. In fact, he was the best boy vocalist in his school. But when he spoke, he ran his words together and overassimilated sounds to that his listeners missed at least half of what he was saying. The speed with which he spoke affected even the quality of his speaking voice. It became muffled. Yet when he sang he articulated very clearly and the quality of his voice was excellent. As he heard the contrast between his singing and speaking voices on a recording, he diagnosed his own difficulty and proceeded to do something about it.

Teaching the Improvement of Voice

Discussing voice and its part in communication makes children aware of their own voices. Children talk about the kinds of voices they like. Almost inevitably, they will discuss how voice reflects personality. They ask themselves whether certain voices suggest friendliness and kindness or whether voices indicate that the person is bored and irritated. Children also talk about the control of pitch, volume, and speed. The individual child then uses a voice that expresses his/her intended meaning and feeling. A recording of voice is an excellent motivation for children to change their voice. (See Chapter 12 for a detailed discussion of voice).

LOUDNESS. Sometimes children have to be reminded to speak

loudly enough to be heard in a classroom. The inability to hear a child justifies interrupting him. One teacher said that he did not like to interrupt Jimmy to ask him to speak louder, because Jimmy was so interested in what he was telling. Jimmy was interested, but at least 16 children in the room were squirming and at least six were talking with one another. They resented the teacher's admonition to them to listen. An early interruption, casually asking Jimmy to speak so that all could hear him, might well have avoided the discourtesy on the part of his audience. Children need to know that rate of speaking and clear articulation are related to ability to be heard. When the teacher insists on each child's speaking loudly enough to be heard, communication is easier. In some instances, the child's speaking too softly may be related to a feeling of insecurity in the room or of general insecurity. Teachers must do what they can to make sure the social atmosphere of the room is conducive to speaking and being heard. If the child is generally insecure, help should be given to modify this situation.

PITCH, QUALITY, AND RATE. Children learn that the rate of speaking and the pitch and quality of their voices show how they feel about what they are reading or saying. Some teachers use puppets or creative dramatics very effectively for this purpose. One child holds the angry puppet who tells the other puppets off. Another holds the sad puppet who speaks slowly of the misfortunes of others. Another holds the happy puppet whose speech is merry. The teacher helps the child to use the pitch, quality, and rate that are most expressive for a particular puppet. The teacher can use creative dramatics for the same purpose. Through setting up particular situations, children realize the importance of pitch, quality, and rate of speaking in their interpersonal relationships. They learn that the expression of different moods and of different meanings requires differences in pitch, quality, and rate.

One teacher uses a single phrase, asking that the children think of as many ways as possible of conveying different meanings with it. One of the phrases is, "Why, Joe and Jill were half an hour late." Children express happiness, sorrow, anger, sarcasm, or sympathy at Joe and Jill's being late. Sometimes they build a story around a particular child's rendition of the phrase.

THE ROLE OF THE SPEECH/LANGUAGE CLINICIAN IN PROMOTING STANDARD ENGLISH

First, speech/language clinicians help teachers to distinguish between cognitive difficulties that are inherent and those that are culturally based. As noted earlier, the clinicians explain the biases of some individuals against nonstandard English and the biases found in many of the present standardized tests. Further, they can show that Black English is useful in many social situations such as in teasing friends and in getting chores completed.

Second, they explain the characteristics of Black English and illustrate them when necessary. Some of these include:

- Lack of agreement of subject and verb, as *They was in the playground.*
- Lack of copula verb, as *He going to the lab.*
- Lack of plural, as *Five minute ago* or *Three boy there.*
- Lack of possessive, as *My brother coat lost.*
- Double negative, as *He aint got no coat.*
- Invariant *be*, as *He be looking.*

They can note for the teachers the dialectical phonological differences such as omitting the /d/, /t/, /ŋ/, /n/ (*He be ole* for *He is old*) such as the substitution of /f/ or /t/ for /ɵ/ and /v/ or /d/ for /ð/ (*bruver* for *brother*). Furthermore, they can call teachers' attention to morphemic deletions of syllabic *l* [l̩] as in *little*, syllabic *r* [ɚ] as in kinder, syllabic *s* and *z* as in *caps* and *cads*, and syllabic *d* and *t* as in *flowed* and *kept.* (*He learn de rope* for *he learned the ropes.*)

Third, clinicians show the teacher how to provide activities and experiences that activate talk in children. This provision for communicative activities is discussed in Chapters 1 and 8.

Fourth, they can provide guidance to the teacher in helping children to use acceptable pronunciations and vocal qualities. This aspect is described earlier in this chapter.

TEACHING THE FOREIGN-SPEAKING CHILD ENGLISH

Schools today have a substantial number of children for whom English is either an unknown foreign language or a limited second language. According to a 1980 issue of *Time,* the city of Los Angeles has more than two million Spanish speaking residents. In fact, of California's 39 million school children, 10 per cent have been defined as limited or non-English speakers. New York City has 80,000 children in bilingual classes, 60,000 of which are Spanish-speaking. Others in New York speak Arabic, Chinese, Greek, Haitian Creole, Hebrew, Korean, and Russian.[8] Grubb (1974) reports that 10 per cent of our school-age children come from homes where English is not spoken. Obviously these limited and non-English-speaking children need to

[8] *Time,* September 8, 1980, pages 64–65.

gain proficiency in the English language in order to succeed in elementary and high schools, colleges, trades, and professions.

Controversy exists as how to bring about this proficiency. The need is obvious, for the drop-out rate of Spanish-speaking children is high throughout the United States. Because of Title VI of the Civil Rights Act of 1964, the Supreme Court ruled unanimously in *Lau* v. *Nichols* in 1974 that the Chinese children in San Francisco have a right to special assistance in acquiring English. This ruling did not specify any particular program or strategies. Federal authorities such as the Department of Education and the Health, Education, and Welfare Department have, however, provided guidelines for compliance with this decision.

In 1975, the Health, Education and Welfare Department issued guidelines that required bilingual programs in districts having 20 or more students from a specific group. An English as a Second Language program was not deemed appropriate. But a 1981 decision by the Department of Education[9] involving the Fairfax County School District in Virginia did not require classes in the students' primary language but rather ruled that the District's courses in English as a second language complied with the intent of the Civil Rights Act of 1964, which forbids discrimination based on national origin. The U.S. Department of Education found that students who took ESL classes were performing at a level comparable with those studying under a bilingual approach. Spokesmen for the bilingual approach believe, however, that Fairfax County's minority citizens were recent immigrants from highly-motivated families of prosperous socioeconomic status and that these facts account for the success of the ESL program.

Some educators argue for maintaining the child's first language until he/she becomes thoroughly proficient in that language. They believe that mastery of one's primary language lays the basis for mastery of English. Further, they believe that this competency in the native language helps the child to build a positive self-concept in that he/she will not feel threatened or uncomfortable in the classroom; as a result, he/she will be successful in learning English. Lastly, since the language spoken at home is his/her native language, the child can communicate effectively at home and will remain an integral part of the family—and perhaps of his/her community.

We believe that local districts can select the programs best suited to deal with their children's second-language problems. Many factors differ in the various districts in which these children reside. The backgrounds of the parents differ; even the foreign languages spoken by

[9] Reported in the *New York Times*, January 1, 1981, p. 20.

the parents differ from one district to another and within the district. In some instances parents of these children speak both English and the foreign language fluently and help their children to develop competence in both languages. For instance, a seven-year-old child arrived in a community of fairly high socioeconomic status speaking only French. She was placed in the first grade based largely on her reading skills in English. However, her mother, who was fluent in English, tutored her and within a few months she was placed in the third grade. But this kind of child and this type of mother are not representative of all foreign-speaking children. In other instances, the child may be a member of a large family with a working father and mother who themselves have a limited knowledge of English. This type of situation is quite different from the one with the seven-year-old French child.

To summarize, since districts differ in available personnel and in philosophy, and since the language backgrounds of children within districts differ, we believe the administrators and teachers within a district are the personnel most qualified to make decisions about programs to help these children speak, write, and read English proficiently. Whereas the reliance on local initiative seems advisable, the Federal Government nevertheless has a responsibility to see that some type of program is provided to help the foreign-speaking child learn English.

The Role of the Speech/Language Clinician in Handling the Foreign-Speaking Child with a Speech/Language Disorder

What is the import of the inclusion in the program for the speech-, language-, and hearing-handicapped of children with limited English or children who know no English? The speech/language clinician needs to be cognizant of the difficulties involved in diagnosing, classifying, and providing therapy for these children. He/she also needs to be aware of the options for overcoming these difficulties.

Hechinger (1979) reports the results of a class action suit on behalf of black and Hispanic children that presented the complaints of denial of educational opportunities as the result of inadequate programs in racially segregated schools and the denial of due process to parents seeking to remove what they believed to be mistaken labels for their children. After a lengthy trial, the Federal District Judge ordered the re-evaluation of all children in the special schools, the introduction of procedures to inform parents of their rights at every step of the child's diagnosis and placement, and a training program for all members of the staffs of the school system to improve their capacity to place children in the "least restrictive, most appropriate system." As a result, a staff development program was initiated under the auspices of the Center for Advanced Study at the City University of New York. This action points to the need of careful assessment and placement of children whose first language is not English.

Admittedly a paucity of testing materials exists for these children. Unless the test is standardized for a particular language and sometimes even for a particular dialect, the assessor's use of norms based on the testing may be far from valid. When the assessor, speaking the language of the testee, translates the test to the child's language, the test may still not be valid, for the test may be based on American culture and not appropriate for the child from a different culture. Holtzmann (1968) notes the existence of subculture variations within a nation, lack of semantic equivalence in instruments and methods of data collection. As just noted, dialectal differences within the native language can occur, as in the Italian language; a child born in South Italy often speaks a somewhat different dialect from one who was reared in North Italy. Or lexical varieties exist. When tests are translated into another language, problems of standardization, semantics, syntax, and phonology arise.

To use a test in a child's current language is often wise. A number of tests involving languages other than English do exist.[10] For example, the Boehm Test of Basic Concepts is available in Spanish. In fact, many of the current language tests are available both in Spanish and in Chinese.

The assessor may be fluent in the child's language; if not, he/she may be assisted by someone who speaks the child's language, such as a paraprofessional. In one instance, at least, a parents' organization provided assistance through volunteer, non-working mothers who understand both the child's foreign language and culture. In addition, the speech/language clinician must determine whether the speech, language, or hearing problem of the child is inherent or is due to the child's present language environment. For example, phonological deviations may be the result of particular phonemes being absent in the child's language. Or the syntax in his/her language may differ as to the order of parts of speech.

Damico, Oller and Storey (1982) compared the effectiveness of pragmatic criteria and traditional surface oriented criteria in the diagnosis of language disorders in ten Spanish bilingual children. Damico,

---

[10] See L. Glass, "Coping with the Bilingual Child," ASHA, 21 (August 1979), page 519.

Oller and Storey studied language samples collected from each child in both Spanish and English and assessed: (1) the method involving use of pragmatic criteria such as general fluency, appropriateness of response, and specificity of referring terms and (2) the method utilizing surface-oriented criteria such as tense marking, syntactic ordering and noun-verb agreement. These two assessments tended to identify *different* individuals exhibiting language disorders; the investigators then determined the accuracy of the diagnostic procedures through pre- and post-testing in academic areas and through teacher ratings. The pragmatic criteria were effective in differentiating genuine language disorders from mere lack of proficiency in certain surface forms whether in the first or second language. In addition, pragmatic criteria used in diagnosing language disorders seemed more effective than the traditional surface-oriented criteria.

Two disorders in children speaking a foreign language are more readily discovered than others: those of hearing and those of voice. Hearing disorders are easily diagnosed through the testing with hearing instruments; however, only an individual fluent in the child's language either administers the tests or assists in its administration. Usually voice disorders, because of their obvious characteristics, are also readily discernible.

Remediation

Sometimes the clinician speaks the language of the child and understands the culture in which he/she has been raised and its implications. Speaking the language, the clinician then knows the rules of phonology, semantics, morphology, and syntax in the child's native language. Then the clinician, when dealing with language problems, begins his/her remediation with those elements of the English language that have elements similar to the native language. Furthermore, since research shows many similarities in the development of different languages, he/she measures the progress readily. Understanding the culture helps the clinician to understand the child, for he/she would know the sociocultural situation of the child's home and some of its implications.

Rarely, however, will the child be part of this particular situation. Rather the speech/language clinician, speaking mostly English, will learn some of the child's vocabulary, gain information about his/her cultural background from teachers and parents, find out some of the basic rules of phonology, morphology, semantics, and syntax in the child's native language, and rely on the assistance of a bilingual paraprofessional or volunteer. The need for such paraprofessionals and volunteers becomes readily apparent when the district requires children to receive all services in their dominant language.

The clinician finds out what strategies are likely to be effective for the specific culture of the child. Some children will be well on their way to being assimilated in Anglo-American culture while others will be traditionally following their ethnic culture. Pickering (1976) summarizes studies showing some of the relationships between different cultures and teaching techniques and strategies. As with all children, the speech/language clinician serves as a counsellor helping individual children discover their feelings about themselves, their communicative abilities, their school, their teachers, and their friends. In addition, the speech/language clinician helps the teacher to understand the communication problems of these children and to suggest ways in which the cooperative efforts of the pathologist and the teacher are useful. Sometimes an English as a Second Language specialist is available, who provides information and strategies for both the teacher and the clinician.

SUMMARY

All human beings need to communicate. Communicative behaviors and responses to them change from situation to situation, from culture to culture, and even from region to region. The responses, often charged with emotional reactions (even to different speech styles) can be as varied as happily accepting or hostile, condescending or sympathetic, and interested or apathetic. The responses are partly the result of language and culture being so closely entwined. As children enter school, they bring with them the language of their culture and attitudes about its particular attributes; at this stage they speak the language of their own culture. But some at a later date are encouraged to speak a classroom standard language. The dialect they learn, sometimes as a second language, is usually representative of the educated members of the community in which they live. Because of school and life demands, children are usually instructed at the appropriate stage to acquire this school dialect. The teacher and the children examine and find ways wherein their voice and articulation better represent their communicative intent. The speech/language clinician often serves as a guide in this area. Some children enter school, however, speaking only a foreign language. These children require special help in one of two modalities: an English as a Second Language (ESL) program or a program of bilingual education. The local school district can best decide which type of program is appropriate—but the Federal government must help to implement it.

Problems

1. Listen for *y'know* in a classroom discussion. How often did it occur? What do you think motivated its use in some of the particular incidents?
2. What is your reaction to a college professor who says:
    a. He don't.
    b. He hardly never.
    c. He done fine?
3. Would you use any of the following phrases? Under what circumstances would you use those phrases?
    a. I wrote a letter.
    b. I put pen to paper and sent it off with a flourish.
    c. I penned a sympathetic note.
4. The word *strategy* is applicable to educational methods. Indicate other uses for the same word. What remains constant in the various uses of this word?
5. *Competencies* and *competence* are used in Chapters 2 and 7. What are the differences and similarities in the two uses of the word?
6. List some of the present-day slang terms for *drunk*.
7. Would you say, "She's a compiler of terminological inexactitudes."? Would anyone say this at any time? If so, when?
8. List ten pronunciations that you have changed over the past few years. Why did you change them?
9. Remember when you met someone from a different region. What were some of this person's pronunciations that were different from yours?
10. Visit a classroom. List either (a) the articulatory errors you hear or (b) the characteristics of the voices that are ineffective in the classroom situation.
11. Indicate the ways in which the teacher of a classroom you have visited helped the children to speak with more pleasant and more effective voices.
12. Read the introductions to two unabridged dictionaries. Tell how the information might prove helpful in your use of the dictionary in the classroom.
13. Listen to your favorite newscaster. What are the characteristics of his voice that made you think him effective?
14. As far as possible, list the influences of parents, school, community, and education upon your own speech.
15. List five sentences, phrases, or words in which assimilation occurs. Indicate the assimilation that may occur.
16. Would you accept the following omissions or transpositions in the pronunciation of the following words?
    > *goverment* for *government.*
    > *childern* for *children.*
    > *liberry* for *library.*
    > *English* (without the *g*) for *English* (with the *g* sound).
    Support your "decision."
17. Questions concerning Black English:
    a. Do you believe that at certain times the teachers themselves should use black English? If so, when?

b. In the classroom should or should not the Black English speaker be encouraged to use both standard and nonstandard dialects appropriately rather than to eradicate the nonstandard speech? Support your answer. (See I. Feigenbaum, *English Now*, New York: New Century, 1970).

c. How can children be made aware that they speak differently from others?

d. How can you show children how different dialects within the classroom are sometimes alike?

18. Questions concerning bilingualism:

Recently bilingual programs have come under criticism. There are those who believe that children must be taught in their native language so that they can keep up with their classmates academically until such time as they learn English. On the other hand, there are those who believe in the English as a Second Language (ESL) Program. As a result, these questions, among others have arisen:

a. For how many years should children be in a bilingual program?

b. Is there research which measures the effectiveness of: the Bilingual Program, the English as a Second Language Program, the High Intensity Language Program?

c. Do we need teachers and specialists who are proficient in more than two languages? Support your answer.

d. How important is teaching the native culture of ethnic groups? Should music, dance, and literature of this group be presented in the classroom?

References and Suggested Readings

Adler, S., *Poverty Children and Their Language: Implications for Teaching and Treating.* New York: Grune and Stratton, 1979. (Describe the language processes of those racially, ethnically, and culturally different children who speak a variant language or dialect and who possess different mores, values, and behavior patterns.)

American Speech-Language-Hearing Association, *Social Dialects: Differences versus Disorders.* Washington, D.C., American Speech-Language-Hearing Association, 1977. (Contrasts speech/language differences and speech/language disorders. Explains identification of social dialects.)

Bailey, B. L., "Some Aspects of the Impact of Linguistics on Language Teaching in Disadvantaged Communities." *Elementary English,* **45** (May 1968), 570–578. (Reports the findings of linguistic research as related to the teaching of English in schools that serve the disadvantaged. Includes phonology, grammar, language programs. Contains many examples of the speech of the disadvantaged.)

Baratz, J. C., "Educational Considerations for Teaching Standard English to Negro Children." In R. W. Fasold and R. W. Shuy, Eds., *Teaching English in the Inner-city.* Washington, D. C.: Center for Applied Linguistics, 1970.

Baskervill, R. D., "The Speech-Language Pathologist—A Resource Consultant for Enhancing Standard English Competencies Among Inner City Children." *Language, Speech, and Hearing Services in Schools,* **8** (1977), 245–249.

Bolinger, D., *Aspects of Language,* 2nd ed. New York: Harcourt Brace Jovanovich, Inc., 1975.

Bountress, N., "Approximation of Selected Standard English Sentences by Speakers of Black English." *Journal of Speech and Hearing Research,* **20** (1977), 254–262.

———, "Comprehension of Pronomial Reference by Speakers of Black English." *Journal of Speech and Hearing Research,* **21** (March 1978), 96–102. (Investigates changes in six linguistic features as functions of age among children who use Black English.)

Cazden, C., *Children's Language and Education.* New York: Holt, Rinehart and Winston, 1972.

Damico, J., J. W. Oller and M. E. Storey, "The Diagnosis of Language Disorders in Bilingual Children," University of New Mexico, Submitted for publication, 1982.

Eisenson, J., *Voice and Diction,* 4th Ed., Chap. 10. New York: Macmillan Publishing Co., Inc. 1979. (Discusses changing speech patterns.)

Evard, B. L., and D. L. Sabers, "Speech and Language Testing with Distinct Ethnic-Racial Groups: A Survey of Procedures for Improving Test Validity." *Journal of Speech and Hearing Disorders,* **44** (August 1979), 271–281.

Fleming, J., "Children's Perception of Socially Significant Speech Variants." *Education and Urban Society,* **3** (1971), 323–331.

Fowler, E. D., "Black Dialect in the Classroom." *Language Arts,* **53** (March 1976), 276–280. (Discusses theory of how to deal with the Black dialect in the classroom and indicates appreciation of dialect differences.)

Frentz, T., "Children's Comprehension of Standard and Negro Nonstandard English Sentences. *Speech Monographs,* **38** (March 1971), 10–16.

Geiger, S. L. and B. R. Greenberg, "The Black Child's Ability to Discriminate Dialect Differences: Implications for Dialect Language Programs." *Language, Speech, and Hearing Services in Schools,* **7** (1976), 28–32.

Giles, H. and K. Farrar, "Some Behavioral Consequences of Speech and Dress Styles." *British Journal of Social and Clinical Psychology,* **18** (1979), 209–210.

——— and P. F. Powesland, *Speech Style and Social Evaluation.* New York; Academic Press, 1975.

——— and R. St. Clair, *Language and Social Psychology,* Baltimore: University Park Press, 1979

——— and J. N. Thakerer, "Language Attitudes, Speech Accommodations and Intergroup Behavior: Some Educational Implications." *Language Arts,* **57** (September 1980), 669–670.

Gonzales, P. C., "How to Begin Language Instruction for Non-English Speaking Students." *Language Arts,* **58** (February 1981), 175–181. (Suggests activities and provides guidelines for working with non-English speaking students.)

Goodman, K. S., "Dialect Barriers to Reading Comprehension," in E. L.

Evertts, ed., *Dimensions of Dialect*. Champaign, Ill.: National Council of Teachers of English, 1967. (Discusses regional variations.)

————, "Dialect Barriers to Reading Comprehension," in J. C. Baratz and R. W. Shuy, eds., *Teaching Black Children to Read*. Washington, D.C.: Center for Applied Linguistics, 1970, 3–25. (Lists alternatives for school programs.)

Grubb, E. B., "The Right to Bilingual Education." *California Journal of Educational Research*, **25** (1974), 240–244.

Hechinger, F. M., "Suit Brings Changes in Special Education." *New York Times*, November 27, 1979, page C4.

Holtzmann, H. "Cross Cultural Studies in Psychology." *International Journal of Psychology*, **3** (1968), 83–91.

Joos, M., "Language and the School Child." In J. Fleming and H. Popp, *Language and Learning*. New York: Harcourt, Brace and World, 1966.

————, *The Five Clocks*. Publication 22, Indiana University Research Center in Anthropology, Folklore and Linguistics, April 1962. (Discusses a wide variety of speech styles—from the most intimate to the most formal.)

Kaiser, R. B., "Wrestling with Meaning and 'Black English.'" *New York Times*, November 27, 1979, page c4.

Kenyon, J. S., and T. A. Knott, *A Pronouncing Dictionary of American English*. Springfield, Mass.: G. & C. Merriam Company, 1944. (Provides an excellent source for the pronunciation of American English words.)

Krescheck, J. D., and L. Nicolos, "A Comparison of Black and White Children's Scores on the Peabody Picture Vocabulary Test." *Language, Speech, and Hearing in the Schools*, **4** (January 1973), 37–40. (Studies the differences between the scores of black and white children on the Peabody Picture Vocabulary Test. Finds a significant difference and suggests differences may be because of cultural bias.)

Labov, W., *Language in the Inner City: Studies in the Black English Vernacular*. Conduct and Communication Number 3, Philadelphia: The University of Pennsylvania Press, 1972.

————, "Stages in the Acquisition of Standard English." In W. Shuy, Ed. *Social Dialects and Language Learning*. Champaign, Ill.: National Council of Teachers of English, 1965.

Levy, B. B., and H. Cook, "Dialect Proficiency and Auditory Comprehension in Standard and Black Nonstandard English." *Journal of Speech and Hearing Disorders*, **16** (December 1973), 642–649.

Light, R. L., "Children's Linguistic Abilities: A Study and Some Implications." *Language Arts*, **56** (February 1979), 132–140. (Studies the reception of standard and non-standard English on children.)

Loban, E., "Teaching Children Who Speak Social Class Dialects." *Elementary English*, **45** (May 1968), 592–599. (Tells how to add a second language to teach a prestigious dialect, established usage, and pronunciation.)

McDavid, R. I., Jr., "Variations in Standard American English." *Elementary English*, **45** (May 1968), 561–564. (Considers regional differences.)

Marwit, S. J. and G. Neumann, "Black and White Children's Comprehension of Standard and Non-standard English Passages." *Journal of Educational Psychology,* **66** (January 1974), 329–332.

Mencken, H. L., *The American Language,* 4th ed. New York: Alfred A. Knopf, Inc., 1946.

Newman, E., *Strictly Speaking.* Indianapolis/New York: The Bobbs-Merrill Company, 1974.

Piché, G. L., M. Michlin, D. Rubin and A. Sullivan, "Effects of Dialect-Ethnicity, Social Class and Quality of Written Compositions on Teachers' Subjective Judgement-Evaluations of Children." *Communication Monographs,* **44** (1977), 60–72.

Pickering, M., "Bilingual/Bicultural Education and the Speech Pathologist." *ASHA,* **15** (May 1976), 275–279.

Pillar, A. M., "The Teacher and Black Dialect." *Elementary English,* **52** (May 1975), 646–649.

Quay, L. C., "Language Dialect, Reinforcement and the Intelligence Test Performance of Negro Children." *Child Development,* **42** (March 1971), 5–15.

Ramsey, I., "A Comparison of First Grade Negro Dialect Speakers' Comprehension of Standard English and Negro Dialect." *Elementary English,* **49** (May 1972), 688–696.

Reed, C. E., *Dialects of American English,* Rev. Ed., Amherst, Massachusetts: University of Massachusetts Press, 1977. (Discusses the concepts of language and dialects and how dialects may be classified. Includes material on Black English and urban dialects.)

Rigg, P., "Dialect and/in/for Reading." *Language Arts,* **55** (March 1978), 285–290. (Tells how to help students deal with dialect differences.)

Shuy, R. W., "Detroit Speech: Careless, Awkward, and Inconsistent, or Systematic, Graceful, and Regular?" *Elementary English,* **45** (May 1968), 565–569. (Shows the distinction between language differences and value judgments about these differences. Talks about collecting the features of pronunciation, grammar, and vocabulary that set off different social groups, races, age groups, and sexes from each other in Detroit. Tells how to gather this information, analyze it, and evaluate its impact on the teaching of English.)

——, ed., *Social Dialects and Language Learning.* Proceedings of the Bloomington, Indiana Conferences, 1964, Champaign, Ill.: National Council of Teachers of English, 1965.

Tabbert, R., "Dialect Difference and the Teaching of Reading and Spelling." *Elementary English,* **51** (November/December 1974), 1097–1099.

Williams, F., ed., *Language and Poverty.* Chicago: Markham Publishing Co., 1970.

——, "Psychological Correlates of Speech Characteristics on Sounding 'Disadvantaged.'" *Journal of Speech and Hearing Research,* **13** (September 1970), 472–488. (Links language and speech features serving as salient clues in the judgmental process with whatever kinds of evaluations or stereotypes appears in the behavior of listeners.)

——, and R. C. Naremore, "Social Class Differences in Children's Syntactic

Performance: A Quantitative Analysis of Full Study Data." *Journal of Speech and Hearing Research*, **12** (December 1969), 778–793. (Determines whether statistically reliable social class differences are found in the degrees and types of syntactic elaboration in the speech of selected blacks and whites, males and females.)

Williams, F., J. L. Whitehead, and L. M. Miller, "Ethnic Stereotyping and Judgments of Children's Speech." *Speech Monographs*, **38** (1971), 166–170.

4

The Speech-Language Clinician and the Communicative Act

The speech/language clinician recognizes that children's acquisition of speech and language patterns is something that occurs not in a vacuum but rather in the context of the total communicative act. The communicative act, involving the clinician and speech/language-handicapped children, possesses certain elements that influence its success or failure. These elements include:

1. The inherent functions of the communicative act.
2. The intent of the message.
3. The interests and knowledge of the participants.
4. The physical environment.
5. The interaction of the clinician and the children.

THE FUNCTIONS OF COMMUNICATION

Different authorities list different functions of language in communication. Allen and Wood (1978) note five: controlling, sharing feelings, informing, ritualizing, and imagining. Sister Winkeljohann (1981) indicates that language serves the following meaningful uses: to convince, to direct, to request, to tell, and to explain; schools, however, stress the informational purpose. Searle (1969) incorporates under *illocutionary acts* (intended to have an impact on the listener) commanding, warning, promising, questioning, stating, imploring, and requesting; and under *perlocutionary acts* (results in modifying the listener's behavior and beliefs) persuading and moving to action. Klein (1979 p. 660) includes the following purposes:

1. To inform—to provide information to another as giving reports or directions.
2. To move to action—to control, manipulate or persuade. (including commands, orders, pleading, justifying, bargaining.)
3. To inquire—to seek information.
4. To enjoy—to tell stories, to speculate, to theorize. (Klein emphasizes that these activities consist of serious contemplations of issues as well as communication to entertain.)
5. To conjoin—to maintain social relationships.

We have already noted in Chapter 1 Halliday's delineation of the functions of language; Pinnell's (1975) research, based on Halliday's classification, revealed that teachers of first-grade children use language first for socialization and then for the giving of information to the children, whereas the first-graders themselves use language in the classroom over half the time for socialization and most of the rest for two functions: controlling another person's behavior, feelings, or attitudes and giving information to others.

Probably during the first grade much of the communication is egocentric. Donaldson (1978, p. 25) says "We are all egocentric through the whole of our lives in some situations and very well able to decentre in others." The decentering may well depend on the age of the child and the degree of difficulty of the task—whether or not what the child is feeling or planning to do is a very fundamental human skill. Donaldson also points out that preschool children are not nearly so limited in their ability to "decenter" or appreciate someone else's point of view as we have been led to believe. Donaldson (1978, p. 56) tells us that we can motivate school children in early grades to begin to reason deductively. She maintains that language-learning skills are not isolated from the rest of the child's growth.

In speech/language intervention sessions, clinicians promote the need for the use of particular functions of language. They make sure that the planned intervention activities involve a variety of communicative purposes related to the children's maturity. It is important that some of the speech/language activities involve the more complex functions requiring such skills as deductive reasoning, for children, as they mature, need to be challenged to use language for meaning and to grow in its use.

The Intent of the Communication

As noted in Chapter 1, children do not communicate in drill words or even drill phrases but in larger contexts. The clinician, therefore, needs to be aware of the importance of making the intent of the message clear and the importance, in addition, of using strategies to get rid of any existing confusion. This pragmatic aspect of language deserves special attention in clinical surroundings. This aspect, along with the phonological, semantic, morphological, and syntactical aspects of language, becomes more sophisticated as children mature.

Leonard, Wilcox, Fulmer, and Davis (1978) point to this growth. They examined four-, five-, and six-year-old children's understanding of indirect requests using forty videotaped interactions between adults. The children were asked to judge the appropriateness of a listener's response to three indirect requests seen on the screen: (1) one involving an affirmative syntactic structure, such as *Can you shut the door?* (2) one involving a negative element, such as *Can't you answer the phone?* and (3) one involving a change in the predicate suggesting a change in behavior, such as *Must you play the piano?* Even the youngest child showed an understanding of the first two indirect requests but only the six-year-olds showed an understanding of a request for a change in behavior as indicated in the predicate. Children base their reactions to a message on their knowledge of its intent; they often understand the conveyed meanings of even indirect requests. Obviously in this study the negative construction requests function as well as the affirmative construction requests. But not until six years of age were the children sophisticated enough to respond to the intent indicated by an indirect request in which the change of behavior was specified in the *predicate.*

Many factors concerning contexts are still to be examined. Parents undoubtedly supply quite different contexts for understanding the import of a message. For instance, a parent may almost never use any of the indirect requests. Rather the father or mother will say to their son or daughter, "Please clear the table now." They may purposively and consistently use the direct approach. Similarly, parents may respond not with a long discussion of why a child should follow certain household rules but rather with, *Because I say so* or even just *Because.* Somehow the child quickly perceives the import of *because* and proceeds to follow his/her parents' rules. On the other hand, a different set of parents say, "You would be helping us by doing the dishes tonight" or "Could you do the dishes now?" In some families lengthy discussions take place about the desired forms of behavior. We know little about the effects of contexts of conversation in different households. The same is true of speech acts in the classroom. But, in all like-lihood, the child's past experiences with intents of communication do play a definite role.

Prutting (1978) cites a paper delivered by Anderson (1977) who asked three-and-a-half-year-olds to role-play a father, a mother, and a child. She found that children learn the roles from both the microsociety (the child's own family) and the macrosociety (the values of the society). Within one family, the context may differ. For instance, mothers seem to vary the intent of the message according to the sex of the child. Cherry and Lewis (1976) studied the communication of 12 upper-middle-class mothers playing with their two-year-olds. They found that the mothers of the girls talked more, asked more questions, repeated their children's utterances more often and used longer utter-ances than the mothers of the boys. The mothers of the male children used more directives than the mothers of the female children.

Parents participate in many speech acts with their children, and, as a result, parents' input into the communicative act involving their children is undoubtedly strong. Moerk (1976) in an analysis of the verbal interactions of 20 mothers with their children who were be-tween 1.9 and 5.0 years old found that these mothers actively taught all aspects of language. In this process, parents adapt their use of lan-guage to the age of the child. Reichie, Longhurst, and Stepanich (1976) found that mothers of three-year-olds use more complex and more copious discussion and modeled interrogation than do mothers of two-year-olds. Obviously both parents and children use functions of language as the child is reared. Moerk (1977, page 147) notes that:

> Nearly from the beginning of his life, the infant has been actively in-volved in manipulating objects and persons in his environment. He him-self has been manipulated in caregiving procedures and has observed other persons manipulating or moving in space and performing acts in temporal sequence.

As a matter of fact, the home may produce an environment condu-cive to more sophisticated communication than the clinical setting. As a result, a sample of a child's language may well be provided by a home communication activity. Scott and Taylor (1978) demonstrate that language samples gathered at home stimulated substantially higher frequencies of past tense and modal verb forms, complex utter-ances and questions than did the clinic samples. The communicative situation of the home setting, which is natural and comfortable, may carry more meaning for the child than the clinical setting. In addition, other stimulants are present in the home—the father, other children, the shared experiences of the mother and child. Undoubtedly, however, different homes provide different communicative settings, some encouraging more communication than others.

The Background of Knowledge and Experience

In any communicative situation, all of us depend upon our past experiences and knowledge to react to a speaker's message. We need knowledge to participate in a discussion effectively. When we find that we are "out of our depth," we keep still. And so it is with children.

Mrs. Currie, a language resource teacher in a N.Y.C. Public School was telling her group of seventh-grade students with language difficulties that she was going on a cruise. She explained that she and her husband would be on a liner, a steamship, and would be sailing over the ocean. The children looked blank. But when she said, "Like the Love Boat on TV," conversation began to flow—revolving around the idea of the big ship, plenty of water, stopping at ports. Television had provided the experience that made her conversation about her intended cruise clear. The basic understandings that the child brings to school either facilitate or hinder acquisition of further understandings. Some children bring to school understandings far beyond their years. For example, a seven-year-old when asked, "What does *secure* mean?" responded with: "When the bad guy is put in prison's he's secure; he can't get out." After a pause, she added, "When my brother glues two pieces of his airplane together, they're secure." Other children bring less understanding. Another seven-year-old, when asked the same question, responded with: "Scure . . . Scure . . . Scure . . . Sewer . . . Sewer. The guy in the sewer."

The gap between these two seven-year-olds represents a gap in knowledge already acquired—probably not only in the meaning of this word but in the meaning of many more words and, furthermore, in ideas and concepts. And in all likelihood, the gap extends to the phonological, morphological, syntactic, and pragmatic aspects of language.

Most children in the primary grades are limited in their cognitive language development. Five- and six-year-olds largely perceive and talk about persons in their immediate environment, about the color, size, shape, and number of objects rather than their use. Children of this age, as a rule, rarely analyze, synthesize, or reason inductively or deductively. Because of such cognitive limitations, the speech of children in the early grades reflects their egocentric stage, and, consequently, communication involving problem solving other than by implication is somewhat difficult. As children reach the third grade, however, their cognitive ability increases so that they become more aware of communication as a speaker-listener activity. As they mature in their cognitive-linguistic abilities, they prepare their messages with the listeners in mind—giving them appropriate forms and symbols to convey meanings and feelings to a particular audience to attain the communicative purpose they desire.

Adams and Collins (1979) note that the spoken text does not carry meaning; rather it provides direction for listeners as to how they should construct the intended meaning using their own previously acquired knowledge. Spiro (1979) says "what we already know will affect what we can come to know." C. J. Hacker (1980) relates this base of experience and knowledge to acquisition of reading skills.

This need for communicative activities to be based on experiences and knowledge already possessed is an important concept for clinicians. For example, when strategies involve workbooks with articulation or language exercises, the child is asked frequently to choose the correct answer from a group of answers. But the material in the exercises may be beyond the ken of the child, who, consequently, may not be the least bit interested. One boy with many articulatory difficulties was deeply engrossed in the makes of different automobiles. The clinician based her therapy on a collection of pictures of many different kinds and makes of cars. Even in his classroom, this boy encouraged his classmates to become experts at recognizing different makes of cars.

The Physical Environment

The room the clinician works in should invite communication. When every nook and corner is filled with playthings, objects, and books, the child is often distracted by the plethora of attention-getting devices. But the room should possess some interesting pictures and objects; these can often be used as the base for beginning a therapy session. For example, one framed picture with nothing in it but a large chair and a cello leaning against it frequently caught the interest of children and often led to their using language imaginatively. The contents of the room should invite talk, but certainly so should the seating arrangement.

The entire cultural environment of the school has an effect on communication. The students, the faculty, the school administration and the locale all contribute to this environment. Some schools have rich, stimulating environments: As you enter the school building, you see pictures drawn by inspired young artists, poems written by imaginative young writers; you hear music, other than the ordinary, emanating from a classroom; you feel your muscles tense as you watch young dancers portraying a riot. In this school, children from all social classes have anticipating, eager looks. Or the school can have a well-ordered, tightly run ship look: The poems are beautifully handwritten. The floors are barren of even a scrap of paper. The rooms are neat and tidy. Almost everyone moves in an orderly fashion.

These are but two examples of school environments. Just as individuals have different life-styles, schools can display a variety of postures, moods, and collections of culture. But these affect the communicative processes of the students, of the teachers, and of the clinician.

Clinicians who travel from school to school often have a "favorite" school, the style of which makes clinical speech/language work profitable. A school with a humanitarian principal, with teachers interested in every child from the gifted to the retarded, with pride in the achievements of each student, with a somewhat permissive attitude but with boundaries firmly established, with an attractive, adequately equipped speech/language clinic room falls into the category of one clinician's "favorite" school. The principal casually commends the clinician on the ability of a once-silent child to communicate with others. A teacher sends a note indicating that one child's mother is ill in the hospital; another, that a child has completed an unusually attractive poster. This school's style fosters effective clinical work.

THE INTERACTION OF THE SPEECH/LANGUAGE CLINICIAN AND THE CHILDREN

The Size of the Communicative Group

The size of the group varies; the clinician may work with one child or with a group. In some instances, because of the severity of the disorder and/or the child's inability to communicate with other children, the clinician sees the child alone; in other instances, group therapy may be more successful because of the input of the various communicators. In deciding on individual or group therapy, one of the factors the clinician considers is the opportunity and incentive to communicate.

The Clinician's Contribution to the Communicative Situation

Hopefully clinicians see themselves in essentially positive ways, as liked, successful, able persons of dignity, worth and integrity. They perceive themselves and their world accurately and realistically, accepting the world as it is. They have deep feelings of identification with other persons; they feel at one with a large number of persons of all kinds and varieties. (Combs, 1965, p. 70) They also perceive their career as being a helping one, a useful one, and one that is respected by the school personnel. They feel positive about their contributions to the school system.

Clinicians' attitudes are closely tied to the success of children in modifying their verbal behavior. Clinicians get their feedback from the children themselves and from their supervisors. Clinicians probably all verbalize that they feel warmth, empathy, and respect for their children, but they need to analyze on what level of effectiveness they are behaving. They need to examine both the feedback from the children and from their supervisor. Klevans and Volz (1974) present three levels of interpersonal relationships for clinicians:

Superior Level	Intermediate Level	Minimal Level
7 6	5 4 3	2 1
Offered empathetic understanding, warmth, and respect to create atmosphere of trust in him and the therapy offered and facilitated sharing of the problem; when appropriate, the clinician shared his own reactions in genuine, self-disclosing, and confronting ways and moved to the problem-solving phase. The clinician was both model and participant in effective interpersonal relationships.	Created somewhat effective atmosphere; responses indicated a concern for client needs. Imprecise use of "helping skills" reduced effectiveness of responding and problem solving.	Generally unable to establish atmosphere of trust and work jointly with client toward therapy goals; difficulty in relating to client on an open, honest level made him an ineffective model for interpersonal relationships; too much therapy time spent on clinician's concerns.

They go on to note that the clinician in the superior category is able to feel warmth, empathy, and respect for the child and to communicate in a way that leads to maximum therapeutic benefits. At the intermediate level of competence, a clinician is aware of the importance of interpersonal skills and does use some of them. Lack of experience and/or training, rather than lack of concern for the children, are the reasons for reduced effectiveness. The clinician at the lowest level may be behaving this way for a variety of reasons, including lack of training, experience, and interest in the children. Clinicians may become aware of their need to modify their behavior by rating themselves on such scales as these and regarding seriously their supervisors' ratings.

Clinicians need to be constantly aware of the importance of communication of all kinds in clinical settings. For example, he/she must remember that learning can be achieved through channels other than hearing—that looking at pictures showing night and day, pantomiming answering the phone or the actions of a bully, feeling a smooth stone as contrasted with a rough stone, or tasting a bitter lemon and a sweet orange all add another dimension of communication to the purely verbal one. Not all modalities are integrated. Often a student possesses a primary modality such as pantomimic action that is a favored one. The clinician then does well to make use of this particular modality—to further communication—to hasten the acquisition of knowledge and language skills.

Clinicians, too, should not use certain types of utterances as they communicate with children who have language disabilities. Blue (1981) lists five types of utterance to avoid:

1. *Sarcasm.* Messages laden with sarcasm require children to possess language skills enabling them to deal with subtle cues. Blue notes that adults seem to detect intuitively that sarcasm has a negative effect and do not use it.
2. *Idiomatic expressions.* Confusion exists when children have acquired the meaning of a word through their daily experiences and then find it used in a far different context. Blue includes these examples: *You turkey. You're a ham.*
3. *Ambiguous statements.* The precise intent is not clear. For example *That's pretty good but* . . . usually means, "You've tried hard —you're coming but you've got a way to go." Blue notes that the child typically repeats the sentence, in order to do "Pretty good" again.
4. *Indirect requests.* These have already been discussed. Obviously children need a certain degree of language development before they understand the intent of the indirect request.
5. *Words with multiple meanings.* Words with multiple meanings cause confusion for any young language learner until the child can

distinguish the literal meaning from a different meaning in context. Blue exemplifies this statement with *Put your toys up*. The child, having learned *up* in a literal sense, was looking for an elevated position for the toys.

Obviously clinicians' abilities to take into account all the communicative factors are important. They must be able to make their messages and their intents clear to their clients, to clear up confusion of meaning, to listen and to respond to the children's responses. Their choice of vocabulary, syntactic complexity, and abilities to make informing exciting, to make a point clearly, to use appropriate voice and pronunciation are all essential. But particularly noteworthy is the ability of the clinician to increase the verbal flow between himself/herself and his/her clients.

As a clinician, you may find yourself dominating the verbal flow. When the communicative act is heavily weighted with your performance, the child does not have a chance to use newly acquired language patterns. Shields and Steiner (1973) studied the effect on spontaneous speech of different interpersonal situations. In checking utterance length, they found that certain adult-dominated conversations reduced the child to a respondent position and markedly restricted the length of the child's utterances, whereas other types of adult-child communication facilitated fluent speech.

Similarly, Woolf (1971) advises on verbal flow in speech interview situations. Where clinicians need specific information, the questions are specific such as, "What does Paul like to do best?" But when clinicians want to encourage verbal output, the interviewer says less and uses open-ended probes such as "Tell me about yourself," or "Anything that comes to your mind."

The Child as Personality

Children's self-concepts affect their ability to communicate. The clinician's influence is important, for his/her evaluation of the child affects the child's self-concept. Davidson and Lang (1960, pp. 107–108) found that children's perception of their teacher's feelings correlated positively and significantly with the self-perceptions of the children. Furthermore, language and self-concept are inexorably entwined: Language is an inherent part of the school culture—for it is a tool that the child uses in thinking, in communicative acts, and in social intercourse. Erwin and Miller (1963, pp. 107–108) say that language is the greatest force for socialization that exists, and that at the same time it is the most potent single factor in the development of individuality.

Language reflects self and self reflects language. Affect related to attitudes engendered by environment and by the clinician influences both the development of a positive self-concept and language. The emergence of the development of language in and out of the classroom and clinic session may signify emergence and growth of self.

The Child's Communication Skills

Children learn to participate in a verbal environment by recognizing purposes of communication, by achieving these purposes effectively, and by listening to and responding to others in a communicative situation. They learn to express themselves in different ways in different situations, to gauge the particular language needs of a particular situation. Consequently, they need to find their own identities and to bring their images of themselves close to reality. The clinical session is a place where each child begins to find a sense of personal worth in life through communication.

The Clinic Session

Every clinic session has a purpose. It may be to improve the child's ability to discriminate between plosive and fricative sounds, to encourage the child to be objective about his/her stuttering, to decrease stuttering symptoms, to improve expressive language in terms of opposites as *hot* and *cold,* to improve ability to hear a particular defective sound. The structure may be tight or loose. In working with some aspects of language development, the structure may be loose as in conversation about growing plants. In other aspects, as when the clinician is teaching the child to build concepts about trucks and their various uses, the structure may be tight.

Today, much of learning is based on systematic instructional goals. We make predictions about the kind of speech and language skills that the child needs to succeed in school and in society. These skills involve decisions about phonology, vocabulary, syntax, and pragmatics. Clinicians follow different learning traditions. Regardless of which tradition is followed, the clinician should ask four questions:

1. What speech and language behaviors would I like each of my students to possess?
2. What evidence exists for the value of each of these behaviors?
3. What strategies can I employ to help each student attain these speech and language behaviors?
4. What evidence do I use to decide whether the student has attained these goals?

The Circular Speech Communication Model

Steck et al. (1973) report on a study that indicates a circular speech communication model: Teacher → Child → Teacher → Child. The results tended to show that clinicians felt rewarded by certain kinds of children's behavior. Appropriate responses, evidence of motivation, independent learning, and compliance to clinicians' requests seemed to provide the most rewarding forms of client behavior. In other words, a reciprocal reinforcement process is at work. This study concludes with two concepts: (1) that some clinicians will tend to hear more responses as appropriate or correct than occur because an inappropriate or incorrect response is as punishing to the clinician as to the child, and (2) clinicians should be aware of their responses to the child's behavior and should monitor them carefully. In this instance, the child may not be working to achieve specific goals in speech and language behavior but rather to attain the approval of the clinician. The clinician is working toward self-satisfaction. The feedback is built into the model but may affect not the child's speech and language change but rather behavior designed to please the clinician.

It is important that the child understand the clinician's intent clearly and honestly and that the clinician understand the child's intent in the same way. Both need to listen carefully; both need to adjust their communicative endeavors to make sure that the circle is complete and effective. For example, a two-year-old went to ask his slightly hard-of-hearing uncle whether he wanted some coffee. He went to the head of the stairs and called "Coffee, Shank?" He got no response. He repeated the question. Still no response. He thereupon changed his query to, "Tea, Shank?"[1] This example provides insight into how a child goes about getting a response and, perhaps, at the same time avoids frustration of not being understood. The adults surrounding a child need to adjust their listening devices to understand the child's language and furthermore, to adjust their communicative focus to understand the nonverbal communication. Responses from both the child and the clinician, based on a true understanding of the intent, are needed to make the communicative circle truly effective.

Thus, the functions of language, the intent of the messages, the interests and knowledge of the participants, and the interaction of the clinician and the clients all play important roles in the communicative act in the clinical situation. The clinical intervention processes will undoubtedly involve more than one function of language; and the cli-

---

[1] Based upon observation of M. Fontana, Queens College, City University of New York.

nician will attempt to increase the number. Again the clinician will use as a base of his/her lesson the experiences and knowledge that the children have already acquired. The speech/language lesson itself will have a structure, selected from many options, and will involve different strategies all designed to introduce or to change certain speech/language behaviors. The children react both to the lesson and to the clinician. The clinician is aware of this reaction through feedback, which monitors a system that signals effective and ineffective communication. As a result, the clinician adapts to the demands of the particular communicative act. Children also are receiving feedback from the clinician and often from the other students in the clinic session.

Problems

1. Read the Shuy (1981) reference. Indicate how his discussion of the blocked functions in the classroom does and does not apply to a clinical situation.
2. Make a list of the functions of language that you believe could be achieved in a particular specified speech/language clinical session. Note the age of the children and the speech/language goals to be achieved. Indicate through what strategies these goals might well be achieved.
3. Visit a clinical session. Note the variety of functions of language used, and whether the clinician had purposively provided activity to include them. (Whether or not they were purposively included will, of course, be a surmise.)
4. Draw up a list of children's books which you believe would motivate communication among seven-year-old delayed-language children.
5. What experiences could you provide a group of ten-year-old language-delayed children that would help them understand what a trip involving mountain climbing involves?
6. Visit a clinical session. Note how the clinician attempts to build the self-concept of the children in a positive way. Be specific.
7. Listen for sarcastic remarks. Evaluate their effect on the particular communicative act.
8. List ways in which you can receive feedback from children in a clinical setting.
9. Note instances when the intent of the message was not received accurately. Indicate how this situation was resolved in one of the instances.

References and Suggested Readings

Adams, M. J., and A. Collins, "A Schema-Theoretic View of Reading." In R. Freedle, Ed., *New Directions in Discourse Processing.* Norwood, New Jersey: Ablex Publishing Corporation, 1979.

Allen, R. R., and B. S. Wood, "Beyond Reading and Writing to Communication

Competence." *Communication Education,* **27** (1978), 286–292. (Notes the functions of communication.)

Anderson, E. S., "Learning to Speak with Style." Paper presented at the Stanford Child Language Research Forum, Stanford University, Palo Alto, California, 1977 cited in C. Prutting, "Process \prǎ|,ses \n: The Action of Moving Forward Progressively from One Point to Another on the Way to Completion." *Journal of Speech and Hearing Disorders,* **44** (February 1979), 3–30.

Auten, A., "Classroom Communication Observation: A Reliable Resource." *Language Arts,* **58** (May 1981), 613–616.

Blue, C. M., "Types of Utterances to Avoid When Speaking to Language-Delayed Children." *Language, Speech, and Hearing Services in Schools,* **12** (April 1981), 120–124.

Cazden, C., V. John, and D. Hymes, Eds., *Functions of Language in the Classroom.* New York: Teachers College Press, 1972.

Cherry, L., and M. Lewis, "Mothers and Two-Year-Olds: A Study of Sex Differentiated Aspects of Verbal Interaction." *Developmental Psychology,* **12** (1976), 278–282.

Combs, A. W., *The Professional Education of Teachers.* Boston: Allyn and Bacon, Inc., 1965. (Chap. 6 describes the self of the effective teacher; Chap. 7 explains the purposes of teachers.)

———, Ed., *Perceiving, Behaving, Becoming: A New Focus for Education.* 1962 ASCD Yearbook, Washington, D.C.: Association for Supervision and Curriculum Development, 1962. (Gives a concept of teaching based on Rogerian psychology.)

Curtis, S., C. A. Prutting, and E. L. Lowell, "Pragmatic and Semantic Development in Young Children with Impaired Hearing." *Journal of Speech and Hearing Research,* **22** (September 1979), 534–552.

Dale, P., "Is Early Pragmatic Development Measurable?" *Journal of Child Language,* **7** (1980), 1–12.

Davidson, A. H., and G. Lang, "Children's Perceptions of Their Teachers' Feelings Toward Them," *Journal of Experimental Education,* **29** (December 1960), 107–108.

Donaldson, M., *Children's Minds.* Glasgow, Scotland: Fontana Collins, 1978.

Egolf, D. B., and S. L. Chester, "Nonverbal Communication and the Disorders of Speech and Language. *ASHA,* **15** (September 1973), 511–517. (Discusses the various facets of nonverbal communication in regard to the message of the clinician.)

Erwin, S., and W. Miller, "Language Development," In *Child Psychology* 62nd Yearbook of National Society for Study of Education. Chicago: University of Chicago Press, 1963, pp. 107–108.

Flynn, P. T., "Effective Clinical Interviewing." *Language, Speech, and Hearing Services in Schools,* **9** (October 1978), 265–271.

Ginsburg, H., and S. Opper, *Paget's Theory of Intellectual Development: An Introduction,* Englewood Cliffs, N.J.: Prentice-Hall, Inc., 1969.

Hacker, C. J., "From Schema Theory to Classroom Practice." *Language Arts,* **57** (November/December 1980), 866–871. (Examines reading comprehension from a schema-theoretic perspective and discusses several education practices that the theory seems to support.)

Hong, L. K. N., "Must Children Know that They Know?" *Language Arts*, **55** (March 1978), 280–284. (Discusses what children need to know about language to meet contextual demands.)

Klein, M. L., "Designing a Talk Environment for the Classroom," *Language Arts*, **56** (September 1979), 647–654.

Klevans, D. H., and H. B. Volz, "Development of a Clinical Evaluation Procedure." *ASHA*, **16** (September 1974), 489–491.

Leonard, L. B., "Modeling as a Clinical Procedure in Language Training." *Language, Speech, and Hearing Services in the Schools*, **6** (April 1975), 78–85. (Advises teaching specific language structures to language-handicapped children making use of a problem-solving set to emphasize the structural relationships of modeled utterances.)

————, M. J. Wilcox, K. C. Fulmer, and G. A. Davis, "Understanding Indirect Requests: An Investigation of Children's Comprehension of Pragmatic Meanings." *Journal of Speech and Hearing Research*, **21** (September 1978), 528–537.

Lindfors, J., *Children's Language and Learning*, Englewood Cliffs, N.J.: Prentice-Hall, Inc., 1980.

Moerk, E. L., *Pragmatic and Semantic Aspects of Early Language Development.* Baltimore: University Park Press, 1977.

————, "Processes of Language Teaching and Training in the Interaction of Mother-Child Dyads." *Child Development*, **47** (1976), 1064–1078. (Studies the practices of mothers in teaching language to their children in one-to-one situations.)

Muma, J. R., "The Communication Game: Dump and Play." *Journal of Speech and Hearing Disorders*, **40** (August 1975), 294–309. (Describes in detail the communication game—dump and play operations in a clinical setting.)

Pinnell, G. S., *Language Functions of First Grade Students Observed in Informal Classroom Environments.* Ph.D. Dissertation, Ohio State University, 1975.

Platt, N. G., "Social Context: An Essential for Learning Language." *Language Arts*, **56** (September 1979), 620–627. (Discusses and exemplifies the pervasive relationship between learning and its context. Parallels are made between the early learning in the home and later learning in schools. Examples are based on visits to English schools.)

Prutting, C. A., N. Bagshaw, H. Goldstein, S. Juskowitz and I. Umen, "Clinical Child Discourse; Some Preliminary Questions." *Journal of Speech and Hearing Disorders*, **43** (May 1978), 128–239. (Describes communicative acts, responses to prior requests, and discourse topics in the interaction between clinician and child.)

Rees, N. S. and M. Shulman, "I Don't Understand What You Mean by Comprehension." *Journal of Speech and Hearing Disorders*, **43** (May 1978), 208–219. (Suggests that the assessment of linguistic comprehension take into account the complexity of operations listeners perform to figure out what speakers mean. Shows that present tests are limited to the literal-meaning aspect of spoken messages and do not measure the listener's ability to determine the speaker's illocutionary intent.)

Reichie, J. E., T. M. Longhurst, and L. Stepanich, "Verbal Interaction in Mother-Child Dyads." *Developmental Psychology,* **12** (1976), 273–277. (Compares aspects of communication between a mother and a two-year-old and between a mother and a three-year-old.)

Rogers, C. R., *On Becoming a Person.* Boston: Houghton Mifflin Company, 1961. (Makes the perceptual viewpoint of psychology clear.)

Schultz, M. C., "The Bases of Speech Pathology and Audiology: What Are Appropriate Models?" *Journal of Speech and Hearing Disorders,* **37** (February 1972), 118–122. (Considers interaction of patient and clinician and the appropriate models for speech and hearing.)

Scott, C. M. and A. E. Taylor, "A Comparison of Home and Clinic Gathered Samples." *Journal of Speech and Hearing Disorders,* **43** (November 1978), 482–495.

Searle, J., *Speech Acts.* Cambridge, England: Cambridge University Press, 1969. (Categorizes speech acts into utterance acts, propositional acts, illocutionary acts, and perlocutionary act. *Utterance acts* refer to uttering words and sentences; *propositional acts* refer to the production of meaningful sentences. The other two we have considered earlier under "Functions of Language.")

Shields, M. M., and E. Steiner, "The Language of Three-to-Five-Year-Olds in Preschool Education." *The Journal of Educational Research,* **15** (February 1973), 97–105. (Examines a sample of spontaneous speech for developmental features and for the effect on language of different interpersonal situations.)

Shriberg, L. D., "The Effect of Examiner Social Behavior on Children's Articulation Test Performance." *Journal of Speech and Hearing Research,* **14** (September 1971), 659–672. (Studies interpersonal variables in the clinical process.)

Shuy, R. W., "Learning to Talk like Teachers." *Language Arts,* **58** (February 1981), 168–174. (Cites language functions. Describes language functions the teachers have but which are blocked to children. They include opening the discourse, closing the discourse, keeping attention, and seeking clarification.)

Spiro, R. J., *Prior Knowledge and Story Processing: Integration, Selection, and Variation.* Urbana, Illinois: Center for the Study of Reading, University of Illinois, August 1979.

Stark, J., "Current Clinical Practice in Language." *ASHA,* **13** (1971), 217–220.

Steck, E. L., J. W. Curtiss, P. J. Troesch, C. A. Binnie, "Clients Reinforcement of Speech Clinicians: A Factor-Analytic Study." *ASHA,* **15** (June 1973), 287–289. (Explores the possibility that certain behaviors consistently reward and others punish speech clinicians who offer therapy.)

Taylor, N. E., and J. M. Vawter, "Helping Children Discover the Functions of Written Language." *Language Arts,* **55** (November/December 1978), 941–945. (Includes a categorical framework for the functional aspects of language—largely based on Halliday and Smith whose categorizations are discussed in Chapter 1.)

Winitz, H., "Problem Solving and the Delaying of Speech as Strategies in the Teaching of Language." *ASHA*, **15** (October 1973), 583–586. (Describes a set of language training principles that have been developed and that reflect the fact that children are able to solve problems of grammatical structure because mothers are skillful in presenting language stimuli.)

Winkeljohann, Sister Rosemary, "How Can Teachers Promote Language Use?" *Language Arts*, **58** (May 1981), 605–606. (Highlights experience and functions of language as the source of children's meaning.)

Woolf, G., "Informational Specificity: A Correlate of Verbal Output in the Diagnostic Interview." *Journal of Speech and Hearing Disorders*, **36** (November 1971), 518–526. (Examines the influence of the clinicians' verbalizations on the clients' verbal output.)

5

The Mechanisms for
Speech and Language

In our later discussion on the development of language we emphasize that the capacity to acquire language by listening and to produce language by "word of mouth" is a form of behavior that is peculiar and specific to human beings. Despite this assumption, it is difficult to localize and identify all of the unique anatomical structures that make oral language as a form of behavior possible. Students of language and speech who are concerned with such matters attribute the behavioral achievement of oral language to differences in the neurological mechanisms that are found in human beings and not even in the other higher forms of living beings. Within the neurological mechanisms, the greatest differences are found in the brain. Primates such as the chimpanzees and the gorillas come closest to human beings in regard to anatomical structures that serve speech. These subhuman primates also come closest to human beings in regard to their capacities to use symbols that parallel if not approximate those employed in human oral and visual linguistic systems.

The overview of the mechanisms for processing and producing oral language that follows is intended (1) to provide insights about their structures and normal manner of functioning, and (2) to describe what, on occasion, may go wrong when children have problems of delay and/or deficiencies in acquiring a proficient oral-linguistic symbol system for communicative behavior.

VOICE PRODUCTION

The human voice-producing mechanism functions in a manner that is roughly comparable to that of a musical wind instrument. The wind or horn instruments employ (1) reeds or the lips of the blower as vibrators or noisemakers; (2) air blown over or through the reeds as the source of energy to set the reeds in vibration; and (3) an elongated tube to reinforce the sound produced by the "vibrating" reeds. The human voice-producing mechanism employs laryngeal folds (vocal bands) for vibrators, air that might otherwise have served only normal respiratory purposes for a source of energy, and the cavities of the larynx, pharynx (throat), mouth, and nose as reinforcers or resonators. These cavities, if we include the trachea or windpipe, may be directly compared to a curved, elongated tube of a wind instrument. The human "elongated tube" is considerably more modifiable than that of any wind instrument, however, and so is capable of producing a wide variety of laryngeal tones that may be modified in respect to pitch, quality, loudness, and duration. The arrangement of the parts of the voice mechanism is indicated in Figure 1.

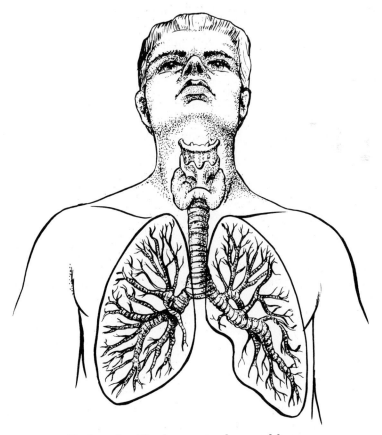

FIGURE 1.   The larynx, trachea, and lungs.

The Larynx

The larynx, commonly referred to as the voice box, is located in the neck between the root of the tongue and the trachea. The outer and largest part of the larynx consists of two shield-shaped cartilages fused together along an anterior line. Together, these fused shields are known as the thyroid cartilage. The reader may locate the larynx at this point by running his/her index finger down from the middle of his/her chin toward the neck. The finger should be stopped by the notch at the point of fusion of the cartilages.

From each side of the larynx, folds of muscle tissue lined by mucous membrane appear as transverse folds that constitute the vocal bands. The upper pair of folds (the paired ventricular or false bands) are relatively soft and flaccid, and not as "movable" as are the true bands below.

In normal breathing, the true vocal bands are separated in a letter V arrangement. To produce voice, the vocal bands must be brought together (approximated or adducted) so that they are close and parallel (see Figure 2).

The Vocal Bands

The vocal bands or vocal folds[1] are small, tough strips of connective tissue, which are continuous with comparatively thick strips of voluntary muscle tissue. Viewed from above, the vocal bands appear to be flat folds of muscle with inner edges of connective tissue. In male adults the vocal bands range from about $\frac{7}{8}$ inch to $1\frac{1}{4}$ inches; in adult females they range from $\frac{1}{2}$ inch or less to about $\frac{7}{8}$ inch.

The opening between the vocal bands is called the glottis. In normal phonation (vocalization) the breath under pressure meets the approximated vocal bands and forces them to move apart. As a result, a stream of air flowing with relatively high velocity escapes between the vocal bands, which continue to be held together (approximated) at both ends. The reduction in pressure beneath the bands, together with the reduced air pressure along the sides of the high-velocity air stream, aided by the elasticity of the bands themselves, brings about recurrent closures after successive outward movements of the bands. Thus vocalization is maintained. If the action or position of the vocal bands fails to produce a "complete" though momentary interruption in the flow of air, the result is a kind of noise or voice quality we identify as breathiness or hoarseness. Figure 2 indicates the position of the

---

[1] Unless otherwise specified, all references are to the true vocal bands. These may also be referred to as the vocal folds or vocal cords.

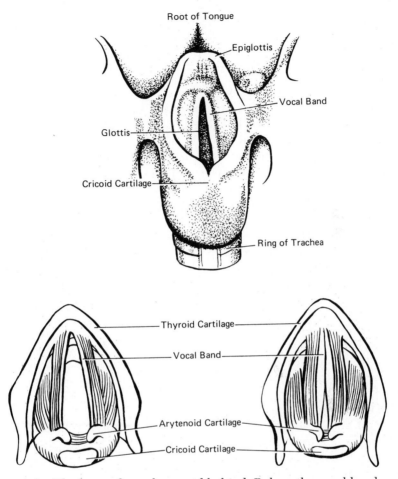

FIGURE 2. The larynx from above and behind. Below, the vocal bands, in position for breathing (left) and for vocalization (right).

vocal bands as they are approximated and ready to be set into motion by the pressure of the air beneath them.

Loudness

The loudness of the voice is directly related to the vigor with which air is forced from the lungs through the larynx, though not to the total amount of air that is expended. Pressure and velocity depend, in part, upon the size of the glottal opening and the length of time the glottis is open. Loudness is, in effect, a result of the pressure of the released pulsations produced by the movements of the bands. Vocal tones are reinforced in the larynx, in the tracheal cavity immediately below the larynx, in the cavities of the throat and mouth, and in the nasal cavities.

Pitch

The fundamental pitch of a vibrating body varies directly with its frequency of vibration. Thus, the greater the frequency, the higher is the resultant pitch. Vocal pitch is a product of factors related to the condition of the vocal bands. The primary factors are the mass or thickness of the bands, their length, and the elasticity of the bands (tension) in relationship to their mass and length. In the process of phonation the vocal bands elongate as they increase in tension. By the same process, the bands are reduced in mass per unit area. The overall effect of the modification of mass-tension factors is to produce a higher rather than a lower pitch when the bands are set into motion. In general, the greater the tension, the higher is the pitch. If tension is held constant, with greater length or mass, the pitch is lower. If length and mass are held constant, the tension of the vocal bands is greater, and the pitch is higher.

Women tend to have higher pitched voices than men because usually they have shorter and thinner vocal bands than men. Our voices become lower in pitch as we mature because maturation is accompanied by an increase in the length and thickness of the vocal folds.[2]

The changes in pitch that we are able to produce under voluntary control take place, as we have indicated, largely by modifications in the degree of tension of the vocal folds. Through these modifications, we are capable of producing tones with ranges of pitch. The ranges may vary somewhat for singing and speaking. Most proficient speakers have a range of about two octaves. Less proficient speakers may have narrower ranges. For most nonprofessional speakers it is probably more important to have good control of a one-octave range than poor control of a wider range. For each individual speaker it is important that voice be produced within the pitch range that is easiest and most effective for him or her. The range will include the optimum pitch level—the level of pitch at which the individual is able to produce the best quality of tone with least expenditure of effort. This is considered later in the discussion of optimum pitch.

---

[2] The average fundamental frequency for male voices is 128 cycles (Hz) per second; it is between 200–256 Hz for adult female voices.

The Arytenoid Cartilages

The vocal bands are attached at their sides to the wall of the thyroid cartilage. At the front, the bands are attached to the angle formed by the fusion of the two shields of the thyroid cartilage. At the back, each of the bands is attached to a pyramidal-shaped cartilage known as the *arytenoid*. The shape and muscular connections of the arytenoid cartilage enable them to move in ways that make it possible for the vocal bands to be brought together for vocalization, partly separated for whispering, or more widely separated for normal respiration. The arytenoids can pivot or rotate, tilt backward, or slide backward and sideways.

The Cricoid Cartilage

The arytenoid cartilages rest on the top of the first tracheal ring. This ring, which has an enlarged and widened back, is known as the *cricoid cartilage.*

The movements of the vocal bands are brought about by the muscular connections of the bands to cartilages, and by the interconnections of the cartilages. Two types of action are important for vocalization. One is for the closing and opening of the bands (adduction and abduction) and the other is for changing the length and tension of the approximated bands to bring about changes in pitch.

The Chest Cavity

The larynx, with its intricate structure of cartilages and muscles, provides the vibrator for phonation. The source of energy that sets the vibrators into motion is found in the chest cavity.

The chest (thoracic) cavity comprises a framework of bones and cartilages that includes the collarbone, the shoulder blades, the ribs, the breastbone or sternum, and the backbone. The diaphragm, as may be noted in Figure 3, constitutes both the floor of the thoracic cavity and the ceiling of the abdominal cavity. The lungs and the trachea are within the chest cavity. In the abdominal cavity directly below are the digestive organs, which include the stomach, the intestines, and the liver.

The Lungs

The lungs consist of a mass of air sacs that contain a considerable amount of elastic tissue. The lungs expand or contract, and so are partly filled or partly emptied of air as a result of differences in pressure brought about by actions of the muscles of the ribs and abdomen,

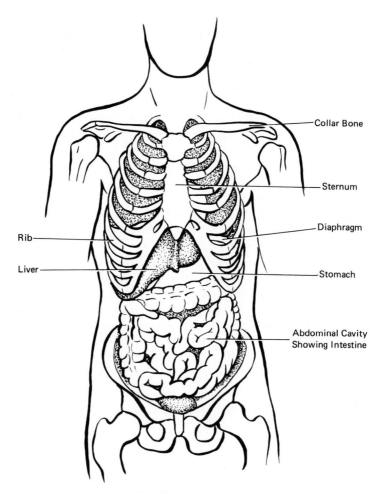

Collar Bone

Sternum

Diaphragm

Rib

Liver

Stomach

Abdominal Cavity
Showing Intestine

FIGURE 3.   The chest and abdominal cavities.

which expand and contract the thoracic cavity. When the muscles of
the ribs and abdomen and the downward action of the diaphragm expand the chest cavity, air is forced into the lungs by the outside air
pressure. When the ribs and the upward movement of the diaphragm
and abdominal muscles act to contract the chest cavity, air is forced
out of the lungs. Through these actions, inhalation and exhalation take
place.

The Diaphragm

The diaphragm is a double-domed muscular organ that separates
the thoracic and abdominal cavities. The right half of the diaphragm

rises somewhat higher—is more dome-shaped—than the left. When the capacity of the chest cavity is increased, air enters the lungs by way of the mouth, nose, throat, and trachea. In this part of the respiratory cycle—inhalation—the diaphragm is actively involved. The contraction of the diaphragm and its downward action serve to increase the volume of the chest cavity. In exhalation, the diaphragm is passive. It relaxes and returns to its former position because of the upward pressure of the abdominal organs. In the modified and controlled respiration necessary for phonation and speech, the muscles of the front and sides of the abdominal wall contract and press inward on the liver, stomach, and intestines. These organs in turn exert an upward pressure on the diaphragm, which transmits the pressure to the lungs and so forces air out of the lungs. Throughout the respiratory cycle, the diaphragm remains roughly dome-shaped. The height of the dome, as may be observed from Figure 4, is greater after exhalation than after inhalation.

Although the diaphragm is passive during exhalation, it does not relax suddenly and completely. Because the diaphragm maintains some degree of muscular tonus at all times, pressure upon it produces a gradual rather than an all-at-once relaxation. Gradual relaxation makes it possible for a steady stream of breath to be created and used to set the vocal bands in vibration. Pressure exerted by some of the abdominal muscles on the diaphragm supplies the extra amount of energy needed for setting the vocal bands in vibration. Without such pressure, exhalation would be passive, and sufficient only for normal respiratory purposes.

Breathing for Phonation

Normal respiration for a person without pathology or anomaly of the respiratory mechanism requires no special thought or effort. Breathing for phonation is different from normal respiratory breathing in at least two respects: (1) the ratio cycle of inspiration to respiration is modified so that there is a considerably longer period for exhalation than in casual breathing; (2) a steady stream of air must be created and controlled at the will of the speaker to ensure the initiation and maintenance of good tone. This type of air flow is usually most easily accomplished by controlling the abdominal musculature and by using small amounts of air rather than by inhaling large amounts of air. Attempts at deep inhalation tend to be accompanied by exaggerated activity of the upper part of the chest. This type of breathing (clavicular) frequently promotes unsteadiness. The result may be a wavering tone and a strained voice quality. Clavicular breathing tends to produce excessive neck and throat tensions, and so prevents free and appropriate

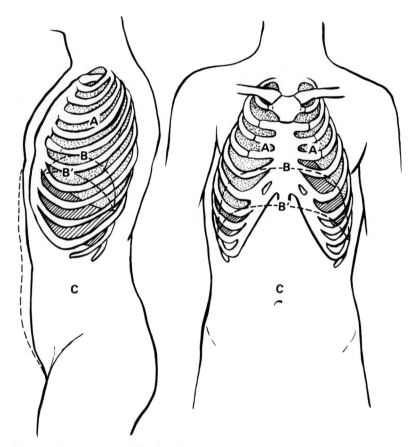

FIGURE 4. Action of the diaphragm and abdomen in breathing.

A. The chest cavity or thorax.
B. The diaphragm "relaxed" when exhalation is completed.
B'. The diaphragm contracted as in deep inhalation.
C. The abdominal cavity. The abdominal wall is displaced forward as
     the diaphragm moves downward during inhalation.

reinforcement of vocal tones in the cavities of the larynx and throat.
Adequate breath supply is difficult to maintain, and the speaker needs
to inhale more frequently than in abdominally controlled breathing.

The Resonating Cavities

The important resonating cavities for the human mechanism are those
of the larynx, throat (pharynx), mouth (oral or buccal cavity), and nose

(nasal cavity). To a lesser but not insignificant degree, the part of the windpipe below the larynx also serves as a resonating cavity. The principal cavities may be located by an examination of Figure 5.

The resonating cavities serve two functions in voice production: (1) they permit us to reinforce or build up the loudness of tones without resorting to constant energetic use of air pressure; and (2) through modification in the tension and shape of the cavities of the mouth, the nasopharynx, and the nasal cavity, we produce changes in the quality of vocal tones. For example, nasality may result when sound is permitted to enter and be emitted through the nasal chambers. This, however, is not the only cause of nasality as a voice quality.

We have little control over the larynx as a resonating chamber. We have most control over the oral cavity and considerable control over the pharynx. The speech sounds we identify as vowels are produced by modifications in the size and shape of the oral cavity. Those sounds we recognize as consonants are produced as a result of changes of the organs of articulation, the lips included, within the oral cavity. Articulatory action will be considered in the chapter on articulation and articulatory disorders.

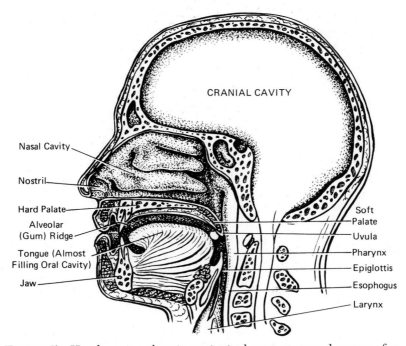

FIGURE 5. Head section showing principal resonators and organs of articulation.

The Nervous Mechanism

Primates such as the apes have oral and respiratory mechanisms that approximate and parallel those of human beings, but with one important exception. The exception is that the nonhuman primates do not have a nervous system capable of the fine and specialized perception of those auditory events that constitute the signals and symbols of oral language. Nor do their systems permit, even on a reflexive level, the production of the variety of sounds that is normal for the infant and young child. Most apes are relatively quiet unless they are agitated. The chimpanzee, the subject of considerable study and training for its possible capabilities for learning a language system, is notably a very quiet animal.[3] So if we proceed on the assumption that, until proven otherwise, only the human being is capable of oral speech, we ought to consider what is unique and functionally different that is associated with this capability.

The Cerebral Cortex

The very special part of the nervous system that endows man with the capability for speech is the cerebral cortex, the outer layer of the brain. The billions of cells of the cortex enable man to perceive, analyze, and synthesize events that come to the cortex through the sensory avenues, and to determine appropriate output in the light of what was received. Particular areas of the cortex are related to different kinds of intake and output. For the purposes of this chapter, there is no need for us to go into detail about cerebrocortical functions. The diagram of the brain (Figure 6) shows some of the areas of specialization in which particular language functions are normally controlled or localized.

Man's cerebral system is significantly different from that of other primates in that the two hemispheres have become functionally different (see Figure 7.) Most important for us in regard to speech is the recently gained knowledge that the left temporal area of the cortex processes speech events for almost all right-handed persons and for a majority of left-handed person's, whereas the right temporal cortex processes auditory intake that is not speech (oral/aural language), for example, musical, mechanical, and other environmental noises.[4] By

---

[3] See References at end of chapter to articles by R. A. Gardner and B. T. Gardner and J. D. Fleming and E. Linden on the recent achievements of chimpanzees to learn to use visual sign-symbol systems.

[4] In general, for about 95 per cent of all persons, symbol behavior and language in particular is processed in the left hemisphere (left hemisphere dominant). The right hemisphere normally has functions such as music, spatial relationships, and the recognition of complex visual patterns for which it is comparably dominant. Among the left-

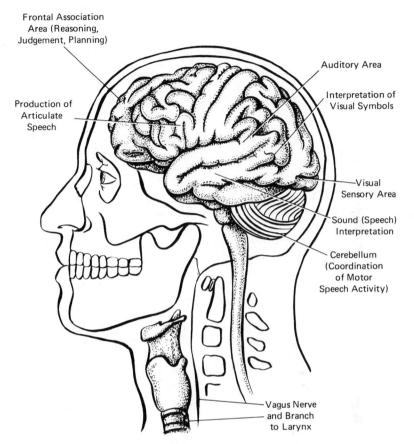

Frontal Association
Area (Reasoning,
Judgement, Planning)

Auditory Area

Interpretation of
Visual Symbols

Production of
Articulate
Speech

Visual
Sensory Area

Sound (Speech)
Interpretation

Cerebellum
(Coordination
of Motor
Speech Activity)

Vagus Nerve
and Branch
to Larynx

FIGURE 6. Localization of some brain functions in relation to speech.

virtue of this specialization, we may say that the left brain (cortex) is
for speech listening. Because those of us who do not have severe impairment in hearing learn to speak by imitating what we hear, the left
brain is also for talking. Damage to the left temporal cortex impairs the
capacity for auditory perception of speech and so results in serious
delay in the onset and development of language. Damage to a child or
an adult who has acquired language will usually result in a breakdown
of language function. Fortunately for the child below the age of 12, the
cerebrocortical system at this stage seems to have sufficient plasticity
for the alternate or nondominant hemisphere to take over the language functions normally controlled by the left or language dominant

handed the differences in the specializations of the cerebral hemispheres is less pronounced than in the right-handed. (Geschwind, 1979, p. 117).

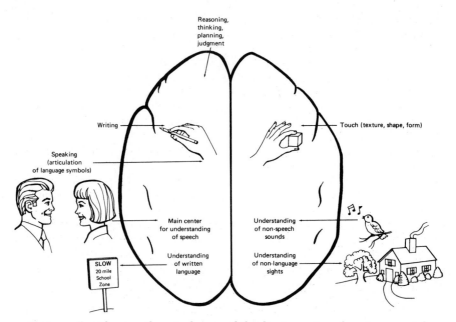

FIGURE 7. The two hemispheres of the brain cortex showing special areas related to language (left half) and non-language areas (right half). Although the hemispheres are virtually twins in superficial appearance, there are anatomical (structural) differences and, as indicated, they have different functions. As may be noted from the diagram, many of the functions are related as to modality of intake.

hemisphere. Unfortunately, this is not so for adults. Impairments of language function associated with brain damage are known as aphasias. We discuss the aphasic child in Chapter 16.

Problems

1. What determines the range of pitch of a musical instrument? What part of the violin reinforces the sounds of the vibrators? What are the essential differences between the sounds of a violin and those of a cello?
2. Is deep breathing necessary for most speech purposes? Why should clavicular breathing be avoided?
3. Read pp. 84–87 of D. R. Boone, *The Voice and Voice Therapy* (Prentice-Hall, Inc., 1977) for a description of types of breathing. What does Boone recommend as most efficient for speaking?
4. What are the functions of the resonating cavities in phonation?
5. Over which resonators do we have the most control? Over which do we have the least control?

6. What is nasality? What is denasality? Is nasal reinforcement always to be avoided? What is the effect of a "stuffed" nose?
7. What cavities does the diaphragm separate? What is the shape of the diaphragm during exhalation? How does the shape of the diaphragm change during inhalation? How are these changes achieved?
8. What is a syrinx? What are the essential differences in sound making between birds and most mammals? How does a parrot manage to sound as if he is speaking? What is the source of the whistling of dolphins?
9. Male and female vocal bands overlap in range of length, yet it is usually easy to distinguish the voices of low-pitched females from high-pitched males. Why?
10. What is cerebral dominance? How is cerebral dominance related to language functioning? Where are nonlanguage auditory events perceived? What is meant by "The left brain is for talking?"
11. Read a recent article on animal language. Is any animal coming close to human beings in learning (acquiring) a language system merely by exposure rather than by being directly taught? What modality seems to be most feasible in teaching language to chimpanzees? Why?
12. Read an article on dolphin communication. Do you think that dolphins have a symbol-language system? Why?

References and Suggested Readings

Denes, P. B., and E. N. Pinson, *The Speech Chain: The Physics and Biology of Spoken Language.* Baltimore: The Williams & Wilkins Co., 1963, Chaps. 2–7. (An introductory but authoritative discussion of the mechanisms for spoken language.)

Eisenson, J., "The Left Brain Is for Talking." *Acta Symbolica,* **2** (1971), 33–36. (A discussion of why the left hemisphere is dominant for language functioning.)

———, *Voice and Diction: A Program for Improvement,* 4th ed., New York: Macmillan Publishing Co., Inc., 1978, chap. 2. (A more detailed but basic consideration of the mechanisms for speech than in the present chapter.)

Fleming, J. D., "Field Report, The State of the Apes." *Psychology Today* (January 1974), 31–50. (An overview of recent accomplishments in teaching sign language and other symbol systems to chimpanzees. Includes an explanation of why chimpanzees are not able to learn to use an oral (word-of-mouth) language system.)

Gardner, R. A., and B. T. Gardner, "Early Signs of Language in Child and Chimpanzee." *Science,* **187** (February 1975), 752–753. (An updated explanation of how two chimpanzees are learning to use signs by exposure to deaf persons who use the American Sign Language.)

Geschwind, N. "Specializations of the Human Brain." In *The Brain,* San Francisco: W. H. Freeman, 1979.

Hardy, J. C., "Neural Processes of Speech and Language." In J. F. Curtis, Ed., *Processes and Disorders of Human Communication,* New York: Harper & Row, Publishers, 1978.

Linden, E., *Apes, Men, and Language*. New York: Penguin Books, 1978. (A rather generous view, at least to the apes, as to their potential for learning a language system.)

Moore, P., *Organic Voice Disorders*. Englewood Cliffs, N.J.: Prentice-Hall, Inc., 1971. (Chaps. 1–3 deal with the mechanisms for voice production. Brief, clear scientific exposition.)

Palmer, J. M., and D. A. La Russo, *Anatomy for Speech and Hearing*. New York: Harper & Row, Publishers, 1965, chap. 8.

Scientific American, *The Brain*. San Francisco: W. H. Freeman, 1979. (This is a special issue of *Scientific American* devoted entirely to the brain. The chapter by N. Geschwind on "Specializations of the Human Brain" is recommended for its clear exposition on language processing and control of language.)

Singh, R. P., *Anatomy of Hearing and Speech*. New York: Oxford University Press, 1980. (Chapters 3, 4, and 5 deal with the mechanisms for breathing and articulation.)

6

The Production of
Speech Sounds

In this chapter we explain how consonants, vowels and diphthongs are usually produced. We recognize that the described positions are merely the conventional ones and that, because our voice-producing mechanisms are adaptable, we produce sounds in ways other than the conventional ones. We also recognize that characteristics of neighboring sounds foster changes in the makeup of a sound as it is spoken in a word or phrase. We attempt also to show characteristics that are shared by a number of sounds because to be able to recognize like characteristics in sounds is important for understanding the development of speech sounds and for the remediation of inaccurate speech sounds. This information helps the clinician to work with children who have articulatory disorders.

Most of this discussion of sounds is based on the writings and research of authorities in articulation and phonologists who work primarily in the discipline of speech communication. You may have studied sounds from a somewhat different point of view—perhaps one which deals with acoustic phonetics. We have included, however, a brief explanation of terms frequently used in research dealing with distinctive features and a summary of such a distinctive feature scheme. Much of articulatory remediation is based on the concept of distinctive features. We have also included one scheme which is representative of others and two schemes devised by authors particularly for use in articulatory remediation.

117

RELATIONSHIP OF SPELLING TO SOUNDS IN ENGLISH

It is hardly necessary to impress the readers of this text with the realization that American English, or British English for that matter, does not consistently represent the same sound with the same alphabet letter. The teacher who has had any concern with teaching children to read has on numerous occasions explained that many words are pronounced in a manner only remotely suggested by their spellings. Perhaps the teacher has been aware that we have 40 or more sound families in our spoken language. If not, the teacher has surely known that we have 26 letters, many of which represent more than one sound, and some of which, according to given words, represent the same sound. So the child has been instructed to memorize the pronunciation and spelling of such words as *though, enough, through,* and *cough* as well as the varied ways in which the sound *sh* /ʃ/ is represented in the words *attention, delicious, ocean,* and *shall.* Vowel sounds, too, have their inconsistencies so that before school children are too far along in their careers they become aware that the sound of *ee* in *see* /i/ may be represented differently in words such as *eat, believe, receive, species,* and *even.* Later, they may be able to accept without too much consternation the spellings of words of foreign derivation such as *subpoena* and *esprit.*

PHONEMES

If you have had a course in phonetics, the concept of the phoneme may have been established. A phoneme is a distinctive phonetic element of a word. It is the smallest distinctive group or class of sounds in a language. Each phoneme includes a variety of closely related sounds that differ somewhat in manner of production and in acoustic end results, but do not differ so much that the listener is more aware of difference than of similarity or sameness. So, for example, the *t* of *tin* is different from the *t* of *its, spotted, button,* and *metal,* and from the *t* in the phrase *hit the ball,* but an essential quality of *t* is common in all these words. Despite differences we have a phoneme /t/.

In this text, phonemes are represented by the symbol of the International Phonetic Alphabet (IPA).

Note that phonetic symbols represent pronunciations as they are made. The same sound and its phonemic variants are represented by a single symbol. This is not the case with diacritic symbols, which, consistently for some vowels and diphthongs, require several representations for the same phoneme.

The Common Phonemes of American English

Key Word	IPA Symbol
CONSONANTS	
1. pat	p
2. bee	b
3. tin	t
4. den	d
5. cook	k
6. get	g
7. fast	f
8. van	v
9. thin	θ
10. this	ð
11. sea	s
12. zoo	z
13. she	ʃ
14. treasure	ʒ
15. chick	tʃ
16. jump	dʒ
17. me	m
18. no	n
19. sing	ŋ
20. let	l
21. run	r
22. yell	j
23. hat	h
24. won	w
25. what*	ʍ or hw
VOWELS	
26. fee	i
27. sit	ɪ
28. take	e
29. met	ɛ
30. calm	ɑ
31. task	æ or a
	depending upon regional or individual variations
32. cat	æ
33. hot	ɒ or a
	depending upon regional or individual variations

* If distinction is made in pronunciation of words such as *what* and *watt; when* and *wen*.

The Common Phonemes of American English (*continued*)

Key Word	IPA Symbol
34. *s*aw	ɔ
35. *o*bey, s*ew*	o or oʊ
36. b*u*ll	ʊ
37. b*oo*n	u
38. h*u*t	ʌ
VOWELS	
39. *a*bout	ə
40. upp*er*	ɚ
	by most Americans and ə by many others
41. b*ir*d	ɝ
	by most Americans and ɜ by many others
DIPHTHONGS	
42. s*igh*	aɪ
43. n*oi*se	ɔɪ
44. c*ow*	aʊ or ɑʊ
	depending upon individual variations
45. m*ay*	eɪ
46. g*o*	oʊ
47. ref*u*se	ɪu or ju
	depending upon individual variations
48. *u*se	ju

If you wish to memorize the phonetic symbols, it may encourage you to know that 16 of the consonant symbols are taken from the English alphabet. They are: p, b, t, d, k, g, f, v, s, z, m, n, l, r, h, and w. The IPA symbols for the vowels, however, vary considerably from their alphabetic representations.

MORPHEMES

The speaker combines phonemes meaningfully to produce what the linguist calls *morphemes*. A morpheme is a minimal unit that carries meaning and is made up of one or more phonemes. Lloyd and Warfel note that "written sentences break up into words, but spoken sentences break up into morphemes" (Lloyd and Warfel 1956, p. 61). When the speaker combines morphemes in meaningful ways, he produces phrases and sentences, or what the linguist calls *utterances*.

This example may illustrate: The word *hit* is a combination of the phonemes /h/, /ɪ/, and /t/. This combination /hɪt/ is a morpheme, for it cannot be broken into a smaller form with meaning. The word *lemon* constitutes a morpheme, for neither the syllable /lɛm/ or /ən/ carries meaning on its own. In the plural form /lɛmənz/, the added /z/ is a morpheme in itself, for it is a minimal unit that does carry meaning.

In this chapter, although we are primarily concerned with phonemes, we wish to emphasize the influence of one sound upon another in context. The following discussion is concerned with how sounds are produced and a description of the parts of the speech mechanism that are employed in articulation.

ARTICULATORY MECHANISM

Speech sounds are produced when the breath stream that comes from the lungs by way of the trachea and larynx is modified in the mouth before leaving the body. Breath may be modified by movements of the lips, teeth, jaws, tongue, and the soft palate (roof of the mouth). Most American-English sounds are produced as a result of lip and tongue activity and resulting contacts with oher organs of articulation. The front part of the tongue (tip and blade) and the part of the mouth at or near the upper gum ridge is the "favored" area for articulatory contact for American-English speech sounds. The sounds *t, d, l, n, s, z, sh* /ʃ/, *zh* /ʒ/, *ch* /tʃ/, and *j* /dʒ/ are all produced by action of the anterior tongue and contact at or close to the upper gum ridge.

As can be seen in Figure 8, the upper gum ridge or alveolar process is the area directly behind the upper teeth. Immediately behind the alveolar process is the hard palate. Posterior to it is the soft palate or velum. The uvula is the most posterior part of the "roof of the mouth."

The tongue lies within and almost completely fills the oral or mouth cavity. The tongue, from the point of view of articulatory action, may be considered as being divided into tongue tip, blade, front (mid), and back, as indicated in Figure 8.

The lips act as articulators for the production of the sounds *p* and *b*. The sound *m* is produced with closed lips. The sounds *f* and *v* are usually produced as a result of action involving the lower lip and upper teeth. The various vowel and diphthong sounds are produced with characteristic lip and jaw movement, though the lips do not make any articulatory contacts for these sounds. The production of American-English sounds is considered later in somewhat greater detail.

Speech sounds may be emitted either through the mouth or through the nasal cavity. In the absence of specific pathology, the

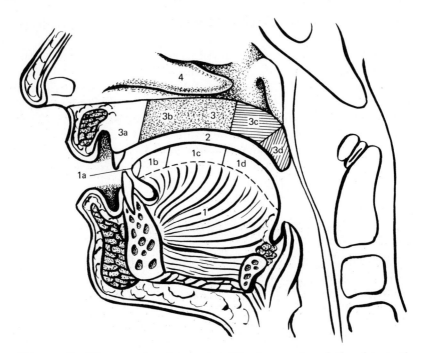

FIGURE 8. Diagram showing parts of the tongue in relationship to the roof of the mouth.

1. Tongue	3. Palate
1a. Tongue tip	3a. Gum or alveolar ridge
1b. Blade of tongue	3b. Hard palate
1c. Front or mid of tongue	3c. Soft palate
1d. Back of tongue	3d. Uvula
2. Mouth (oral) cavity	4. Nasal cavity

speaker is able to determine the avenue of sound emission. Most American-English sounds are emitted through the mouth. The sounds *m*, *n*, and the consonant usually represented in spelling by the letters *ng* are emitted through the nasal cavity.

Sounds usually are categorized as (1) consonants, (2) vowels, and (3) diphthongs. A consonant is a sound that results from the action of articulating agents somehow interrupting the expiring breath, with the vocal bands sometimes vibrating, sometimes not. A vowel is a sound with little or no stoppage of the breath stream, whose quality comes from the vibration of the vocal bands and from the shape and size of the resonating chambers in the throat and mouth. Diphthongs are combinations or rapid blends of two vowels—usually beginning with one vowel and gliding into another.

CONSONANTS

As you say *pat, bat,* and *mat,* you hear three distinct words, because the first consonant in each of these three words is different. However, as you say the three words, you find that in each instance you have made the sounds with your two lips. Another likeness exists in /p/ and /b/. In these sounds, you have held the sound briefly and quickly released it. /p/ and /b/ are called *stops.* How, then, do /p/ and /b/ differ? /p/ is made without voice, /b/ with voice. How, then, do /b/ and /m/ differ? Both sounds are voiced but /p/ is held and quickly released without nasal emission, whereas /m/ is continued and is emitted nasally. Thus, the manner of production of /m/ results in acoustic features that enable the listener to distinguish it from /p/.

From this discussion we can then classify the consonant sounds according to (1) manner of production, (2) place of articulation, and (3) the vocal component.

Manner of Production

STOPS. When you say the /p/ and /b/ in *pat* and *bat,* you use your lips but you also make the sounds by compressing the breath and suddenly releasing it. These sounds are therefore called *stops.* Other stops are /t/, /d/, /k/, and /g/.

CONTINUANTS. All other sounds are *continuants,* which in turn are classified as (1) *frictionless consonants* or *semivowels* and (2) *fricatives.* The continuant /m/ that you hear in *mat* is emitted nasally by lowering your velum and by directing the air through the nose. The other two nasal sounds are /n/ and /ŋ/ as in *sing.* The lateral /l/ and the glides are also classified as semivowels. /l/ is made with the sound being forced over two sides of the tongue. The glides, /r/ as in *run,* /j/ as in *yell,* /w/ as in *won,* and /ʍ/ as in *what,* are made by the movement of the articulatory agents from one position to another. All these sounds are frictionless. Other continuant sounds called fricatives, however, have a frictionlike quality, which is caused by the release of sound through a narrow opening between the organs of articulation. A stream of breath is maintained with some pressure to make the sound continuous. These sounds are /f/, /v/, /s/, /z/, /h/, /θ/ as in *thin,* /ð/ as in *this,* /ʍ/ as in *what,* /ʃ/ as in *she,* and /ʒ/ as in *treasure.*

AFFRICATES. Lastly, American-English sounds include affricates or the consonantal blends, as /tʃ/ in *check* and /dʒ/ in *jump.* Thus, each sound achieves some of its characteristic acoustic quality by its manner of production.

Place of Articulation

The classification of consonants just given was according to manner of articulation. Consonants may also be classified as to which articulators are used and the position they are in during the act of sound production. The following is a classification of consonants as to position of articulators:

LIPS. Sounds are produced as a result of the activity of the lips. The sounds /p/, /b/, /m/, /ʍ/, and /w/ are bilabials.

LIP-TEETH (LABIODENTAL). Contact is made between the upper teeth and lower lip for the production of labiodental sounds. The sounds so produced are /f/ and /v/.

TONGUE-TEETH (LINGUADENTAL). Contact is made between the point of the tongue and the upper teeth or between the point of the tongue in a position between the teeth. The *th* sounds /θ/ and /ð/ may be made either postdentally or interdentally. Most mature speakers are likely to produce these sounds postdentally.

TONGUE-TIP ON GUMS (LINGUA-ALVEOLAR). The region of the mouth at or near the gum ridge is the "favored place" for the articulation of American-English sounds. The sounds /t/, /d/, /n/, and /l/ are produced with the tip of the tongue in contact with the upper gum ridge. The sound /r/ is most frequently produced with the tongue tip turned back slightly away from the gum ridge. The sounds /s/, /z/ are produced with the blade of the tongue making articulatory contact a fraction of an inch behind the gum ridge.

TONGUE-HARD PALATE (LINGUA-PALATAL). The sounds sh /ʃ/, zh /ʒ/, ch /tʃ/, j /dʒ/ are produced by raising the blade of the tongue toward but not touching the alveolar ridge and arching the tongue upward toward the soft palate. The sound y /j/ is produced by arching the tongue high near the hard palate. /r/ is sometimes made by raising the middle of the tongue toward the line between the hard palate and the velum with the tip remaining low.

TONGUE-SOFT PALATE (VELAR). The sounds /k/ and /g/ are usually produced with the back of the tongue in contact with the soft palate. In some contexts /k/ and /g/ may be produced with the middle of the tongue in contact with the hard palate. The reader may check his/her place of articulation for the /k/ in *car* compared with /k/ in *keel*. He/she may also wish to compare the /g/ of *get* with the /g/ of *got*.

The sound of *ng* /ŋ/ is most likely to be produced with the back of the tongue in contact with the soft palate.

GLOTTAL. One American-English sound, /h/, is produced with the breath coming through the opening between the vocal folds and without modification by the other articulators. The /h/ is referred to as a glottal sound.

The Vocal Component of Consonants

A third classification of sounds is according to the presence or absence of voice. Consonants produced without accompanying vocal-fold vibration are referred to as *voiceless* or *unvoiced;* those produced with accompanying vocal fold vibration are called *voiced.* The voiceless consonants of American-English speech are /p/, /t/, /k/, /ʍ/, /f/, *th* of *th*ink /θ/, /s/, *sh* /ʃ/, and /h/. The voiced consonants are /b/, /d/ /g/, /m/, /n/, *ng* /ŋ/, /v/, *th* of *this* /ð/, /z/, *zh* /ʒ/, /w/, /r/, *y* /j/, and /l/.

A resumé of the multiple classification of American-English consonant sounds is presented in the chart that follows.

Production of American English Consonants

Involvement of Articulatory Agents							
Manner of Production	LIPS (BILABIAL)	LIP-TEETH (LABIODENTAL)	TONGUE-TEETH (LINGUADENTAL)	TONGUE TIP ALVEOLAR RIDGE (LINGUAALVEOLAR)	TONGUE AND HARD PALATE (LINGUAPALATAL)	TONGUE AND SOFT PALATE (VELAR)	GLOTTIS (GLOTTAL)
Voiceless stops	p			t		k	
Voiced stops	b			d		g	
Voiceless fricatives	ʍ	f	θ	s[1]	ʃ[2]	ʍ[4]	h
Voiced fricatives		v	ð	z[1]	ʒ[2]		
Nasals	m			n		ŋ	
Lateral semivowel				l			
Glides	w			r[3] j		w[4]	
Voiceless affricate					tʃ		
Voiced affricate					dʒ		

[1] In /s/ and /z/, the channel is narrow.
[2] In /ʃ/ and /ʒ/, the channel is broad.
[3] The tongue tip in many instances is curled away from the gum ridge to the center of the palate.
[4] In /ʍ/ and /w/, both the lips and the back of the tongue are involved.

Assimilation

Seldom are sounds uttered singly. Rather they are part of a phrase or a sentence. This onward flow of speech then results in *assimilation*, the modification of pronunciation because of adjacent sounds. In Chaucer's day the past tense of verbs was pronounced with an *ed* syllable; now it is pronounced either with a /d/ or a /t/. For example, whereas the past tense of *grabbed* is pronounced with /d/, the past tense of *tapped* is pronounced with /t/. The final sound in *grab* is voiced; consequently the *ed* occurs as /d/, which is also voiced. But the final sound in *tap* /p/ is unvoiced; as a result, the *ed* occurs as an unvoiced /t/. A similar influence exists in plurals of nouns. *Caps* is pronounced with a final unvoiced sound /s/ whereas *cabs* is pronounced with a final voiced sound /z/. The use of /z/ rather than /s/ is due to the voicing influence of /b/. Assimilation, an integral part of the onward flow of speech, makes for ease and economy of utterance.

Assimilation is *contiguous* if the consonant causing the assimilation is immediately adjacent to the one affected, as *bwown* [bwaun] for *brown* [braun] and *noncontiguous* if it is further removed, as [dɔd] for *dog*. Assimilations are further classified as *regressive, progressive*, and *reciprocal. Regressive assimilation* is assimilation where a sound influences the preceding sound. The change of /n/ in the prefix *con to ng* /ŋ/ in the words *congregate* and *conquer* exemplifies this type of assimilation. Another example is the use of [gɔg] for [dɔg]. In *progressive assimilation*, a sound retains its identity but influences the following sound. *Open the door* may become [opm̩ðədɔr]. /p/, being made with both lips, has influenced /n/ to become /m/, also a bilabial sound. The example given earlier of the pronunciation of [bwaun] for [braun] is also an example of progressive assimilation. In *reciprocal assimilation*, both forward and backward influences are at work; two sounds influence each other so that a third sound, a compromise between the two is introduced. [tʃit] or [dʒit] for *did you eat* is an example of reciprocal assimilation. The /t/ or /d/ and the *y* sound /j/ interact in such a way that the /tʃ/ or /dʒ/ results.

Distinctive Features (Binary Contrasts) of Consonants

If we apply the term *distinctive features* to the system just described, we may base our distinctions on the differences in consonants on manner of production, place of articulation, and the vocal component. For example, let us contrast /p/, /b/, and /m/. The feature distinguishing /p/ and /b/ is the vocal component. On the other hand, /m/ has three features to distinguish it from /p/: it possesses voice, is made with nasal resonance, and is a continuant, whereas /p/ does not possess these three characteristics.

The term *distinctive features* as applied in the literature refers to features presented as binary contrasts. The feature is present [+] or absent [−]. If we put the distinguishing features of /p/, /b/, and /m/ as just discussed in this form it would appear as:

Distinctive Features of /p/, /b/, and /m/

	Voice	Nasal	Continuant	Labial
p	−	−	−	+
b	+	−	−	+
m	+	+	+	+

So far we have been talking about strictly articulatory features. But in describing systematic phonemes, a more general categorization is used. This categorization is appropriate in describing the phonological rules of the languages of the world. As noted previously distinctive features are binary in form; that is, each feature is present [+] or absent [−]. This structure can be helpful in noting the rules of phonology. An example from assimilative processes follows: Assimilative processes are at work in the word *small*. Normally /m/ possesses the feature [+ voicing]. But the /m/ in *small* is preceded by /s/ with its feature [− voicing] and this /m/ then changes its feature to [− voicing], because of the influence of the feature of [− voicing] in /s/. Or where an unvoiced sound as /t/ in *better* is surrounded by two sounds /ɛ/ and /ɚ/ with the feature [+ voicing], the /t/ tends to change the [− voicing] feature to [+ voicing].

The following scheme used in articulatory therapy based on distinctive features mixes the criteria from both articulatory and acoustic phonetics. Its origin is hybrid; for example, *high* is a physiologic term, whereas *strident* refers to *quality*. The terms used in this scheme[1] and their definitions appear on p. 128.

Telage's Classification (See p. 129)

A somewhat different classification of distinctive features is that of Telage (1980). Telage's primary objective in classifying distinctive

---

[1] For other examples of distinctive feature schemes, see L. V. McReynolds and D. L. Engmann, *Distinctive Feature Analysis of Misarticulation;* Baltimore: University Park Press, 1975, H. Winitz, *From Syllable to Conversation,* Baltimore: University Park Press, 1975, or S. Singh and K Singh, *Distinctive Features: Principles and Practices,* Baltimore: University Park Press, 1976.

Terms Used in Distinctive Feature Analysis

Term	Characterized by
Consonantal	Interference of breath stream and abrupt movements of formants.
Vocalic	No interference of breath stream and steady or slow moving formants.
High	Front or back of tongue being raised from neutral position.
Low	Front or back of tongue being lowered from neutral position.
Back	Back of tongue being retracted from neutral position.
Anterior	Production in the front position of mouth, tongue, or lips.
Coronal	Involvement of the tip or blade, which is raised from neutral position.
Continuant	Partial obstruction of air stream, which continues to flow.
Voicing	Accompanying vocal fold vibration.
Nasal	Lowering of the velum with the air stream passing through the nose.
Strident	High degree of turbulence or noisy sound where articulated.
Sonorant	Absence of any interference with flow of glottal sound.

Distinctive Features of Various Phonemes

Feature	p	b	t	d	k	g	tʃ	dʒ	f	v	θ	ð	s	z	ʃ	ʒ	m	n	ŋ	r	l	j	h	w	ʍ
Consonantal	+	+	+	+	+	+	+	+	+	+	+	+	+	+	+	+	+	+	+	+	+	−	+	−	+
Vocalic	−	−	−	−	−	−	−	−	−	−	−	−	−	−	−	−	−	−	−	+	+	−	−	−	−
High	−	−	−	−	+	+	+	+	−	−	−	−	−	−	+	+	−	−	+	−	−	+	−	+	+
Low	−	−	−	−	−	−	−	−	−	−	−	−	−	−	−	−	−	−	−	−	−	−	+	−	−
Back	−	−	−	−	+	+	−	−	−	−	−	−	−	−	+	+	−	−	−	−	−	−	−	+	−
Anterior	+	+	+	+	−	−	−	−	+	+	+	+	+	+	−	−	+	+	−	−	+	−	−	+	+
Coronal	−	−	+	+	−	−	+	+	−	−	+	+	+	+	+	+	−	+	−	+	+	−	−	−	−
Continuant	−	−	−	−	−	−	−	−	+	+	+	+	+	+	+	+	−	−	−	+	+	−	+	+	+
Voicing	−	+	−	+	−	+	−	+	−	+	−	+	−	+	−	+	+	+	+	+	+	+	−	+	−
Nasal	−	−	−	−	−	−	−	−	−	−	−	−	−	−	−	−	+	+	+	−	−	−	−	−	−
Strident	−	−	−	−	−	−	+	+	+	+	−	−	+	+	+	+	−	−	−	−	−	−	−	−	−
Sonorant	−	−	−	−	−	−	−	−	−	−	−	−	−	−	−	−	+	+	+	+	+	+	−	+	−

Some authors use [č] for [tʃ]   [j] for [dʒ]   [š] for [ʃ]   [ž] for [ʒ]   [y] for [j]

features is to point out those of the client's articulatory behaviors that contribute most significantly to his/her pattern of misarticulation. Telage emphasizes that whereas other systems may be concerned with the universality of phonological acquisition, his system represents the functional dynamics of consonant production at the syllabic level. He believes that the speech/language clinician's purpose for analyzing the distinctive features of clients should dictate the features to be used and the categories to be included. After critically reviewing the applicabilities of present systems, he devised the following:

Telage's Classification

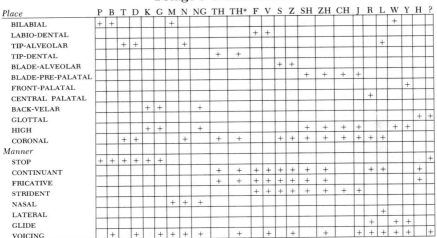

Place	P	B	T	D	K	G	M	N	NG	TH	TH*	F	V	S	Z	SH	ZH	CH	J	R	L	W	Y	H	?
BILABIAL	+	+					+															+			
LABIO-DENTAL												+	+												
TIP-ALVEOLAR			+	+				+													+				
TIP-DENTAL										+	+														
BLADE-ALVEOLAR														+	+										
BLADE-PRE-PALATAL																+	+	+	+						
FRONT-PALATAL																							+		
CENTRAL PALATAL																				+					
BACK-VELAR					+	+			+																
GLOTTAL																								+	+
HIGH					+	+			+							+	+	+	+			+	+		
CORONAL			+	+				+		+	+	+	+	+	+	+	+	+	+						
Manner																									
STOP	+	+	+	+	+	+																			+
CONTINUANT										+	+	+	+	+	+	+	+			+	+	+			
FRICATIVE										+	+	+	+	+	+	+	+								
STRIDENT												+	+	+	+	+	+	+	+						
NASAL							+	+	+																
LATERAL																					+				
GLIDE																				+		+	+		
VOICING		+		+		+	+	+	+				+		+		+		+	+	+	+	+		+

* A binary production feature matrix used for computer analysis of omission and substitution errors. A blank cell denotes a minus. From K. M. Telage, "A Computerized Place-Manner Distinctive Feature Program for Articulation Analyses," *Journal of Speech and Hearing Disorders,* **45** (November 1980), page 483.

Telage also makes clear the capability of computers to assess a large data input rapidly and to organize the results in a meaningful way. Data based on such a system could simplify the process of identifying an individual's underlying pattern of misarticulation. Implied, then, is that these data would also permit clinicians to focus therapy on the critical articulatory behavior. This aspect will be discussed in the chapter on articulatory diffculties.

Numerical Values

Bryans, McNutt and Lecours (1980) advocate still another classification, which allots numerical values to feature differences in consonants. Their consonant difference measures were found to be significantly related to children's substitution errors and to account for more than half of the variance in data on normal consonant acquisition. They believe that a classification based on articulatory variables is the most suitable for the analysis of overt speech behavior. They describe their classification:

In the present binary articulatory classification, voicing is listed as the first variable and is followed by two place variables, *Pre-Alveolar* and

Post-Alveolar. The bilabials, labio-dentals, and dentals are assigned 1 for Pre-Alveolar, and the palatal, velar, and glottal sounds are assigned 1 for Post-Alveolar. Consonants produced in an intermediate position are characterized by zero on both variables (Alveolars) or, in the case of the affricates, by a zero on one variable and ½ on the other.

The traditional manner categories are specified by the remaining three binary variables. The first, *Nasal*, is marked 1 for sounds produced with a lowered velum. The two final variables refer to the degree of constriction at sites other than the velopharyngeal port. Thus, glides are marked 1 for Minimal Constriction whereas stops and nasals are assigned a 1 for Complete Constriction. Sounds involving an intermediate degree of constriction are characterized by a zero on both variables (fricatives) or by a zero on one and ½ on the other (affricates). (Bryans, McNutt and Lecours, 1980, pp. 348–349)

This classification is intended to permit quantitative estimates of differences among consonants with respect to manner, place, and voicing and to provide a framework for an initial rather than an exhaustive analysis of articulatory data. The classification follows:

Binary Articulatory Descriptions of English Consonants[1]

	Consonant																							
	p	b	t	d	k	g	m	n	ŋ	f	v	θ	ð	s	z	ʃ	ʒ	h	tʃ	dʒ	j	r	l	w
ARTICULATORY VARIABLE																								
Voicing	0	1	0	1	0	1	1	1	1	0	1	0	1	0	1	0	1	0	0	1	1	1	1	1
Pre-Alveolar	1	1	0	0	0	0	1	0	0	1	1	1	1	0	0	0	0	0	0	0	0	0	0	1
Post-Alveolar	0	0	0	0	1	1	0	0	1	0	0	0	0	0	0	1	1	1	½	½	1	0	0	0
Nasal	0	0	0	0	0	0	1	1	1	0	0	0	0	0	0	0	0	0	0	0	0	0	0	0
Minimal Constriction	0	0	0	0	0	0	0	0	0	0	0	0	0	0	0	0	0	0	0	0	1	1	1	1
Complete Constriction	1	1	1	1	1	1	1	1	1	0	0	0	0	0	0	0	0	0	½	½	0	0	0	0

[1] Variables characteristic of a given consonants are indicated by 1 or ½. Those that are not characteristic are shown by a zero. (From B. Bryans, J. McNutt and A. R. Lecours, "A Binary Articulatory Production Classification of English Consonants with Derived Difference Measures," *Journal of Speech and Hearing Disorders*, **45**, August 1980, p. 348.)

In addition, this classification provides for measures of production differences—between two consonants and between a particular consonant and all other consonants. The Overall Difference Measure is obtained by adding the Paired Difference Measures for all pairs that involve the selected consonant. The Overall Difference Measures are listed on the right of the table appearing on p. 131.

This system, obviously, does not have the advantage of the Telage system, which has a more complete description of the consonants' properties. Bryans *et al.* (1980) point out, however, that this system may permit greater accuracy in the description of the stable character-

Measures of Articulatory Difference Between Consonant Pairs (PDMs) and Overall Articulatory Difference Between Each Consonant and All Others (OADM)

	Paired-Difference Measure (PDM)	Overall Difference Measure (OADM)
	p b t d k g	
p	0	60.0
b	1 0	54.0
t	1 2 0	52.0
d	2 1 1 0	46.0
k	2 3 1 2 0	60.0
g	3 2 2 1 1 0	54.0
	m n ŋ	
m	2 1 3 2 4 3 0	72.0
n	3 2 2 1 3 2 1 0	64.0
ŋ	4 3 3 2 2 1 2 1 0	72.0
	f v θ ð s z ʃ ʒ h	
f	1 2 2 3 3 4 3 4 5 0	56.5
v	2 1 3 2 4 3 2 3 4 1 0	50.5
θ	1 2 2 3 3 4 3 4 5 ½ 1 0	56.5
ð	2 1 3 2 4 3 2 3 4 1½ 1 0	50.5
s	2 3 1 2 2 3 4 3 4 1 2 1 2 0	48.0
z	3 2 2 1 3 2 3 2 3 2 1 2 1 1 0	42.0
ʃ	3 4 2 3 1 2 5 4 3 2 3 2 3 1 2 0	56.5
ʒ	4 3 3 2 2 1 4 3 2 3 2 3 2 2 1 1 0	50.0
h	3 4 2 3 1 2 5 4 3 2 3 2 3 1 2½ 1 0	56.5
	tʃ dʒ	
tʃ	2 3 1 2 1 2 4 3 3 2 3 2 3 1 2 1 2 1 0	52.0
dʒ	3 2 2 1 2 1 3 2 2 3 2 3 2 2 1 2 1 2 1 0	46.0
	j r l w	
j	5 4 4 3 3 2 5 4 3 4 3 4 3 3 2 2 1 2 3 2 0	66.0
r	4 3 3 2 4 3 4 3 4 3 2 3 2 2 1 3 2 3 3 2 1 0	58.5
l	4 3 3 2 4 3 4 3 4 3 2 3 2 2 1 3 2 3 3 2 1½ 0	58.5
w	3 2 4 3 5 4 3 4 5 2 1 2 1 3 2 4 3 4 4 3 2 1 1 0	66.0

From B. Bryans, J. McNutt and A. R. Lecours, "A Binary Articulatory Production Classification of English Consonants with Derived Difference Measures," *Journal of Speech and Hearing Disorders,* **45** (August 1980), p. 350.

istics of each phoneme since many variations of a sound occur in the context of a phrase or sentence.

Such schemes are but the beginning of distinctive feature articulatory generalizations. More research and study will likely bring about refinement in the categories and in their descriptions. For example, in the literature we find some questioning of the assignment of the feature *stridency* to /f/ and /v/ but not to /θ/ and /ð/. Bolinger calls this assignment "rather arbitrary" (Bolinger 1975, p. 80).

Applying Distinctive Feature Analysis

An examination of some of the present systems of distinctive features classification reveals that their proponents do not agree on either the nature or the number of distinctive features. Each has his/her own scheme depending on which system he/she prefers to use and for what purpose. The concept of distinctive features was originally devised as a theoretical approach to language analysis, useful to characterize some of the universal properties of language at an abstract level. Today speech/language clinicians frequently use such systems for the purpose of describing actual articulatory behavior. Admittedly some features, such as stridency, which has an acoustic rather than an articulatory base, are included. The advantage of the use of a system of distinctive features is that two phonemes can be defined quantitatively by the number of features on which they differ.

From your newly acquired knowledge of the presence or lack of voice, the articulatory agents involved and the manner of production of consonants, examine the following changes and indicate what happens. For example, *tense* often becomes [tɛnts]. The insertion of /t/, which is made with approximately the same articulatory agents as /s/ and /n/, takes place because the morpheme becomes easier to utter with the /t/ inserted. Why, then, does *something* become [ˈsʌmpˌθɪŋ], tenth [tɛntθ] and *dance* [dænts]?

1. As you say *tackle* and *gargle,* the /k/ and /g/ are aspirated laterally. Explain why.
2. As you utter *at the store* and *add the numbers,* the /t/ and /d/ are made with the tongue on the teeth rather than on the alveolar ridge. Why?
3. In *let out the dog, little, city mouse, cutting the grass,* /t/ takes on some of the voiced characteristics of /d/. Why?
4. In *grandmother* and *handsome,* speakers frequently omit /d/. What characteristic of the /n/ influences the omission of /d/?
5. In *campfire* and *obviate,* the /f/ and /v/ are made by some speakers with both lips, causing the sounds to become labial fricatives. Why does this happen?
6. In rapid speech, you are likely to omit /θ/ in *fifth* and *seventh.* Explain in terms of the place of articulation.
7. Why in the speech of one individual do two pronunciations of *with* occur—*with Dan* [wɪð dæn] and *with Tom* [wɪθ tam]?
8. Why, in terms of the articulatory agents involved, does *Captain* become [kæpm̩]?

VOWELS

Whereas consonants are important because they help bring intelligibility to the message, vowels, through their variables of quality, pitch, time, and loudness bring emotion and feeling to the message. The word *no* printed singly carries some meaning as a written symbol, but *no* spoken singly carries more meaning and feeling. Spoken with loudness and a downward inflection, it conveys one kind of meaning and feeling; spoken softly with a rising inflection, it carries another kind of meaning and feeling. The vowel /o/ is what makes the difference in the message—the phonemic–semantic value permits the expressions of feeling in the speaker's message.

Vowels are more variable than consonants; neighboring sounds influence vowels more than consonants. For example, in *no* and *sing*, the vowels in both words are usually nasalized because of the influence of /n/ in *no* and /ŋ/ in *sing*. And the effect of the continuing movement of the vocal articulators during the utterance of a vowel in a word or phrase makes for differences both in acoustic results and articulatory movements. Although we describe vowels according to the previous discussion, you must remember that these characteristics are based on norms and that many individual variations exist.

Vowel sounds share the following characteristics in their manner of production: (1) All vowels are voiced, unless for special purposes the entire speech content is intentionally whispered; (2) all vowels are continuant sounds in that they are produced without interruption or restriction of the breath stream; (3) changes in the place of production, height of tongue, muscle tension, lip rounding, and degree of stressing are responsible for differences in acoustic end results.

Place of Production

All vowel sounds require activity of the tongue as a whole. It will be noticed, however, that each of the American-English vowels is produced with one part of the tongue more actively involved than the remainder of the tongue. For example, in the production of the vowel of the word *me*, the tip of the tongue remains relatively inactive behind the lower teeth while the front of the tongue is tensed and raised toward the hard palate. In changing from *me* to *moo*, we may note that the front of the tongue is relatively relaxed while the back is tensed and elevated toward the roof of the mouth. The vowel of *me*, because of its characteristic tongue activity, is considered to be a *front vowel;*

similarly, the vowel of *moo*, because of the back-of-the-tongue activity, is considered to be a *back vowel*.[2]

Height of Tongue

Now, let us contrast the production of the vowels of *me* and *man*. Both of these are produced with front of the tongue activity, but the tongue is higher for the vowel of *me* than it is for the vowel of *man*. Similarly, the tongue is higher for the back vowel of *moon* than it is for the vowel of *mock*. In the words *mirth* and *mud*, where middle-of-the-tongue activity is characteristic, we may also note that the vowel of *mirth* is produced with the tongue higher in position than it is in *mud*. The difference in height of tongue position, however, is not as great as for the other pairs of words.

Thus far, we have seen that vowels differ somewhat in individual production according to the part of the tongue that is most actively involved and the height of the tongue. We may also have noted that the change in the height of the tongue is likely to be accompanied by a change in the position of the lower jaw. That is, the jaw drops as the tongue drops, in going from a "high" to a "low" vowel. A third aspect of vowel production is now considered.

Muscle Tension

If we compare the vowels of *tea* and *tin*, we should be able to sense that the tongue is more tense for the vowel of *tea* than it is for the vowel of *tin*. Similarly, the vowel of *moot* is produced with more tongue tension than the vowel of *mock*. Further analysis will show that the differences in tension are not confined to the muscles of the tongue. The muscles of the chin also differ in degree of tension. A third muscle difference may be felt by observing the changes in the position of the apex of the larynx—the "Adam's apple." When the tongue and under part of the chin are tense, the apex of the larynx is elevated and moves toward the front of the chin as it does in the act of swallowing. When the tongue and the under part of the chin are relatively relaxed, the larynx drops back to its normal position of rest as in quiet breathing.

---

[2] In some contexts, the positions we have described may be more theoretic than real. The descriptions may sometimes be more accurate for the isolated vowel than in the flow of speech. Nevertheless, we think that when a child has difficulty in producing the vowels of English, training that follows these descriptions should be helpful. The reservation about tongue positions also holds for the other features of vowel production.

On the basis of our discussion thus far, we may arrive at a threefold classification for vowels sounds.

1. Vowels differ as to place of production. They may be produced either in the front of the mouth, with the front or blade of the tongue most active; in the middle of the mouth, with the midtongue most active; or in the back of the mouth, with the back of the tongue most active.
2. Vowels differ as to height of tongue position.
3. Vowels differ as to degree of muscle tension.

Front Vowels		*Midvowels*		*Back Vowels*	
	PHONETIC SYMBOL		PHONETIC SYMBOL		PHONETIC SYMBOL
m*ee*t	i			b*oo*n	u
m*i*lk	ɪ			b*oo*k	ʊ
m*a*y	e	M*i*rth	ɜ or ɝ	b*oa*t	o
m*e*n	ɛ	*a*bout	ə	b*a*ll	ɔ
m*a*t	æ	upp*er*	ɚ	b*o*g	ɒ
*a*sk[1]	a	m*u*d	ʌ	b*a*lm	ɑ

[1] When the speaker compromises between the vowels of *mat* and *balm*.

Lip Rounding

A fourth feature that distinguishes some vowels from others, especially when the vowels are produced as isolated sounds, is lip-rounding. Back vowels, with the exception of the *a* of *calm*, are produced with the lips somewhat rounded. The vowel of the word *pool* is most rounded. There is lesser rounding for the vowels in *pull*, *boat*, *ball*, and *cot*. For persons who do not distinguish between the vowels of *cot* and *calm*, there will be no lip-rounding for either.

In the lists of words in the preceding section, the first column contains front vowels, arranged in order of highest to lowest tongue position. The second column contains midvowels, and the third column contains back vowels, arranged in the same order.

The tongue positions for the vowels of these words are shown in Figure 9. The dotted area represents the high points of the tongue.

Degree of Stressing

Vowels with greater stress tend to be longer than those with less stress; in fact, the stressed vowel often becomes diphthongized.

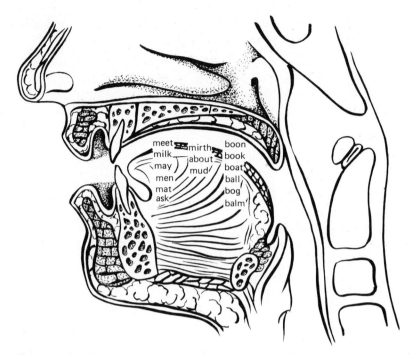

FIGURE 9.   Representative tongue positions for American-English vowels. In actual speech there is considerable individual variation from these positions according to speech context.

Where /e/ is stressed as uttered in the list of words, *vague, day, rain,* it is diphthongized. But when it is not stressed, as in the first syllable of *vacation* and in the last syllable of *mandate,* it is not dipthongized. Context is also important in the degree of stress. When you say, "Give me Kay's address," you are likely to use the monophthongal /e/. But when you say, "Are you meeting Kay?" you are likely to use the diphthongal /eɪ/. A second example involves /o/. When you say *obey,* the /o/ not being stressed is usually /o/, whereas in *row,* the /o/ being stressed is usually /oʊ/. When you stress *throw* in "Throw it out," the /oʊ/ is diphthongal. But when you do not stress *throw* in "Did Johnny throw away today's paper?" the /o/ tends to be the monophthongal /o/.

Defective Vowel Production

Defects of vowel production do not occur as frequently as those for the production of consonants. The intensity of the vowels and possibly the visible aspects of their articulation help to make it comparatively easy for most children to learn to produce them accurately. Difficulties are sometimes experienced by the child who has hearing loss in the low-pitch ranges. A child exposed to foreign language influences may also experience some difficulty in the production of American-English vowels. We should be careful not to confuse defective vowel articulation with differences in vowel production on the basis of regional variations.

From our discussion of vowels, we can hypothesize that vowel phonemes will never contrast in voice but that they *will* contrast in such features as where the tongue is raised or bunched, whether it is high or low in the mouth, and whether the vowel is rounded or unrounded and lax or tense. Some of these features coexist. No front vowel is rounded; back vowels tend to be rounded.

On the basis of the characteristics of vowels just discussed (height of tongue, raising or bunching of tongue), explain what has happened in the following changes. For example, *Patricia* is sometimes pronounced with an /i/ not an /ɪ/ in the second syllable. The /ɪ/ used by most speakers has been raised to become /i/.

1. Why does *keel* become [kɪəl]?
2. What happens as *milk* is pronounced [mʊlk]?
3. The final sound in *Monday, Tuesday, Wednesday* is usually pronounced /ɪ/. How is this different from the final sound being pronounced /e/?
4. Southerners sometimes pronounce *pen* and *pin* alike. In terms of the characteristics just discussed, what is happening?
5. What has occurred in these changes?
   [frʌm] for *from* in *from the farm.*
   [e haʊs] for *a house*
   [ði dɔg] for [ðə dɔg].
   [rʊf] for [ruf].
   [tʊrɪst] for [turɪst].
6. In *tomato salad* and *I bought a tomato,* what is the change in the last sound in *tomato?*
7. Some Southerners say [ra:t] for [raɪt]. What change has occurred?

DIPHTHONGS

Diphthongs, like vowels, are produced as a result of modifications in the size and shape of the mouth and position of the tongue while vocalized breath is being emitted without obstruction of the breath stream. Diphthongs are voice glides uttered in a single breath impulse. Some diphthongs, such as the one in the word *how*, are blends of two vowels. Most diphthongs originally—as far as the history of the language is concerned—were produced as "pure" vowels but "broke down" to what is now a strong vowel gliding off weakly to another vowel lacking distinct individual character. The diphthongs in the words *name* and *row* are examples where the first element is emphasized and readily recognizable and the second element is "weak" and somewhat difficult to discern.

The following list of words includes the most frequently recognized diphthongs in American-English speech. Most phoneticians would limit the *distinctive* diphthongs to those in the words *aisle, plough, toil,* and *use.*

*ais*le	ba y
plou gh	ho*e*
toi l	de*a*r
f*ai*r	*su*re
fo*r*t	*u*se

Problems

1. Distinguish spelling representation from sound representation:
   a. Pick out all words with the sound [ɪ] as in *hit* in *Women are undependable. Their so-called stability is but a myth.*
   b. List as many different spellings for these sounds as you can think of: /i/ as in *tree*, /eɪ/ as in *jail*, /aɪ/ as in *try.*
2. Note slight differences within these groups of phonemes:
   /k/ *cool, key*
   /t/ *stop, tape, rat*
   /p/ *paid, spray, apt*
   /ʌ/ *but, cut.*
3. Note the similarities and dissimilarities in terms of articulatory agents involved, manner of production, and vocal components in the final sounds of *tank, tack; rat, race; lamb, can; taps, tabs; cough, five; truth, bathe; call, car.*
4. The following are pronunciations of other cultures as reported in various articles. What are the changes from a phonetic standpoint?
   duty [dʒutɪ]
   forget you [fəgɛtʃu]
   have [hæb]
   chicken [ʃɪkən]
   record [rɛkət]
   them [dɛm]
   man [men]
   set or sat [sɑt]
   ice [is]

    pig [piɪg]
    storm [tɔrm]
    lets [lɛs]
    lumber [lʌmɚ]
    children [tʃɪrən]
On the whole do the preceding substitutions make more phonetic sense than the following:
    cat [tæk]
    squirrel [gɝdl̩]
    run [bʌn]
    look [lik]
    Sam [ræt]
    mule [mel]
What substitutions would make sense in the preceding words?

5. Why, in teaching /s/, would you use the phrases *can sing* and *right song* rather than *bath soap?* The explantion is a phonetic one.

    Why, in correcting the substitution /f/ for /θ/, would you use the phrase *right through the door* rather than *come through the door?*

    Why, in correcting the substitution of /w/ for /l/, would you use the phrase *the cat's long hair* rather than *blow long and hard?*

    Why, in correcting the substitution of /w/ for /r/, would you use the phrase *turn red* rather than *barn door?*

6. A child makes the following substitutions:
    /t/ for /k/ as in [tæt] for [kæt]
    /f/ for /θ/ as in [bof] for [boθ]
    /d/ for /g/ as in [do] for [go]
    /θ/ for /s/ as in [θi] for [si]

Chart these substitutions in terms of distinctive features. Note changes in features and whether there is any consistency in the change of features in the four substitutions.

References and Suggested Readings

Amerman, J. D., R. Daniloff, and K. L. Moll, "Lip and Jaw Coarticulation for the Phoneme [æ]," *Journal of Speech and Hearing Research,* **13** (March 1970), 147–161. (Investigates the extent of coarticulation and the synergy of two articulatory gestures, lip-rounding and jaw-lowering, for the vowel [æ].)

Bolinger, D., *Aspects of Language,* 2nd ed. New York: Harcourt Brace Jovanovich, Inc., 1975, Chaps. 3 and 4.

Bronstein, A. J., *The Pronunciation of American English.* New York: Appleton-Century-Crofts, 1960.

Bryans, B., J. McNutt, and A. R. Lecours, "A Binary Articulatory Production Classification of English Consonants with Derived Difference Measures." *Journal of Speech and Hearing Disorders,* **45** (August 1980), 357–377. Reprinted by Permission.

Catford, J. C., *Fundamental Problems in Phonetics*. Bloomington, Indiana: Indiana University Press, 1977. (Described by its author as "a survey of the sound-producing potential of Man and an outline of the parameters which appear to be needed for a systematic universal phonetic taxonomy." Classifies sounds; provides a basis for categorizing newly discovered sounds, the prelinguistic sounds of infants and the deviant sounds uttered by those with articulatory disorders.)

Chomsky, N., and M. Halle, *The Sound Patterns of English*. New York: Harper & Row, Publishers, Inc., 1968.

Denes, P. B., and E. N. Pinson, *The Speech Chain*. New York: Bell Telephone Laboratories, 1963, Chap. 4. (Outlines anatomy and physiology of speech production.)

Gimson, A. C., *An Introduction to the Pronunciation of English*, 2nd ed., London: Edward Arnold & Co. 1970.

Harms, R. T., *Introduction to Phonological Theory*. Englewood Cliffs, N.J.: Prentice-Hall, Inc., 1968. (Introduces the student to generative phonology.)

Ladefoged, P., *Preliminaries to Linguistic Phonetics*. Chicago: University of Chicago Press, 1971.

LaRiviere, C., H. Winitz, J. Reeds, and E. Herriman, "The Conceptual Reality of Selected Distinctive Features." *Journal of Speech and Hearing Research*, 17 (March 1974), 122–133.

Lehmann, W. P., *Descriptive Linguistics: An Introduction*. New York: Random House, Inc., 1971. Chap. 2: "Articulatory Phonetics," Chap. 3: "Acoustic Phonetics."

Liberman, A. M., K. S. Harris, H. S. Hoffman, and B. G. Griffith, "The Discrimination of Speech Sounds Within and Across Phonetic Boundaries." *Journal of Experimental Psychology*, 54 (November 1957), 358–368.

———, K. S. Harris, P. Einas, L. Lisker, and J. Bastian, "An Effect of Learning on Speech Perception: The Discrimination of Duration of Silence with and Without Phonemic Significance." *Language and Speech*, 4 (October–December 1961), 175–196.

Lloyd, D. J., and H. R. Warfel, *American English in Its Cultural Setting*, New York: Alfred A. Knopf, Inc., 1956.

McReynolds, L. V. and D. L. Engmann, *Distinctive Feature Analysis of Misarticulation*. Baltimore: University Park Press, 1975.

McReynolds, L. V., and K. Huston, "A Distinctive Feature Analysis of Children's Misarticulations." *Journal of Speech and Hearing Disorders*, 36 (May 1971), 155–156.

Mackay, I. R. A., *Introducing Practical Phonetics*. Boston: Little, Brown and Company, 1978. (Includes material on the anatomy of speech, the physics of sound, acoustic phonetics, word stress, assimilatory processes, and the phoneme.)

Menyuk, P., "The Role of Distinctive Features in Children's Acquisition of Phonology." *Journal of Speech and Hearing Research*, 11 (March 1968), 138–146.

Parker, F., "Distinctive Features in Speech Pathology." *Journal of Speech and Hearing Disorders*, 41 (February 1976), 23–39.

Singh, S. and K. Singh., *Distinctive Features: Principles and Practices*. Baltimore: University Park Press, 1976.

Telage, K. M., "A Computerized Place-Manner Distinctive Feature Program for Articulation Analyses." *Journal of Speech and Hearing Disorders*, **45** (November 1980), 481–494. (Describes how to use a computer in a distinctive feature program; includes a classification for this purpose.) Reprinted by permission.

Tiffany, W. R. and J. Carrell, *Phonetics: Theory and Application*. New York: McGraw-Hill Book Company, 1977. (Explains the physics, physiology, and linguistics of phonetics.)

Van Riper, C. G., and D. E. Smith, *An Introduction to General American Phonetics* 3rd ed., New York: Harper & Row, Publishers, 1979. (Introduces the symbols of the International Phonetic Alphabet. Explains the effects of coarticulation and non-distinctive features of English. Makes clear the basis of distinctive features.)

Winitz, H., *From Syllable to Conversation*. Baltimore: University Park Press, 1975, Chap. 2. (Describes in some detail distinctive features and their role in articulation therapy.)

7

The Development of
Language in the Child

As indicated earlier, we consider that the ability to speak—to learn to understand and produce an oral/aural code—to be a human-species-specific function. The particular code that is acquired is, of course a learned function related to a given culture. Almost all human beings acquire speech, or learn a given language code, because they are born with the capacities for this particular type of learning. Spoken language is a system of symbols, a code, which normally is produced by articulatory activity that associates sounds (utterances) and meaning in particular ways.

Children may be said to be speaking, to be using an oral/aural linguistic system when they demonstrate by their productions that their utterances conform to the conventions of other speakers in their environment. These conventions include the acquisition of a phonemic or sound system, a morphemic system (the combination of sound elements into words), a semantic system (acquisition of verbal meanings) associated with a syntactical system (the combining of words into "strings" or formulations that approximate the utterances of the mature members of their culture).

Deaf children and other who learn to use a visible code or sign system are exceptions in regard to the use of the oral/aural code. A visible code may, however, be acceptable within our definitions of speech and language. We believe that the American Sign Language (*ASL* or Ameslan), though it does not incorporate the equivalent of phonemic and morphemic subsystems, nevertheless constitutes a linguistic symbol system. Signing Exact English (*SEE*) adds English morphemes to

142

Ameslan and tries to bring this sign system closer to full-fledged morphemic code in function if not in design features (Gustason *et al.*, 1972). Signed English (Bornstein, 1974) represents an attempt to develop a manual sign system that includes a syntax (grammatical features) similar to that of spoken English. For a review of these and other visible sign systems, see Silverman (1980, Chapters 3 and 4).

CRITERIA FOR LANGUAGE ACQUISITION

Some time between the last quarter of the first year and the middle of the second year of life, the vast majority of children begin to speak. The development of language (language acquisition) is a continuous process throughout life. Normally, comprehension precedes production and exceeds production from the beginning to the end of life. We may, however, consider the following to be the criteria for the establishment of sufficient competence in comprehension and production to permit us to identify a child as one who has acquired language. Children may be said to be competent users of an oral/aural linguistic code:

1. When they understand—decode and derive meanings from—a conventionalized system of audible and/or visible symbols.
2. When, without specific and direct training, they can understand verbal formulations to which they never before have been specifically exposed. Children are then *listening creatively.* They understand what people say based on past understandings of what people have said.
3. When they can produce verbal formulations, new utterances that they never before have tried, and have the utterances understood by others. Children are then *talking creatively.*

Criteria (2) and (3) reveal that the child is capable of generalizing from the specific words and utterances individually learned "directly" to the comprehension and production of an indefinite number of new utterances. In a very real and important sense, the child has become a linguistic generalizer and generator. Children indicate that they have learned the rules of their language, and are applying these rules—the conventions of older and presumably proficient speakers—to what they hear and what they want to say. Children are likely to make many errors that are products either of overgeneralizing or of correct generalizing where a linguistic system has exceptions, for example, saying *sheeps* and *childs* as plurals for *sheep* and *child* or *foots* as plural for *foot.* Children may make errors because they have not really caught on to the rules but are moving in that direction. Such errors are good positive indicators that a given child is linguistically normal, and has become a verbal being and a member of a verbal culture.

Although children begin to speak because they are born with the capacities for this achievement, their accomplishments as verbal beings will vary with a variety of innate and environmental factors. The *onset of speech* appears to be unrelated to the particular language a child will speak, only roughly to his/her level of intelligence (unless the child is severely subnormal), or to the talkativeness of members of the family or other key persons in the environment, providing, of course, that these persons *do* talk. An individual child's proficiency as a speaker, including language development, is determined by a number of factors that we consider later.

THE FUNCTIONS OF LANGUAGE

Primarily, the function of language is to permit the child to behave like a human being in the variety of ways in which human beings behave. More specifically, language is used for talking to and with others, to signal needs, intentions, feelings, and thoughts. Language is also used for self-talking (thinking), and for controlling and directing one's own behavior, as well as for controlling and directing the behavior of others. Language is used for deception and even for self-deception, for saying many nothings to avoid a vacuous existence and to becoming an accepted, socialized, and civilized human being. Language is used to disarm or delay nonverbal hostility, and for engaging and instigating hostility. In time, the maturing child will learn that not only does man have a way with language but that language has a way with man.

In time the child will both experience and learn how important it sometimes is to "string pretty words that do not have to make sense;" to use words to bridge distances as well as to create chasms and voids; that there are words without thoughts, but only rarely are there thoughts without words. With good fortune the child may also learn that though some words are "like razors to a wounded heart," other words can heal; that words may be "nimble and full of subtle flame." But above all, the child may learn along with Lytton Strachey that "perhaps of all the creations of man, language is the most astonishing." And if the child learns this, then may also come the realization that he or she is ever involved in creating this recurring miracle. This, we appreciate, is a restatement of the functions of language presented in Chapter 1.

In the discussion that follows we consider the levels or stages of language development and some of the correlated maturational factors in these stages of "the most astonishing creation."

THE STAGES OF LANGUAGE DEVELOPMENT

Prelingual Stages

Before a child speaks first words—produces verbal signals with intended meaning—the girl or boy normally goes through a series of stages in vocalic and articulatory productions that are characteristic and universal. That is, regardless of the particular language a given child will begin to use during the second year of life, children are almost all likely to engage in some amount of vocal "behavior" that is peculiar to human infants. We assume, even though it is not clearly established, that these stages are necessary precursors for later speech sound production. In our review of the stages we speculate as to their implications for later language acquisition. Our discussion will be about children who are born after a full-term normal pregnancy without any pre-, para-, or immediate postnatal factors to suggest any likelihood of abnormality.

Undifferentiated Crying

Babies cry, and parents, especially if they are new in this role, wonder why. Although we offer no philosophic speculation as to the reason for the early cries, we do know that babies enter the extrauterine world with a cry. Should a baby fail to do this, the attending physician is likely to give him or her a sharp slap on the tender backside to elicit such a cry. Perhaps the cry is a reflexive expression of the pain that comes initially with the baby's having to take care of its own breathing. If we cannot say positively that the child cries because of discomfort, we can certainly observe that the child cries when uncomfortable. In any event, the birth cry and the crying during the first few weeks of life are considered reflexive manifestations of discomfort. The cries are *undifferentiated,* in that the nontrained adult ear cannot distinguish or associate the nature of the discomfort with any features of the crying. The crying may be described as nasal, shrill wailing. It is essentially the same whether the child is hungry, thirsty, cold, in pain, or needs a change of linen. Students of infant crying may recognize differences. Most of us cannot.

We regard the first cry, and the subsequent undifferentiated crying, as reflexive expression of physiological (chemico-neuro-muscular) internal ongoings. The occurrence of crying indicates that for the time being the respiratory and laryngeal mechanisms are functioning normally. The child is responding normally to internal changes. The child can approximate (bring together) the vocal bands, and they can be set into action as air on intake and breath on output is forced between them. If there are any identifiable sounds in reflexive crying, they are likely to be nasalized vowels.

We should point that our observations about the child's crying are based on assumptions relative to the changes that take place when an adult does something because the child is crying. Thus, we conclude that the child who stops crying after being fed must have cried initially because he/she was hungry, or that the child who stops crying after being given additional covering must have cried because he/she was cold. These may well be likely cause-and-effect changes in behavior. It is possible, nevertheless, that the child's cessation of crying may be the result of being handled and receiving some direct human physical contact. The actual cause of the child's crying may not, however, have been alleviated. Perhaps that is why the child so quickly resumes crying when the adult leaves.

Comfort Sounds

A few infants may vocalize during noncrying periods in states we consider comfortable, for example, after a feeding and burping. Most infants are silent, awake or asleep, when they are not crying. Comfort sounds become considerably more evident during the second and third month. This is also the period of differentiated crying and more generally of differentiated vocalization.

Differentiated Vocalization

Beginning in the second month, most children become differentiated vocalizers, when crying or when otherwise engaged in sound production. In regard to crying, most mothers can tell when a child is hungry, not just because the child is crying when the mother thinks it is time to be hungry, but because the cry sounds characteristically different at such a time compared with times when there is evidence that a diaper change is needed or that the child is cold. There is a crescendo pattern to the child's hunger cry that is not present under other discomfort conditions.

The differences in crying constitute an early signal system for parents. Parents who tune in are able to make associations between a kind of condition and a form of vocalization. We are not suggesting that the child has any intention or awareness about the vocalization. The productions are still reflexive. However, because the infant's neuromuscular system has matured, the unwitting evocations become increasingly differentiated. The child is a reflexive producer, but those who attend may become interpreters of varying states. Differentiated vocalization thus permits a one-way communication for the sensitive listener-respondent, usually the mother.

Cooing, gurgling, and "squealing," and sounds that approximate consonants are soon added to the vowel-like sounds in the child's inventory of sound production. Lenneberg (1967, p. 128) observes that beginning at 12 weeks of age, vowel-like (cooing) sounds may be sustained for 15–20 seconds. The infant is well on the way to becoming a proficient sound maker. At this stage, the infant is an internationalist in sound making. The products are by no means restricted to the language or languages of the home. We may, according to our prejudices, recognize front vowels in the child's squealings, and mid- and back vowels, *ah*, *uh*, and *oo*, in the child's cooing. We may also identify sounds that suggest *m*, *b*, and *g* and *k*.

By 16 weeks of age, the child begins to make definite responses to human sounds and sound makers. The child, on hearing a voice, turns toward the speaker. The infant's eyes begin to scan and search for the sound maker. If the child is engaged in vocalization, the initial response is likely to be an interruption of the effort. On making visual "contact" with the other speaker, the child may then respond by smiling or cooing. Vocal play may be maintained by an interchange of sound making between the child and another vocalizer. The evidence is strong that infant vocalization is reinforced by the presence and stimulation of an adult. Research on the sound making of children brought up in orphanages as well as on their early true speech development—Goldfarb (1954), Lenneberg (1967, p. 137)—reveals that these children engage in less sound play than do those of peer age who are brought up in homes and receive parental attention.

It is possible to overwhelm the child by too much stimulation. Some children respond to adult efforts by ceasing their own vocalization. The wise adult can be guided by what needs to be done by observing the effects of what is done. If the child responds to adult sound play by more vocalization then the play should be continued. If the child stops vocalization, then the adult should cease too. We are not suggesting that the adult should refrain indefinitely from stimulating the child. The effort should certainly be resumed at a later time, and the results observed. A 16-week-old child may welcome stimulation that was rejected a week or two earlier or even an hour or two earlier. Few normal children will long deprive adults or themselves of the enjoyment of vocal interchange.

The first three months take the infant from undifferentiated, reflexive crying to differentiated vocalization. Even the objective observer may conclude that the child's sound play, the cooing, gurgling, and more discernible oral products, is fun. There are, however, some silent children who cry very little and with no suggestion of feeling or enthusiasm. Though some of these ultimately will become adequate if not loquacious speakers, a few will be among the small number who will grow up as nonverbal children. These, whom parents retrospectively recall as "very good" infants, whose cries were token whimpers, may later be identified as autistic children. Not only in their failure to respond to human speech, but in other aspects of their behavior, they are essentially silent and nonrelating children. They rarely smile in response to stimulation that produces smiles or laughter in most children.

Babbling

The period from three to six months of age is one characterized by a considerable increase in vocalization that includes identifiable sounds that are used in speaking. Some of these sounds, and combinations of sounds, are reduplicated. So we may hear "ga-ga" and "ug-ug" and "bah-bah." There is also a marked increase in the child's responses to the nonverbal behavior of members of the environment. The child may squeal with apparent pleasure at the sight of mother, or when given a toy, or when picked up for play by a parent. The child may respond with crying to loud sounds, or any suggestion of "No" or scolding in the voice of someone from whom warmth and friendliness are usually expected. By six months of age most children have reached the prelingual stage we designate as babbling.

We consider babbling an exceedingly important stage in speech development.[1] Innate drives toward vocalization and sound play may be reinforced or discouraged. Environmental factors—the influence and effects of external stimulation—become determinants of what the child will be doing as a future sound maker. The child seems to be aware that sound making is pleasurable, both as an accomplishment in itself and as a technique for giving pleasure to others. We agree with Lewis (1959) that the primarily innate forces that bring the child to babbling will be enhanced and sustained by the nature of his/her environment. The child needs a favorable climate, with attentive but not

[1] Not all students of child language agree with our position. For a review of differences in point of view, see Clark and Clark (1977, pp. 389–391).

A psychologist concerned with the development of language behavior reports that some children have begun to speak without going through the prelingual stages normal to almost all children. E. H. Lenneberg, *Biological Foundations of Language* (New York: John Wiley & Sons, Inc., 1967), pp. 140–141.

overwhelming adults, to be sustained in continued speech and language development.

By about the sixth month, differences in the vocalizations of deaf and hearing children may be discerned by a sophisticated listener. For the most part, these differences are more readily apparent in the deaf child's responses to the vocalization of others than in his own spontaneous efforts. The deaf child now seems to have a more limited repertoire of sounds than does the peer who can hear. Lenneberg (1964, p. 154) observes:

> the total amount of a deaf child's vocalization may not be different from that of a hearing child, but the hearing child at this age will constantly run through a large repertoire of sounds whereas the deaf children will be making the same sounds sometimes for weeks on end and then suddenly change to some other set of sounds and "specialize" in them for a while. There is no consistent preference among deaf children for specific sounds.

The voice of the deaf child in spontaneous utterance is no different from that of the hearing child. In response to inner drives, the deaf child's voice is as true an indicator of feelings as is the voice of the hearing child. The internal physiological mechanisms that create the neuromuscular state for vocalization are the same for the deaf child as for the one with normal hearing. So, too, the product is of the same variety. It is only when the deaf child's voice is part of a voluntary effort that differences appear and the high-pitched, poorly modulated voice of the deaf begins to be heard. Amplification of the deaf baby's early sound-making may sustain the normal process of language development, late babbling included.

Later Babbling (Lalling)

By eight months of age, most children engage in a considerable amount of self-imitation in their sound making. We can begin to hear clear "ga-ga," "da-da," and "ma-ma" utterances, often accompanied by intonation patterns that resemble those in the child's home. The child's voice will make it quite clear to the listener that something is wanted *now*, or that the child is pleased or displeased with what is going on at the moment. During this stage of development the child is not as random a sound maker as in earlier infant babbling. The child makes fewer sounds, but has better control of the oral products. The child is listening to and monitoring the oral products produced, and so is able to control them. Sound replication is an expression of such control. Some of the sound combinations such as "da-da" and "ma-ma" resemble words. However, parental pride to the contrary, very few children who say "ma-ma" at eight months of age assign any meaning to their utterance. But many children do associate sound (what they hear) and meaning by eight months of age, and parental pride may not always be misplaced. Most children need a few months before they really mean what they say. Part of this time is devoted to responding to what they hear with their own echolalic, imitative utterances.

Deaf children are not likely to enter spontaneously into the lalling stage. All too frequently, without the ability to hear and to feel the results of their articulatory play, they tend to become silent children. When provoked or extremely uncomfortable, deaf children may make sounds as in the babbling stage. However, it is possible for some deaf children to progress from babbling to lalling if they can see themselves in a mirror when they are engaged in sound play. In more than one way reflexive action may produce reflective behavior. If deaf children can be motivated to keep their oral mechanisms in shape, they can also be motivated to listen and so continue to use their residual hearing. Virtually no deaf child is "stone deaf." Mechanical amplification of sound may help to maintain vocal efforts, self-imitation included.

Imitative (Echoic) Utterance

Sometimes preceding and often accompanying their first words to label or identify objects and events in their environment, children imitate the articulatory efforts of others. Earlier, children demonstrate echoic ability in their imitations of vocal contours. Now they expand their imitative ability by including articulation. Through this achievement children indicate continued maturation of their linguistic motor systems. Some of the imitations are so proficient that it is difficult for many parents to distinguish between echoic utterances and true oral language.

Some children are echoic for a month or two before producing utterances that are labels or identifiers for key objects, persons and events about them.

Yasuko and Owada (1973) report on a longitudinal study of echoic utterances of Japanese children ages one through three. They found that some of their subjects developed imitative utterances along with true language up to two years of age and others up to two years and six months of age. Yasuko and Owada observe that "The patterns of growth and decline of echoic utterances could be regarded as indicators of the child's developmental level of expression."

In another sense, however, the baby is acquiring language. We may note an increasing amount of differential behavior to specific utterances directed to the child. An appropriate gesture may be made when the child hears "bye-bye." We may also observe anticipatory action such as reaching when the child is asked "Do you want your dolly?" When, perhaps between 10 and 12 months of age, and not uncommonly before the age of 15 months, the child says "doddy" or "da da" or just "da" when presented with a doll, we do have the onset of speech.

Some children seem to become arrested at the echolalic stage. Such children include the severely mentally retarded (intelligence quotients below 50 or 60) and the autistic. However, some autistic children may be able to mimic long strings of words with accurate articulation and vocal intonation. They sound as if they are talking except that they give no indication of expecting anything in particular to happen as a result of what they seem to have said.

Except under conditions of stress or fatigue, we do not consider it normal for children to maintain echoic utterances beyond age three. This exception does not include occasional echoic responses that almost all of us produce when we are not certain of what we have heard and so "rehear" before we organize an answer.

Deaf children do not go beyond the early lalling stage unless extraordinary measures are taken to make maximum and effective use of their residual hearing and their ability to see what people do when they speak.

Identification Language (Labeling)

Before they produce their first "intelligible" words, most children indicate some of their needs by gesturing (pointing) accompanied by sound making. The sounds may be "uh-uh" or an articulated product that suggests a later first word.

By the beginning of the second year and usually by 15 months of age, most children have words to identify objects, persons, and some satisfying events in their environment. However, because echolalic utterances are likely to continue, one-year-old and post one-year-old children will seem to speak some words for which they have no apparent meaning. Their first words—ones with apparent meaning—are likely to be reduplicated syllables, such as "dada" and "mama." The child is now able to obey verbal "commands," such as pointing to the nose, ears, and so on, in response to directions. "Show me your nose," "Where is baby's nose?" and so forth. The child may also play "Peek-a-boo," or bang a cup when an adult says "cup." In these situations the child's utterances, as well as the nonverbal actions, are used to identify events. Unless somewhat on the precocious side, the child is not likely to be using words initially to bring about an event—to get the doll or a bottle of milk, or to call for mother when any one of these is not in view.

Anticipatory Language: Demands and Commands

By the middle of the second year, most children are able to use language to bring about an event, to get something or someone not physically in view and/or to "command" something or someone in view. During this stage the child's utterance may be accompanied by a change in posture or "motor set" that is consistent with an appropriate reaction to what is expected to happen. Thus, the child not only says "up" but gets ready to be picked up. When the child says "mama," the words are accompanied by looking to the door through which mother is supposed to make her appearance. Words at this stage have a "magical" power for the child. Words are a way of getting people to do one's bidding, of satisfying one's needs physically and psychosocially.

At this language stage most children have productive vocabularies of from three to 50 or more words, and much larger comprehension vocabularies. They are definitely "with it" linguistically, and ready for more complex verbal behavior. Some verbally precocious children may have several hundred words in their productive lexicons, and several thousand that they are able to comprehend.

The child's single-word utterances are, in effect, sentences. The intended meaning of the utterance is indicated by the manner of intonation. Thus, "mama," depending on intonation, may mean an empiric "Mother, come here!" or "Where is mother?" or even, "Mother, I've had enough of you now." Similarly, "cup" may mean "Fill it up" or "I've had my fill of it." If we accept intonation as a form of syntax, then we may consider that the child's variously intoned words are complete sentences, which may have as many meanings as adults regularly give to the word forms "yes" or "no" or "uh-uh."

Children who later will be designated as severely intellectually retarded may not go beyond the stage of identification language, even though they may have a small vocabulary for naming (identifying) some objects and persons in their environment. A few retarded children may develop single-word or two-word utterances to bring about events, but growth of vocabulary is slow, both for comprehension and production of language. Retarded children have fewer words than their normal age peers, and fewer meanings for the words they know. Moderately intellectually retarded children will shadow the linguistic development of normal and bright children. Severely retarded children (those with intelligence quotients below low-grade idiocy) may be totally nonverbal or almost completely so.[2]

Some children are slow in onset but not at all slow in their understanding of speech. These children may not say their first words until they are two years of age, and a few, happily a very few, do not speak until they are 30 months old. These children go through the prelingual stages on schedule and show that they understand what is said to them in games they play with adults. They can even carry out spoken directions to "fetch and carry" and yet make no verbal responses of their own. Some of these children come from families of late talkers, especially on the father's side. Most of these children catch up quickly once they begin to talk. They do manage to give their parents, and more particularly their grandparents, a difficult and anxious time. Just why these children are well within normal range for understanding spoken language and yet slow to start speaking remains a mystery. It is, however, important to distinguish these children from others who are both slow to talk and slow to understand what others say to them.

Syntactic Speech

By two years of age the child is likely to have a vocabulary of between 50 and 100 words. Some children may be able to name all the familiar objects in their environment. The most distinctive achievement is the combination of words from their inventory into phrases that, though lacking in the conventional markers of syntax, nevertheless constitute sentences. The form of the words used may be two nouns—for example, *cup* and *milk* to mean "Give me a cup of milk" or "I want milk" or, in the adult usage, an adverb + noun, for example, "more milk" with the meaning apparent. There is little value in trying to determine whether the child's vocabulary has a preponderance of nouns and some adjectives and a few conventional verbs that function as sen-

---

[2] Here we may be dealing with circuitous thinking, with the effect as well as the cause of retarded onset of language. A child of three or more who has not begun to speak may get less stimulation than a normal child. If the severely retarded child is institutionalized, he may indeed never get around to speaking. E. H. Lenneberg *in Biological Foundations of Language* (New York: John Wiley & Sons, Inc., 1967), p. 154–155, reports on a population of 54 Down's Syndrome children who were raised at home (age range six months to 22 years). These children were observed over a period of from two to three years. At the end of the study period, 75 per cent of the children had reached a stage of at least identification language. The children had small vocabularies and could execute simple verbal commands. Lenneberg notes that progress in language development was noted only in the children who were below 14 years of age.

Weiss and Lillywhite (1981, p. 184) note ". . . in the custodial retardates, communication may never develop beyond the briefest vocalization."

tences. Any of the child's words may be used contextually to indicate a variety of meanings. Frequently one word is used recurrently as a pivot (Braine, 1963), so that we get such phrases as "here cup," "here shoe," "here doll," as well as "doll here" and "kitty here." We may also have such phrase-sentences as "more milk" and "more up." The significance of this accomplishment is that the child is developing a sense of word combination, which in time will be modified by conventional word order and markers of syntax.

At two years of age an increasing number, perhaps 50 per cent, of the child's utterances are sufficiently intelligible to be comprehensible to persons who are not members of the child's family. Of great significance is the ability of most two-year-old children to combine words into novel sentences of their own making. These sentences begin to follow the grammatical rules of the language of older members of their environment but are not word-for-word replications. Many two-year-old children now speak creatively in that they are formulating sentences based on their individual word inventories, yet are obedient to the rules or conventions of the syntax of their language. At first, the "syntax" may be just one of word order. So, from "baby up" a child may go to "dolly up" or "mommy up." Some children will begin to show an ability for transformations, if only one of word order. Thus, we may hear "up baby," "up mommy," and "up ball."

When children achieve a vocabulary of 50 or so words, some of which are commands as well as labels, they are likely to begin to combine words into two word phrase-sentences such as the type just indicated. Then, as children progress and build up their word inventories and increase the length of their spontaneous utterances, syntactical features become incorporated into their phrase-sentences and later into more clearly identifiable sentences. Interestingly, there is a fair amount of regularity as to the syntactical features that accompany the increases in length of children's utterance. Thus, correlations have been worked out between Mean Length of Utterance (MLU)[3] and syntactical structure based on samples of normal children's early speech.

Ingram and Eisenson (1972, pp. 148–188) provide samples of five basic levels beyond the single word stage of syntactic constructions in

---

[3] Mean Length of Utterance (MLU) can be determined by taking a sample of a child's spontaneous utterances and dividing the total number of words spoken by the number of utterances. Thus, if the sample consists of 100 utterances and the total number of words is 300, the MLU is 3. A second and more frequently used method is to add the total number of words and the total number of morphemes and divide this number by two for a word-morpheme count. Then, divide this total by the number of utterances. So 300 words + 450 morphemes divided by two = 375, divided by 100 (number of utterances) gives us an MLU of 3.75.

the language acquisition of young children. These levels are based on an investigation by Morehead and Ingram. Language samples[4] were taped and analyzed for mean length of utterance and for syntactical constructions employed in spontaneous speech.

Some examples of the constructions in the Ingram-Eisenson levels follow.

[4] Tyack and Gottsleben (1974) have published a manual on the technique of language sampling.

Bloom and Lahey (1978, pp. 454–491) describe their approach to language sampling by "content and form" and other approaches to "sampling" a child's language when therapeutic intervention is considered likely or necessary.

Ingram-Eisenson Levels

*Level I—Average Utterance Range 2.0–2.5 Words**

hit ball	kick box
big girl	small cat
John candy	Mary cookie
boy walk	girl eat
that kitty	that mommy
doggy hear	kitty there
put in truck	look in box
in small box	in big house
hit it	throw it
it walk	it jump

Level II—Average Utterance Range 2.5–3.0 Words

boy drink water	girl eat(s) candy
throw small can	kick(s) big ball
kick Tom ball	See Mary doll
this ball	that doll
on table	in truck
put on box	put on table
on red table	on green box
Bobby put on table	Mary sit(s) on chair
a boy	a doll
the cat	the doll
boy eat a cookie	Mary see(s) the ball
boys (plural contrast with singular)	girls
hit ball	eat candies
mommy wear shoes	boy hold(s) books
boy eating	girl swimming

* Note that child constructions at level I do not include grammatical markers. So we have *it walk* and not *it walks*.

Ingram-Eisenson Levels (*continued*)

Level II—Average Utterance Range 2.5–3.0 Words

---

boy catching ball	girl riding bike
Bobby put in box	Dick jump(s) on box
Mary eating cookies	girls feeding birds
What that	Where boy
Where girl run	Where boy go

Level III—Average Utterance Range 3.0–4.0 Words

---

boy open door	girl feed(s) cat
put kitty in box	sit dog on chair
going (gonna) eat cookie	going (gonna) ride bike
Mary put doll in wagon	Mommy put(s) baby in bed
John is boy	Cathy is girl
Bobby is here	baby is there
Man is big	Dolly is small
But ball in box	Put candies in box
gonna throw balls	gonna eat candies
Baby is crying	Girl is jumping
Man is pulling wagon	Mommy is driving car
put the box on table	throw the ball in box
boy and girl	baby and mommy
at home	at park
Go to school	Go to park.
Girl is at home.	Mommy is at store.
Boy run to house.	Girl run to school.
She eat cookie.	They play ball.
He hold her.	She carry him.
She is here.	He is there.
He is in wagon.	She is in car.
She gonna (going to) drink milk.	He gonna eat cookie.
They carry cookies to mommy.	They carry ball to park.
Girl gonna go to school.	Boy gonna kick ball in park.
Boy is running to school.	Man is walking to store.
What is that?	What the girl doing?
Where that?	Where the mommy going?
Dog is running.	Baby is eating.
I put the ball in box, OK?	I eat cookies, ok?

Level IV—Average Utterance Range 4.0–5.0 Words

The mommy hold(s) the boy.
The doggy dig(s) the hole.
The girl put(s) a candy in the box.
The boy throw(s) the red ball.
The mommy gonna feed the baby.

Ingram-Eisenson Levels (*continued*)

Level IV—Average Utterance Range 4.0–5.0 Words

The big dog runs.
Tommy is a boy.
That is a dog.
The boy is in a wagon.
Tommy goes to school with Billy.
That is Bobby('s) ball.
That is her cat.
That is Billy('s) dog.
The ball hit Tommy.
You and I laugh.
Daddy see us.
You and I eat cookies.
The dog is running.
This is a bird.
The man is big.
You are laughing.
John eats a candy.
Mommy drives a car.
I see the girl's bike.
The bird has to fly.
I have to (hafta) run home.
What's this?
What is the man reading?
Will Tommy run?
Will the mommy see the baby?

Level V—Average Utterance Range 5.0–6.0 Words

The girl won't run.
The boy can't go.
The baby won't drink the milk.
The airplane flies over the house.
The ball is under the table.
The dog is near the wagon.
The kitty climbs up the tree.
The dog is running.
The baby cried.
The boy jumped.
This is their wagon.
This is our car.
The girl reads the book that she likes.
Won't the dog run?
Who is driving the car?
Who is sleeping on the bed?

Syntactic Transformations

We indicated earlier that when children "realize" that they can say either "up baby" or "baby up" they have learned a simple transformation, or two ways of communicating essentially the same meaning. How the child learns this way we do not know. Nor do we know how a child learns that when asked "Do you want candy?" the answer may be simply "yes" or, more rarely, "No." It may also be "Yes, I (or me) want candy?" Now we have an example of a nominal transposition, another kind of transformation. The *you*, if the child is normal, is replaced by *I*. (It may also be replaced by *me*, but either *I* or *me* represents a transformation.) A question form is reconstructed into a simple declarative statement. Later the child will learn that one may say either "Bobby held mother's hand" or "Mother's hand was held by Bobby." Again, the meaning of the two sentences is essentially the same. Perhaps, less similar are the sentences "Johnny kicked Mary" and "Mary was kicked by Johnny." Some children feel that when "Johnny kicked Mary" the pain was greater that when "Mary was kicked by Johnny." However, the underlying meaning if not the full impact continues to be the same.

Most transformations involve the use of grammatical forms and structures that permit children to understand new meanings and, in turn, to express new meanings. These include how to make distinctions between singular and plural; to use tense endings to indicate the present, past, and future; and to deal with the hypothetical in the past as well as in a possible future. They also learn to make negative statements and to ask questions. The first questions children ask are those that may be answered by "Yes" or "No." Later they learn to ask questions that begin with interrogative (*wh*) words—*where, what, whose, who, why, when, which,* and *how*.

In the later stages of syntactic acquisition, children learn to combine two or more single statement sentences into a single complex sentence. So the sentences "John is my big brother. He will take me to the zoo tomorrow." may become "John, my big brother, will take me to the zoo tomorrow." Also, sentences such as "The girl sees the bird. The bird is flying." may become "The girl sees the bird that's flying."

We are avoiding a discussion of the theory of transformational grammar at this point. We believe that the kinds of transformational forms that children learn *and understand* are associated with their cognitive (intellectual) state. A child will have no use for future tense without an ability to project from present to future, or to use a subjunctive "If I were" form without a capacity to deal with the hypothetical. Some of these forms, however, may be used on an imitative basis, without true comprehension. So, we may have performance (production) without understanding. It is probable, as Carol Chomsky (1969) has found, that children still have much to learn about syntax beyond the age of five and quite likely up to and a bit beyond the age of ten.

The following table, Fourteen English Morphemes, reveals how much most children learn of word structure and the modification of words to express meanings through their knowledge of grammar, specifically, how to use markers to indicate tense, plurals, possession, and the role of prepositions, articles, and conjunctions in multiword utterances. These achievements, in the approximate order of acquisition, usually take place when children are between two and three years of age. Language sampling shows that children who use these morphemes have M.L.U's that range between 2.25 and 7 morphemes.

Fourteen English Morphemes (Suffixes and Function Words) and Their Likely Order of Acquisition by Children

Morpheme (Form)	Likely Intended Meaning	Example
1. Present progressive *-ing*	Ongoing action.	Joe is eati*ng* lunch.
2. Preposition: *in*	Containment.	The cookie is *in* the box.
3. Preposition: *on*	Support.	The cookie is *on* the box.
4. Plural: *-s*	Number (more than one).	The bird*s* flew away.
5. Past irregular: e.g. *went, ran*	The event took place earlier (before the time of the speaker's utterance).	The boy *went* away. The boy *ran* away.
6. Possessive: *-'s*	Possession.	The girl*'s* dress is red.
7. Uncontracted form of the verb to be (copula) e.g. *are, was*	Plural number; past tense (earlier in time).	These *are* cookies. It *was* a cat. It *was* on the tree.
8. Articles: *the, a*	Definite and indefinite article.	Bob has *the* stick. Bob has *a* stick.
9. Past regular: *-ed*	Event happened earlier in time.	Tom jump*ed* (over the fence).
10. Third person regular *-s*	Third person, present action.	He *walks* fast.
11. Third person irregular, e.g. has, does	Present state (situation). On-going action (third person).	He *has* a ball. She *does* the cooking.
12. Uncontracted auxiliary be: e.g. *is, were*	An ongoing action; past action.	Bob *is* eating. They *were* fishing.

Fourteen English Morphemes (Suffixes and Function Words) and Their Likely Order of Acquisition by Children (*continued*)

Morpheme (Form)	Likely Intended Meaning	Example
13. Contracted form of of *be:* e.g. -'s, -'re	State of being (existence).	It's a kitty. We're at home.
14. Contracted auxiliary to *be:* e.g. -'s,)'re	Time: an ongoing action.	He's going. They're eating lunch.

Sources: Brown (1973) and H. and E. V. Clark, (1977).

Communicative Intent

As indicated above, by two-and-a-half years of age most children include functional words—prepositions, articles, and conjunctions—in their utterances. In other respects, too, their formulations approximate those of the older speakers to whom they are exposed. They begin to speak grammatically, or agrammatically, usually depending upon how those in their surroundings speak. Three- to four-word sentences are frequent. Between the age of two-and-a-half and three years, the child's increase in vocabulary is likely to be greater proportionately than for any other equal time period in his/her life. Between 24 and 30 months of age, the child's intention to communicate, to speak with the expectation both of being understood and responded to, becomes clear. If the child is not understood, frustration may be evidenced. Fortunately, the normal three-year-old not only shows control of syntax but control as well of most of the sounds of his/her language. So-called infantilisms, such as "wawa" for "water," decrease. The child's phonemic or articulatory proficiency is usually good enough for most of what is produced to be readily intelligible.

Literally, the three-year-old speaks as a self, using "I" in contexts that a few months before contained "me." The child understands and distinguishes between "I," "we," "me," and "you." The three-year-old can usually transform the "you" of a question addressed to him or her, for example, "Do you want a cookie?" to "I want a cookie." Interestingly, autistic children, even when they begin to speak, are slow to make the distinction and transformation of "you" to "I" or "me." Characteristically, autistic children refer to themselves in the manner in which they are addressed. Thus, "Do you want a cookie?" is likely to be answered by "You want a cookie," or by a repetition of the entire sentence.

Three to Four—The Emergence of an Individuolect

No attempt is made here to discuss, in any detail, the language development of children beyond the age of three. Most children beyond this age progress with giant strides in their ability to use conventional syntax. For the most part they have both the words and the word structures to express their thoughts and they can suit their actions to their words. Yet this is the age of considerable hesitation and repetition in speaking. These disfluencies, we think, suggest that some children have thoughts or the beginnings of thoughts for which they have no immediate or adequate verbal formulations. On the other hand, some post-three-year-olds will talk quite glibly and use both words and structures that makes it evident to a discerning and critical listener that the youngsters do not really know what they are saying. But a few precocious ones do!

In general, we may conclude that children in the three-to-four age range who began to speak by 15 months of age are well along the way to adult syntactic proficiency. However, as previously noted in the reference to Chomsky's (1969) findings, a child of this age still has a way to go. Perhaps by age ten or eleven, most children will have reached adult proficiency in their syntactical usage.

Although the language development of four-year-olds is far from completed, in many ways they are mature speakers. Most show clear evidence of having developed individual rhetorical styles, and have favorite words and favorite ways of turning phrases. Some are verbose and others are on the quiet side. Four-year-olds speak for themselves and about themselves as *selves*. Each is an individual and each, in manner of speaking, is developing an *individuolect*.

THE ACQUISITION OF THE SOUND SYSTEM: PHONEMIC DEVELOPMENT

Thus far in our discussion we have emphasized the lexical (vocabulary) and syntactic aspects of language development. Neither, of course, can take place without the acquisition of the phonemic or sound system of the linguistic code. Many children take longer to establish completely proficient control of the sounds of their language than to acquire a vocabulary of 1,000 words or more and much of the syntax of their system. As infants engage in sound play, many sounds are produced that will not be controlled voluntarily and articulated intentionally until the child is six or seven years of age. Children also show great variability in their phonemic proficiency. Some, especially girls, may arrive at an almost adult level of control by age four or five. Most children, however, need at least a year or two longer before they arrive at this level of proficiency.

Children's errors in phonemic production are not random. Children make their words out of the sounds they are able to control. These, as we have noted, begin with vowels, nasals, and labials (lip sounds). The young child also engages in reduplication. So, with the few sounds under control, the child builds a word inventory. Words such as *mama* present no problem. A *kitty* is, however, likely to be pronounced *kicky* because the child can usually produce a /k/, before he/she can a /t/. So the child substitutes one stop sound for the other and, economically, uses the same sound twice. The production of *bummy* for *bunny* may be explained by the fact that /m/ is a bilabial, as is /b/. The child beginning a word with one bilabial finds it easier to include a second /m/ rather than to introduce a tip-tongue nasal /n/. How would you explain *doddy* for *doggy?*

Characteristics of Early Phonemic Development

Though some children are laws unto themselves, most do follow well established tendencies in their speech sound (phonological) development. Following are some general observations of typical "errors" or, more appropriately, *characteristics of early child speech sound production.*[5]

WEAK SYLLABLE DELETION.   Many children delete an unstressed (weak) syllable in a polysyllabic word. So, the word *elephant* may be pronounced as *elfant* or *hefant*. Even shorter words, such as *belong* and *away*, may be reduced to *bong* [bɔŋ] and *way* [weɪ].

SYLLABLE REPETITION.   Words such as *cracker* and *paper* may become *kaka* [kæ kæ] and *paypay* [peɪ peɪ]. *Dada* [dædæ] or [dada] for *daddy* is an early example of syllable repetition. We should, of course, not confuse this with the syllable or sound repetition (disfluency) that characterizes much early child speech.

CLUSTER SIMPLIFICATION.   Many children do not achieve control of cluster (sound blend combinations) until age five or six, and some

[5] These observations are based on an article by D. Ingram, Phonological Rules of Young Children," *Journal of Child Language*, 1974, 49–64. See also Ingram 1981, Chap. 7.

do not do so until age seven. English has many sound clusters, such as *bl, pl, cl, cr, gr, dr, st,* and triple clusters, such as *str, sks,* and *sts.* Some of these, such as *sts* and *sks,* continue to be troublesome even for adults. Young children tend to simplify sound clusters by dropping out one or more of the sounds, almost always those not yet under comfortable control, and retaining the sound under control. So, the word *cracker* shows both cluster simplification and syllable repetition when the child pronounces it as [kæ kæ]. The pronunciation of *please* as *pease* [piz] and *spoon* as *poon* [pun] are examples of cluster simplification.

ASSIMILATION. Assimilation is the tendency for one sound to be modified in production as a result of proximity to another sound. Young children show a general tendency to produce (substitute) a sound under control for one not yet controlled. So we may hear *doddy* for *doggy* if the *d* is under control. Later we may get *goggy* if the *g* is controlled. Finally, when both the *d* and *g* are secure and controlled in any position within a word, we get *doggy.* Similarly, *kitty* may go from *kiky* [kɪkɪ] to *titty* [tɪtɪ] before it becomes a more mature *kitty.*

Phonemic Discrimination and Production

Differential Sound Perception

If we are tuned in to infant sound production and base our judgments on the first words infants produce, we might come to the conclusion that most infants hear (perceive and differentiate) very few sounds. First words such as *mama, dada, ba-ba* (a form of bye-bye), *doddy* (dolly), *up, mow* (more), *nuh nuh* (no-no) require the production of either a nasal plus a vowel or a stop plus a vowel. Yet there is evidence that even in the first two or three months of life, infants respond differentially to consonants as close together acoustically and in manner of production as /b/-/p/, /m/-/n/, and /k/-/g/. Infants also respond differentially to the different vowel sounds.[6] How do we account for differential reactions in the first months of life and so limited a productive phonemic inventory when the child begins to talk, a year or so later? One explanation is that reflex or conditioned noncognitive responses call for different nervous system capabilities than do cognitive responses. Another possible explanation is that though ultimately our perceptions and productions become intimately related, initially

[6] Eimas and his associates in "Speech Perception in Infants," *Science,* **171** (1971) found that infants from one to four months of age responded differentially when exposed to voiced and voiceless cognate sounds such as /b/ and /p/.

we can perceive differences we cannot produce. So, children may reject an adult's pronunciation of *wawa* for *water* though maintaining the pronunciation for a while themselves.

What, then, do children perceive—differentially and cognitively process—of the speech sounds they hear? Do they follow basic principles or rules? Is there a chronological order or expected sequence in their speech sound discrimination? The answer to each of these questions is "Probably, yes." However, we should not expect invariable or slavish observation on the part of children. Individual exceptions are always possible, expecially for children who present problems in language acquisition.

Shvachkin (see Slobin 1967) studied phonemic perception in early childhood (11 to 23 months of age). Specifically, Shvachkin investigated Russian children's comprehension of words that differed by a single phoneme. On the assumption that speech sound (phonological) discrimination as well as speech sound production remain the same regardless of the language the child is acquiring, we can apply Shvachkin's observations to a child learning English.[7] The following pattern then emerges:

Pattern of Phonemic Development (Distinctions)

1. The presence or absence of consonants in syllables: [bɑk] and [ɑk], [vek] and [ek].
2. Stop and fricative sounds with sonorants (nasals, vowel-like consonants): *b-m, d-r, g-n, v-y/j/.*
3. Nasal and liquid sounds: *m-l, m-r, n-l, n-r, n-y, m-y.*
4. Intranasal distinctions: *m-n.*
5. Intraliquid distinctions: *l-r.*
6. Fricative and nonfricative: *z-m, v-n.*
7. Labial and nonlabial: *b-d, v-z.*
8. Stop and fricative: *b-v, d-z, k-f.*
9. Lingual and velar: *d-g, t-k.*
10. Voiceless and voiced cognates: *p-b, t-d, k-g, f-v, s-z.*
11. Blade and groove sibilants: s-sh /ʃ/, z-zh /ʒ/.
12. Liquid and glide: *r-y, l-y.*

[7] R. Jakobson, in *Child Language, Aphasia and Phonological Universals* (The Hague: Mouton & Company, 1968), p. 46, states without reservation: "Whether it is a question of French or Scandinavian children, of English or Slavic, of Indian or German . . . every description based on careful observation repeatedly confirms the striking fact that the relative chronological order of phonological acquisitions remains everywhere and at all times the same."

Production

Production, as we suggested, follows perception and discrimination for the sounds of a language system. Articulatory development has been a subject of considerable study for many years. Rather than review "older" studies, we confine our considerations to a few studies published since the middle 1950s. The older studies generally found later ages for articulatory control than do more recent ones. Though it is possible that our population is changing and that children are becoming almost as precocious as their grandparents believe, it may also be that our standards of proficiency are more lenient. Though lenient, they may nevertheless be more realistic. The table that follows, based on Templin's data (1957, p. 43), summarizes her findings for the phonemic development of children ages three to seven. This table should be compared with the next one that presents data for children ages two to four. The Prather, et al. (1975) observations begin at an earlier age than Templin's. Templin could have made similar observations for children below age three. However, though we find age differences that indicate earlier age for phonemic proficiency, order of development for the most part is the same. Note also the correspondence in order for the pattern of phonemic distinctions and the Templin and Prather observations for sound production.

Speech Sound Proficiency Based on Templin's (1957) Data and Criteria of 75 Per Cent Correct Production[1]

Sound	Age	Sound	Age
m	3	r	4
n	3	s	4.5
ng	3	sh	4.5
p	3	ch	4.5
f	3	t	6
h	3	th	6
w	3	v	6
y	3.5	l	6
k	4	th (voiced)	7
b	4	z	7
d	4	zh	7
g	4	j	7

[1] 75 percent of the subjects were correct in their productions of the sounds at the indicated ages.

In a more recent statement, Templin (1966) states that "Cross-sectional normative studies have quite consistently shown that seven- to eight-year-old children can satisfactorily utter all the phonemes of English." Fry (1966) observes that "The rate of speech development varies greatly among individual children, but in the normally hearing child one can expect that by five to seven years of age the phonemic system will be completely and fairly well established."

Sander (1972) argues that the "older" criteria for mastery (proficiency) for speech and control were arbitrary and, as we have suggested, possibly unrealistic. Sander considers that a realistic criterion may be correct articulation for a sound in two out of three word positions. He also considers 50 per cent of correct performance to be a rea-

Comparison of Order of Sounds (Articulation Development) in Children[1]

Ages Two to Four Years

SOUND	AGE PRATHER, HEDRICK, KERN	TEMPLIN	SOUND	AGE PRATHER, HEDRICK, KERN	TEMPLIN
m	2	3–0	s	3	4–6
n	2	3–0	r	3–4	4–0
h	2	3–6	l	3–4	6–0
p	2	3–0	ʃ (sh)	3–8	4–6
ŋ (ch)	2	3–0	tʃ (ch)	3–8	4–6
f	2–4	3–0	ð (voiced th)	4	7–0
j (y)	2–4	3–6			
k	2–4	4–0	ʒ (measure)	4	7–0
d	2–4	4–0	dʒ (jump)	4+	7–0
w	2–8	3–0	θ (voiceless th)	4+	6–0
b	2–8	4–0			
t	2–8	6–0	v	4+	6–0
g	3	4–0	z	4+	7–0

[1] Adapted from E. M. Prather, D. L. Hedrick, and C. A. Kern, "Articulation Development in Children Aged Two to Four Years," *Journal of Speech and Hearing Disorders*, **40** (1975), 179–191.

sonable expectation. The observed order of speech sound development is presented in the following table based on Sander's criterion.

Again, we may note differences in the sequence of the sounds compared with Templin's observations. However, there is an over-all correspondence between Sander's order (page 167) and those of Templin.

Order of Consonant Sound Proficiency Based on Sander's (1972) Criteria[1]

Age	Sounds
2	h, m, n, w, b, p, t, k, g, ng, /ŋ/, d
3	f, y /j/, s, r, l
4	ch /tʃ/, sh /ʃ/, j /dʒ/, z, v
5	voiceless th /θ/, voiced th /ð/
6	zh /ʒ/

[1] Correct articulation of a sound in two of three word positions and 50 per cent correct performance.

SPEECH READINESS

A review of semantic and syntactic acquisition (see the table that follows on Maturational Milestones), indicates that the child makes great spurts at particular periods in his life, for example, the great (proportionate) increase in vocabulary at about 30 months of age; the development of syntax at about two years; the control of consonant clusters (blends) between five and six years of age. These may be considered periods of readiness during which basic skills are incorporated and the child then becomes ready for the next stage of development. Perhaps even more striking is the universal onset of speech, regardless of what language the child will speak, between 12 and 18 months of age. We indicated at the opening of this chapter that we consider speech to be a specific function of the human species. Children are born with the potential to speak if the opportunity is provided. The opportunity, so far as the onset of speech is concerned, is exposure to persons who speak. The rate at which children progress from their beginnings is determined by a combination of innate factors such as the integrity of the child's neurological and sensory systems, native intelligence, *and* cultural-environmental factors, which, for the most part, are those that exist *within* each *family*. We now consider some of these factors.

Maturational Milestones: Physical and Cognitive

Piaget, a Swiss investigator of the intellectual (cognitive) development of children, considered it essential to view changes as expressions of a gradual evolution through qualitatively different stages. Piaget held that action rather than language was the source of thought in young children. We recommend the book *Piaget's Theory of Intellectual Development* by Ginsburg and Opper (Prentice-Hall, 1979) as an excellent introduction to Piaget's concepts of the developmental psychology of children. Piaget's position on the development of language and the relationship of language to thought and logical reasoning are presented in *The Psychology of the Child* (Piaget and Inhelder, 1969, Chap. 3).

The acquisition of language is associated with motoric and cognitive milestones that are summarized in the tables that follow. It is important to appreciate that all of the stages or milestones are approximate as related to "usual" age of expected achievement. For a given child the range of difference may vary by as much as three to six months. The tables are intended as a guide but not as a rigid measure.

Maturational Milestones: Motor Correlates and Language Development[1]

Age	Speech Stage	Motor Development
12–16 weeks	Coos and chuckles	Supports head in prone position; responds to human sounds by turning head in direction of sound source
20 weeks	Consonants modify vowel-like cooing; nasals and labial fricatives are frequently produced	Sits with support
6 months	Babbling, resembling one-syllable utterances; identifiable combinations include *ma, da, di, du*	Sits without props using hands for support
8 months	Lalling and some echolalia	Stands by holding on to object; grasps with thumb apposition
10 months	Distinct echolalia, verbal imitation, which approximates sounds heard; responds differentially to verbal sounds	Creeps efficiently; pulls to standing position; may take a side step while holding on to a fixed object
12 months	Reduplicated sounds in echolalia; possible first words for identification; responds appropriately to simple commands	Walks on hands and feet; may stand alone, may walk when held by one hand, or even take first steps alone

Maturational Milestones: Motor Correlates and Language Development[1] (*continued*)

Age	Speech Stage	Motor Development
18 months	Has repertoire of words (between three and 50); some two-word phrases; vocalizations reveal intonational patterns; great increase in understanding of language	Walks with stiff gait; may build two-block tower; begins to show hand preference
24 months	Vocabulary of 50 or more words for naming and for bringing about events; two-word phrases of own formulation	Walks with ease; runs, can walk up or down stairs, planting both feet on each step
30 months	Vocabulary growth proportionately greater than at any other period in life; speaks with clear communicative intent; conventional sentences (syntax) of three, four, and five words; articulation still includes many infantilisms; good comprehension of speakers in his surroundings	Can jump; stand on one foot; good hand and finger coordination; can build six-block tower
36 months	Vocabulary may exceed 1,000 words; syntax much like that of older persons in his surroundings; most of his utterances are intelligible to older listeners	Runs proficiently; walks stairs with alternating feet; hand preference established
48 months	Except for articulation (phonemic production) the linguistic system increasingly resembles that of the adults in his surroundings. He/she may begin to develop own "rhetorical" style of favorite words and phrases	Can hop on one foot (usually right); can throw a ball to an intended receiver; can catch a ball in his/her arms; can walk on a line

[1] Adapted from E. H. Lenneberg, *Biological Foundations of Language* (New York: John Wiley & Sons, Inc., 1967), pp. 128–130.

The Cognitive Stages of Piaget—Birth to Seven Years

Piaget Developmental Stage	*Linguistic Stage*

SENSORI-MOTOR PERIOD (From birth to approximately 24 months)

Movements related to sensory intake (perceptions). Toward end of period children arrive at notion of object permanence (out of sight is *not* out of mind).

1. Prelinguistic sound production, crying, vocal play, babbling, lalling echolalia, and first words. Gesturing, mostly pointing and pulling, but also evidence of anticipatory movements in response to caretaker language.
2. Toward end of stage, single word productions for labeling and commanding; for many children, two-word utterances.

EARLY PRECONCEPTUAL PERIOD (24 to 48 Months)

Beginnings of symbolic representations. In the early months most mental activity is about the ongoing present— the here and now. In the later months the child is able to appreciate (comprehend and deal with) the past and the future. Considerable evidence of symbolic play.

1. Two-word utterances, usually without grammatic features.
2. Gradual increase to three and four word and longer utterances that incorporate grammatic features of work order and syntax; verbal productions approximate those of older speaker and are likely to be well constructed, simple sentences. in keeping with adult standards.

EARLY INTUITIONAL PERIOD (From approximately 4 to 7 years)

Tasks are solved by immediate perceptual responses. Toward end of stage, the child begins to appreciate the concept of reversibility[1] Social play begins to replace ego-centric play.

Begins to use complex sentences including relative clauses. The phonetic system of the child's language, including "difficult" sounds and sound blends becomes increasingly under control and is likely to be completely or almost completely controlled by age 7.

---

[1] Reversibility implies the capacity to apprehend the essence of a problem so that it—the problem— can be followed through mentally. If required, the "direction" of the problem can be reversed to its starting point, e.g. $2 + 4 = 6$; $6 - 4 = 2$. Reversibility is markedly accelerated between the ages 7.0–12.0.

The Neuromotor System

Children's nervous systems must be capable of doing their bidding and of providing them with feedback as to what and how well they are doing. Their nervous systems must be adequate to make them sensitive to the sights and sounds in their environment, and to permit them to make differential responses to different conditions. They must not only be able to hear but to discriminate between speech sounds and other auditory events. It is possible, as we learn later in our discussion of brain-damaged children in Chapter 16, for a child to be able to discriminate, perceive, and make appropriate responses to nonspeech signals and yet not be able to perceive speech as a different form of sounds. Such a child may hear, and yet not learn to speak, for what the child hears does not include the auditory perceptual capacities necessary for speech.

Cerebral-palsied children are, as a total special population, markedly retarded in speech development. Those cerebral-palsied children who are also mentally retarded by virtue of their brain damage are likely to be retarded in all aspects of speech development. In a study of the articulatory proficiency of cerebral-palsied children, Irwin (1952, pp. 269–279) found that these children at five and a half years of age are at a proficiency level equivalent to that of the 30-month-old child. The problems of some cerebral-palsied children are further complicated by hearing loss of both a peripheral and a central nature. Central hearing loss, as a consequence of damage to the auditory area of the brain, makes it difficult for the child to perceive speech differentially from other audible environmental events.

Weiss and Lillywhite (1981, Chap. 9) review articulatory and other communicative disorders related to cerebral palsy. Hardy (in Curtis, 1978, pp. 237–243) describes the principal neuromotor characteristics of the cerebral palsied and their associated speech and language problems. We also recommend MacDonald and Chance (1964) for an overall survey of the multiple problems of and treatment approaches for the cerebral palsied.

The Auditory System

As previously suggested, the auditory system must permit the reception as well as the perception of speech events. That is, the speech signal must reach the brain (reception) and be processed differentially in the brain (perception). Children with hearing loss severe enough to impair reception are slower in speech development than hearing children. Deaf children are those whose receptive impairment is so severe that they cannot learn to speak through the auditory mode. However, some mildly or moderately hearing-impaired children, especially if their impairment is recognized early in life, may speak quite competently if given appropriate attention and training. The perceptually impaired (aphasic-dyslogic child) is considered at some length in Chapter 16. In Chapter 14 we consider in more detail the implications of hearing loss on speech.

Cerebral Dominance and Laterality Preference

Human motor development is characterized by the preferential use of a paired organ—hand, foot, eye, or ear. This preference is an expression of laterality. Most of us are right-handed and right-footed *and* right-eyed. That is, given an opportunity to reach or grasp, to hop or stand on one foot, to view something with one eye, we are likely to use the same organ for the task—the one on the right side of the body— with great consistency. About 7 to 10 per cent of us are left-sided. However, mixed preference, that is, the combination of right-handedness and left-eyedness, is quite common. A small percentage of us are ambilateral, that is, there is less consistency as to which hand will be used for reaching, or grasping, or executing some task that requires only one hand, or where one hand exercises a skill with the aid of the other hand. Among the ambilateral we have some who are also *ambidextrous,* who are equally skilled with either member of paired organs. Usually such skill is expressed in manual (hand) skills. Ambilaterality does not imply ambidexterity. Among children who are intellectually and maturationally retarded, we have a considerable amount of ambilaterality accompanied by ambi-nondexterity. The truly ambidextrous are a chosen few, most of whom are probably innately left-handed (sinistral) and who have developed more dexterity in the use of the right hand than innately right-handed persons are likely to develop in the use of the left.

The expression of laterality—let us use "hand preference" as an indicator of such expression—parallels critical stages in the development of speech. By 18 months of age, when most children have uttered their first true words, they have also begun to indicate hand preference. By three years of age, when much of syntax is acquired, hand preference, foot preference (standing or hopping on one foot), eye preference, *and* ear preference are also normally established. These laterality expressions mean that one hemisphere of the brain is dominant or controls a function.

Speech, however, employs paired organs for intake (reception) as well as production. For example, the tongue consists of two halves which receive nervous innervations from both hemispheres of the brain. Usually, we listen with both ears and we take in visual events with both eyes. However, as noted in chapter 5, the perceptual appreciation of linguistic events—the interpretation of what we hear or of what we read—is normally processed in the left hemisphere for at least 95 per cent of those of us who are right-handed and about 60 per cent of the left-handed. We may generalize therefore that *the vast majority of human beings have cerebral dominance for language behavior in the left hemisphere.* Such dominance is normally established by three years of age (Kimura 1967). Cerebral dominance is delayed in the moderately and severely mentally retarded and in brain-damaged children. Nonspeech events, the noises of our environment, and the perception of music are normally processed in the right hemisphere. Thus, as we indicated earlier, it is possible for a child to respond appropriately to the barking of a dog, or the ringing of a bell, and even to listen to music, and yet not be able to make the discriminations and perceptions that are necessary to understand and acquire speech. This very special capacity—the processing of speech signals—is associated with cerebral dominance and the functioning of the temporal lobe of the left cerebral hemisphere. (See Figure 7 in Chapter 5 on "The Mechanisms for Speech").

Intelligence

The factor of intelligence is so intimately related to language development that we must be careful to avoid circuitous thinking. There is little doubt that intelligence is positively related to vocabulary growth and, perhaps to a lesser degree, also to syntactic competence (sentence length and complexity). Templin's study (1957, p. 117) is representative of most findings. She reports a correlation of .50 between intelligence and vocabulary growth in young children. Virtually all verbal intelligence tests for children, for example, the Stanford-Binet and the Wechsler Intelligence Scale for Children, include a vocabulary test as part of the scale because of the established relationship between language development, as measured by vocabulary, and intelligence.

The implicit assumption of the authors of vocabulary tests such as the Peabody Picture Vocabulary Test (Dunn and Dunn, 1981), The Pre-School Language Scale (Zimmerman, Steiner, and Evatt, 1969) and The Expressive One-Word Picture Vocabulary Test (Gardner, 1979) is that it is possible to estimate a child's verbal intelligence on the basis of his/her acquired vocabulary. For example, Gardner states

"The purpose of this test is to obtain a basal estimate of a child's verbal intelligence by means of his acquired one-word expressive vocabulary . . . ." The Peabody Test makes the assessment through receptive vocabulary. The Pre-School Language Scale assesses both receptive and expressive vocabulary.

One of the concomitants of being born with good native intelligence is the likelihood that one's parents and other members of the family may also be intelligent, and may provide an environment where proficient language usage will stimulate and encourage more of the same. Further, we have a likelihood that such a background will have books as well as parents for reading, for storytelling, and for the other social advantages that go along with good language development.

Sex

Though studies vary in their findings, early investigators found that up to age eight or nine, girls are somewhat more advanced than boys of like age in overall language development. McCarthy (1954, pp. 492–630) reports such an advantage for girls over boys. Templin (1957), based on much the same procedures for collecting data as McCarthy, found smaller differences than those detected in earlier studies. Templin notes that whereas on overall language competence girls do tend to be somewhat superior to boys, the differences for specific language achievements are not consistent and are usually not great enough to be statistically significant. Girls do seem to be about a half year ahead of boys in articulatory proficiency. Boys, however, may exceed girls in word knowledge. Templin explains her findings of reduced differences between the sexes on the basis of changes in child rearing during the past few decades. We have changed from bringing up little girls as girls and little boys as boys to a single standard in child care and training (Templin 1957, p. 147). This observation is supported by the findings of Winitz (1969) on a study of the language development of kindergarten children. Winitz found no significant differences between the sexes in regard to such language measures as length of response, the number of different words used, the structural (syntactic) complexity of the child's utterances, vocabulary skill, and articulatory proficiency.

As of the present, we may conclude that differences in language proficiency between girls and boys are minimal. However, as we shall note later, there are marked differences in speech and language disorders, most notably in regard to stuttering.

Environmental Factors

It is not possible to disassociate factors, such as intelligence, both child and parental, parent-child relationships, and "talkativeness" of key members in a family setting, from other presumably nonlinguistic aspects and influences on a child's language development. Cazden (1972, pp. 130–136) reviews some of the pertinent literature on environmental influences on early child language development. She summarizes the indirect effects as follows (p. 130):

> Non linguistic aspects of the child's environment can be influential in at least three ways: differences in who speaks to the child, differences in the characteristics of the context or situation in which the conversation takes place, and differences in attitudes of the speaker toward language and toward the child.

Cazden cites investigations that indicate that families differ in the amount of talking directed to the young child compared with speech between parents or directed to older siblings. Mothers usually do considerably more talking to a young child than do fathers. Cazden also observes (pp. 105–107) that talking directed to infants, whether by parents or older siblings, tends to be more simplified in syntactic structure than adult-to-adult talking. Thus, the young child may have fewer and less complicated constructions to decode.

Our inclination is to emphasize the importance of the home and the relationship of members of the family within the home as the most important factors for language acquisition in the early stages. Children's potentialities for language development, from onset until the time they begin to spend more of their working hours away from home than at home, are nurtured by key members of the family. The key members may be older siblings or grandparents. Usually, parents are the key members, and mothers the dominant ones and the most significant influences on the child's language development. If we consider an individual child, born without physical or sensory disability or any primary emotional handicap, the following assumptions are positive for normal onset and development of language.

1. The mother has normal maternal drives and enjoys and wishes to interact with the child. Similarly, the father has a normal paternal drive and parallel wishes.
2. The parents enjoy talking to the child, even if in the prelinguistic stage of language acquisition they may be talking *at* the child. In any event, when the child indicates readiness, the parents will provide opportunity for interaction, whether it be for sound play in re-

sponding to early verbal demands, or later by answering questions with relevant answers, or extending a child's remarks without overelaborated explanations.

3. These assumptions imply an underlying one that the child will have an older speaker or speakers with whom to identify and whose speech, in time, will be decodable.

4. The home is not so noisy, with either human or electronic noise (radio and television included), that the child cannot hear and attend to the parent or other key family members.

Given a home where these assumptions prevail, the great likelihood is that the child will start speaking by 15 months of age. If these assumptions do not prevail, development of language, both qualitatively and quantitatively, may be delayed. We believe that unless the child's environment is grossly abnormal, initial onset and acquisition of speaking is less likely to be delayed than is the child's subsequent language development. Parents who have little or no time to talk to their infants, and who provide no surrogate for language stimulation, cannot expect normal language development from their children. We have interviewed fathers who admitted that they had no real interest in their infant children until their little ones began to talk. Fortunately, most mothers do not share this attitude. Fortunately, also, this attitude on the parts of fathers is becoming rare.

Bilingualism

A bilingual child is one who is exposed to *two different language systems* before either has become firmly established. Bilingualism should not be confused with bidialectism, which refers to exposure to two dialects of the same language. This may be any two regional dialects of Americn English or Black English and another dialect of American English. It may also mean any two dialects of British English as well as a dialect of British (regardless of geographic area) and American English.

Some bilingual children are exposed to and acquire two languages simultaneously. These children are brought up in homes where two languages are spoken, or are brought up in an environment where one language is spoken in the home and another is spoken outside of the home. Other bilingual children are exposed to and learn one language, presumably in the home, and then a second language, either in the home or at an early (preschool or primary school) age outside of the home.

What are the effects of bilingualism, either simultaneous or sequential, on language development? Unfortunately, our information is relatively sparse. Many reports on bilingual children are biographical and deal with exceptional homes and so, presumably, potentially exceptional children. On the other hand, some reports lack objectivity because they are generated to prove, rather than to find out, what factors, other than sociopolitical ones, are related to the acquisition and development of language in children who are brought up in bilingual environments. Many questions and issues involved in bilingualism are objectively reviewed by Cazden (1972, pp. 175–181), who says in her closing statement: "In the United States . . . through its influences on children, teachers, and parents—bilingual education can affect both speech behavior and attitudes toward language. . . ."

Early studies, such as Smith's (1949), indicated that bilingual children had below-age expectancy vocabularies in English. The children studied were of Chinese ancestry and lived in Hawaii. Smith also observed that for only two-fifths of the 30 Hawaiian children in the study did the combined vocabularies of words they knew in Chinese and in English exceed the age norms. When words of the same meaning in both languages were subtracted from the combined Chinese and English vocabulary, only one-sixth of the children exceeded the norm.

Smith's study, which we will refer to again, is an "older" one, and her findings may have been influenced by social factors as well as by educational opportunity. For much of the Western world, English is a second if not a first language. We have no evidence to indicate that children in Switzerland or in India or in Israel who learn English as a second language (usually but not invariably sequentially) suffer from any ill effects on their first language.

Our position is that the vast majority of children can learn two languages through either simultaneous or sequential exposure, and that such children are likely to be the richer, linguistically and culturally, for this achievement. On the other hand, if a child is slow in language acquisition and reveals confusion as a result of bilingual exposure, the family should make a choice as to which language the child is to be exposed to and hear—which language is to be directly addressed to the child. If even overhearing a second language produces delay or confusion, then as far as possible a child should hear only one language.

Most Americans, unfortunately, are so accustomed to a monolingual environment that they tend not to know the extent of bilingualism around the world. Much of the Southwestern part of the United States is bilingual, as is much of Eastern Canada. Pertinent issues of bilingualism are considered by Macnamara (1967) and by Ervin-Tripp (1973). See also our references in Chapter 9 on "Delayed or Retarded

Language Acquisition and Development" and our discussion of bilingualism in Chapter 3.

Social Class (Socioeconomic Level and Social Linguistic Status)

What can we project and predict about language development in relationship to the social class and socioeconomic status of the family? On an individual basis for a family, or even for a given child, expectations should be made with caution and reservation. Especially in a mobile and rapidly changing society, social status is not necessarily linked to economic status, to intellectual potential, or to educational achievement. Nevertheless, there are overall correlations that tend to hold for total subpopulations, which we consider with full awareness of the numerous exceptions.

Templin (1957, p. 147) concluded that children from families in upper socioeconomic levels tend to be more advanced in language development than children from lower socioeconomic families. Templin observed that there are consistent differences in language measures such as articulatory proficiency, phonemic discrimination, word recognition, mean length of utterance, and complexity of syntactical constructions. Insofar as socioeconomic status is positively correlated with factors such as intellectual level of parents, educational level, cultural opportunities, and parental attention, as well as attitude to language usage for the young child, the expectations projected by Templin are likely to hold. However, there are economically poor homes that are rich in culture, love, and understanding of children, as well as wealthy homes that are impoverished in factors that nourish children intellectually, emotionally, and linguistically.

Bernstein (1961) has attracted considerable attention by his observations and generalizations in regard to the differences between the "quality" of language used by working-class parents in lower socioeconomic levels compared with middle- and upper-socioeconomic classes. Bernstein uses the terms *restricted* and *elaborated codes* to indicate the differences between the lower and middle and upper classes in regard to language usage. In effect, if we were to take Bernstein literally and accept his generalizations more seriously than he probably intended, we would conclude that persons of lower economic classes use language as emotional expression rather than for the communication of ideas. Their language, as constructed in terms of vocabulary and syntax, is essentially noninformative. In contrast, persons in the middle and upper economic class are more likely to use language that is informative, more detailed, and at the same time more abstract. For critical comments on this position see Cazden (1972, pp. 132–134) and Labov (1972, pp. 204–240).[8]

Our position is to view both what Bernstein states and his critics' evaluations with considerable reservation. We consider any sweeping generalization as both unscientific and dangerous. On the other hand, we believe that some of the critics, including Labov, protest too strongly and go beyond the intentions of persons they criticize. What is important to the child, what matters in regard to language acquisition and development, is the nature of the particular environment in which the child is reared. Sociopolitics sometimes gets out of hand and influences the interpretation of the findings of sociolinguistics. To deny that some children from one kind of environment may need more help than children from another kind of environment is to deny these children their opportunity for social, intellectual, and educational achievement. On the other hand, to assume that any socioeconomic status is invariably associated with any specific factors is to be perceptually defensive and too busy with prejudices to attend to specific facts and their implications. A true concern for the child should help to put matters in proper perspective in the interest of the child, even where dialects and cultural groups are at issue.

Muma (1978, pp. 123–140) reviews the sociolinguistic issues relative to bidialectism with particular reference to Black English as a nonstandard dialect. Muma warns against confusing differences with deficits. His review, we believe, reflects a true concern for the child. In closing his discussion Muma (p. 140) reminds the language clinician that

> They should realize that communication is not just an active speaker talking to a passive listener, nor an encoder producing a series of linguistic codes, but a complex dynamic matrix of various kinds of codes. Realization of these kinds should convince clinicians that assessment and intervention endeavors should be derived primarily from actual communicative events.

Stimulation to Speak

So strong is the human desire to speak, to express the unique capacity to learn to understand and to produce a complex linguistic code, that only the most severe deprivation will prevent some degree of linguis-

---

[8] Labov, in *Language in the Inner City* (Philadelphia: University of Pennsylvania Press, 1972), takes strong exception to Bernstein's position as well as to the teaching programs that accept the position that lower-class children have poor language and need to be taught Standard English in place of their non-Standard dialects. Labov is particularly concerned with black children and their use of Black English.

tic acquisition. On the other hand, positive stimulation, if not ill-timed and overwhelming, enhances a child's potentials as a speaker and listener. In Chapter 8 on "Stimulating Language Development" we will consider some positive stimulating factors and approaches, particularly in regard to what can be done for children in the primary school grades.

LANGUAGE ASSESSMENT

The Limitations of Formal Assessment

We wish it were possible to observe the principles enunciated by the psychologist Bronfenbrenner (1977), that clinical assessment should be concerned with *an individual* as he or she functions in natural contexts, and that the testing procedures should deal with systems and procedures directly relevant to natural behavior. Philosophically, we agree with Muma (1978, p. 211) that "There are no definitive tests in the behavioral sciences because behavior is relative, conditional, complex, and dynamic. Assessment should deal with the patterns of behavior of an *individual* in various cognitive-linguistic-communicative systems." We also agree with Muma that "At best, assessment is probabilistic." So, we strongly recommend Muma's chapter on "Assessment Principles" in his *Language Handbook* (1978) for his philosophy as well as for alternative procedures to the usual approaches to evaluating a child's ability and potential for language behavior.

However, and we say "however" with reluctance, laws and school regulations often mandate assessment by published instruments that usually have standardized procedures and scoring systems. Accordingly, we will review several of the more widely used tests and procedures to acquaint the reader with a token selection of instruments. We will include comments as to the special features, strengths and weaknesses of the tests. But first we will suggest several guiding principles for both assessment and interpretation of results.

Guidelines for Assessment
1. Whenever an assessment is undertaken it is essential that the child first be given a "dry-run" session to get acquainted with the assessor and, if possible, the instruments and procedures to be used.
2. To whatever degree possible, assessment should be considered and made a communicative situation but not an adversary encounter.
3. For all procedures it is essential that the clinician-assessor observe

and note how a result was obtained as well as what was obtained. Evaluations, even if they cannot be translated into scores, should take account of Piaget's principle that there are no wrong or incorrect responses; there are only the *different* responses that a given child in a given situation provides for evaluation.

4. No assessment procedure should be undertaken without clear evidence that the child has no *sensory* or *motor* limitation that would to any degree interfere with optimum performance.
5. The physical environment of the assessment should be free of interfering sights or sounds, and yet not be "cold" or "sterile."
6. All assessment results at best indicate what the child did at a given time and under a given set of circumstances; all test results for whatever reason are tentative. If the clinician feels that the child was not at his/her best, or the conditions were not what they should have been, additional assessment at a different time is in order.
7. Our field and our profession is not suffering from a lack of tests and procedures. If anything, there are too many. Many of the instruments should be regarded as "first order attempts" to respond to a need and have found willing publishers before the tests themselves have had sufficient field testing to meet criteria for validity and reliability.

Testing Auditory Discrimination and Perception

A test of auditory discrimination and assessment for spoken language should incorporate items that call for discriminative responses to oral linguistic events presented in varying quantities and at varying rates, including those for normal utterance. As of this writing we do not believe that there is such a published instrument. We do have respectable attempts in this direction. Among the most frequently used are the Goldman-Fristoe-Woodcock Test of Auditory Discrimination— (TAD)— and the Wepman Auditory Discrimination Test—(ADT).

THE GOLDMAN-FRISTOE-WOODCOCK TEST OF AUDITORY DISCRIMINATION. (Goldman, Fristoe, and Woodcock; Circle Pines, Minn: American Guidance Service, 1970) was designed to assess speech sound discrimination under quiet (favorable) conditions and under controlled noise (unfavorable) condition. The TAD is intended for subjects from 3 years 8 months to "older" adults.

Test results produce scores that may be converted into percentile ratings or standard scores provided by the Test Manual.

Vetter (in Darley, 1979) notes that if the TAD "is used as a test of an individual subject's auditory discrimination ability, interpretation should be made with caution." Vetter indicates the need for more test data to permit further evaluation of the TAD.

The Goldman-Fristoe-Woodcock team also have published tests for *Selective Attention* and *Auditory Memory* and a *Sound-Symbol Test*. For critical evaluations see Darley (1979, pp. 148–161).

THE WEPMAN AUDITORY DISCRIMINATION TEST—(ADT). (Wepman, J., Palm Springs, Calif.: Language Associates, 1973) is included in Wepman's battery for assessing perceptual behavior. The ADT, one of the most widely used instruments in our field, consists of 40 single-syllable word pairs, 10 identical, e.g., *ball-ball*, and 30 which differ by a single phoneme, e.g., *bum-bun*. Subjects indicate whether a presented pair is the *same* or *different*. The ADT has two equated forms to permit retesting, either to check for progress or if the initial test results are considered not indicative of the subject's ability for the test.

The ADT has been used extensively for children who have problems in language acquisition, articulation, and/or reading. For a critical evaluation of the ADT see Locke in Darley (1979, pp. 124–127).

Cognitive Assessment

We believe that Piaget's approach to assessing cognitive abilities, if not taken too literally and with due awareness that all stages are approximate, is probably a better indicator of a child's potential for language than most published "standardized" instruments. Nevertheless, there are some tests that have been in wide use and deserve the respect they receive.

Our token selection will be limited to those instruments that are intended primarily for young children and assess cognitive potential for language acquisition.

THE BOEHM TEST OF BASIC CONCEPTS—(BTBC). (A. E. Boehm, New York: Psychological Corporation, 1971) This test is designed for children in the early grades who are underachievers. The test assesses the child's mastery of concepts that are commonly found in preschool and primary grade instructional materials, which are essential to understanding and responding to instruction in the early grades. The concepts belong in four categories: spatial, quantitative, time, and miscellaneous. For example, the concepts in Book I are *top*, *three*, *away from*, *next to*, *inside*, *some*, *not many*, *middle*, *few*, *farthest*, *around*, *over*, *widest*, *most*, *between*, *whole*, *nearest*, *second*, *corner*, *several*, *behind*, *row*, *different*, *after*, *almost*, and *half*.

The BTBC is a screening device for cognitive functioning that is intended to help a teacher to determine where a given child is cognitively and what needs to be taught to bring the child up to age-grade level. Norms are provided in percents and percentiles for grades and socioeconomic levels.

The BTBC is better suited for children with mild to moderate delay in language than for those with severe language impairment.

THE ILLINOIS TEST OF PSYCHOLINGUISTIC ABILITIES—ITPA. (Kirk, McCarthy, and Kirk, rev. ed. Urbana: University of Illinois Press, 1968)

The ITPA, despite recent negative criticism, continues to be a widely used instrument that presumably assesses three different dimensions of cognitive abilities. The ITPA represents an attempt to arrive at separate measurements through auditory-vocal, auditory-motor, visual-motor, and visual-vocal modalities (circuits). The assessment profile is intended to provide guidelines for determining individual remedial programs.

The ITPA manual includes norms for children two and a half to ten years of age. However, the authors acknowledge that the greatest usefulness of the Test is for children in the four-to-eight-year range.

In answer to recent criticism, Kirk and Kirk (1978) emphasize that the ITPA was developed to be a clinical indicator to help in determining differential abilities and disabilities among perceptual, memory, and cognitive functioning in young children. The authors caution that "One of its greatest abuses is to consider it a solution to all problems and to use scores as a final diagnosis instead of another possible aid to clinical judgment."

We wish this caution had been publicized at the time the ITPA was first published.

More Generalized Tests

We shall briefly note but not review other tests and test batteries that are considered to be well standardized and are used by psychologists rather than language clinicians to assess intellectual potential. Such tests include:

THE STANFORD-BINET INTELLIGENCE SCALE, FORM L-M. (Terman, L. M. and Merrill, M. A., Boston: Houghton-Mifflin Company, 1960) This is a revised edition of a well standardized test that assesses intelligence with verbal and nonverbal items.

THE MERRILL-PALMER SCALE—MPS. (Stutsman, Chicago: Stoelting, 1948) Assesses children in the age range two to five years.

Most of the items can be administered by pantomime. The MPS is not suitable for any child who has manual-motor impairment.

THE WECHSLER SCALES. (New York: Psychological Corporation) Wechsler has a series of scales that are structured to include verbal and performance items in separate subscales. For school-age children the Wechsler tests included the *Wechsler Preschool* and *Primary Scale of Intelligence* (WPPSI) for the age range four to six and a half years and the *Wechsler Intelligence Scale for Children*, Revised as WISC-R (1974). The Performance items of the WISC-R were standardized for deaf children (Anderson and Sisco, as *A Standardization of WISC Performance Scale for Deaf*, Gallaudet College, Washington, D.C., 1977).

Nonverbal Tests

Nonverbal Tests may be administered through the use of pantomime or by demonstration. Such tests include:

*   *The Porteus Maze* (Porteus, New York: Psychological Corporation, 1965) for children in age range 3 to 12 years.
*   *The Raven Coloured Matrices* (Raven, London: Lewis, 1962)
*   *The Leiter International Performance Scale*—LIPS (Leiter, Washington, D.C.: Psychological Service Center, 1948) Our experience with the LIPS suggests that it is a more useful instrument for assessing cognitive potential of non-verbal or linguistically moderately impaired children above five or six years of age rather than those who are below age 5.
*   *The Columbia Mental Maturity Scale*—CMMS, 3rd ed. Burgmeister, Blum, and Lorge; New York: Psychological Corp., 1972) This scale is intended for children in the age range three and a half to ten years. The test may be administered through pantomime. We consider the CMMS to be one of the better instruments for assessing the intellectual potential of preschool children.

Receptive Language Tests for Assessing Intellectual Potential

Tests in this category are frequently administered by language clinicians as well as clinical psychologists. Basically, these tests require the child to point to a picture (one of several on a card) that is appropirate for the test word—e.g., "Show me the———." Among the widely used tests are:

THE FULL-RANGE PICTURE VOCABULARY TEST. (Ammons and Ammons; Missoula, Montana: Psychological Test Specialists, 1958)

The line drawings and some of the key words are not as representative as we would like them to be for a contemporary population of children.

THE PEABODY PICTURE VOCABULARY TEST—PPVT-R. (Dunn and Dunn; Circle Pines, Minn: American Guidance Service, 1981) The PPVT-R, a revision of the widely used Peabody Picture Vocabulary Test, is intended for persons in the age range two and a half years to adult. Two forms (L and M) are available.

We, as well as the Dunns, consider the PPVT-R a guide to where more extensive assessment should be undertaken.

Language Tests and Scales

THE PRESCHOOL LANGUAGE SCALE—PLS. (Zimmerman, Steiner, and Evatt; Columbus, Ohio: Charles E. Merrill, 1969) assesses both receptive and productive verbal ability of children in the age range one year five months to seven years. In effect, the PLS is two separate scales. One, the receptive, requires pointing; the other, the productive, requires the child to identify (label) something or to respond to an instruction verbally.

ASSESSMENT OF CHILDREN'S LANGUAGE COMPREHENSION— ACLC, REV. ED. (Foster, Giddan, and Stark; Palo Alto, Calif.: Consulting Psychologists Press, 1973) The ACLC is intended to assess children's comprehension of syntactic units. The age range for the test is three through seven years.

The ACLC employs a vocabulary of 50 common words to arrive at a measurement of a child's receptive vocabulary, the number of *critical* elements (informative words) a child can process, and the pattern in the breakdown (failures) of critical sequences.

The present (1973) edition of the ACLC provides norms based on the responses of 365 children in the 3.0–6.5 year age range.

NORTHWESTERN SYNTAX SCREENING TEST—NSST. (Lee; Evanston, Ill.: Northwestern University, 1969) The NSST is a quick screening instrument for the child who may be so delayed in syntactic acquisition as to warrant further study. The NSST assesses the child for both receptive and productive syntactic constructions.

The NSST presumes that a child has been primarily exposed to Standard American English. It is, as the name implies, a screening instrument.

TEST FOR AUDITORY COMPREHENSION OF LANGUAGE—TACL. (Carrow; Boston: Teaching Resources Corporation, 1973) The TACL is intended to assess children in the age range three through six years for auditory comprehension of vocabulary and linguistic constructions. The TACL, including a brief form, has both English and Spanish versions.

The manual for the TACL provides norms based on populations of children from a middle-class socioeconomic background.

CARROW ELICITED LANGUAGE INVENTORY—CELI.   (Carrow; Boston: Teaching Resources Corporation, 1974) The CELI, like other elicited imitation tests, is based on the assumption that a child's imitative production of a presented linguistic structure reveals a child's proficiency in language. The CELI is intended to assess the grammatical (syntactic) productions of children in the age range three through eight years.

The CELI takes from 20 to 30 minutes to administer and about twice as long to score. It does yield useful information about a child's understanding and use of grammatical constructions.

Language Sampling —(L.S.)

Language Sampling is a relatively new approach to assessing a child's proficiency for language. Ideally, the sample of language should be of a child's spontaneous production recorded without the subject's awareness. Practically, the usual procedure is to elicit responses from the subject-child through conversation, pictures, toys, or play activities.

An L.S. is supposed to provide a clinician with information about the language a child uses and so, presumably knows, of language. There is no present consensus on the optimum size an L.S. should be to be considered adequate and representative of a child's language production. However, for practical purposes, the usual samples range from 50 to 100 utterances. The usual procedure is to record the child as inconspicuously as possible.

To adjust for the possibility, perhaps probability, that the absence of a linguistic structure may sometimes be a product of circumstances rather than of a child's limited knowledge, an elicited imitation procedure such as Carrow's CELI may be used as a supplement.

Earlier we have made reference to the Tyack and Gottsleben (1977) *Language Sampling* procedure and to the Bloom and Lahey (1978) approach.

Language Sampling is likely to be more time-consuming than most formal testing. Learning how to take and analyze a language sample requires a greater investment in time than learning to administer most published tests. However, we consider it an excellent investment in time and effort because Language Sampling yields considerably more information about a young child's language proficiencies, articulation, and phonological systems, included, than do separate formal assessments.

Problems[9]

1. What is meant by the statement: "Speech is a human species-specific function?" Do you agree with this statement? How close do the chimpanzees come to language usage? Do the "talking" chimpanzees meet the criteria? Compared with a normal child, at what level are chimpanzees "talking?"
2. What are the criteria for true speech?
3. Record the free speech of a boy and a girl at each of the following age levels: two, four, and six years. Note the differences in articulatory proficiency, vocabulary, and sentence length. Are there any consistent differences between the sexes? Are there differences in syntactic complexity?
4. Make the same observations as in No. 3 for a child whom you consider bright and for one you consider to be of average intelligence.
5. Listen to children in the kindergarten and to children in the third grade. What language factors distinguish the two groups?
6. Ask a three-, a four-, and a five-year-old child to repeat the sentence: "Tomorrow Mommy, Daddy, and I will go on a picnic, if it doesn't rain." Note the difference in their elicited imitations.
7. Read and report on two of the references from the list of references and suggested readings that follows.
8. Find a provocative picture in a magazine (one that is likely to induce a story). Ask a five-year-old and an eight-year-old to make up a story based on the picture. Note the differences in use of vocabulary, length, and complexity of each sentence, and in the total length of the story.
9. What are the issues involved in bilingual education? What is your position? Does it agree with Labov's?
10. Define bidialectism. Give three or four examples of differences in dialects for names of things. Give examples of three differences in syntactic forms for plurals, tense endings, progressive verbs in Black English, and a standard regional dialect of American English. What is your regional dialect?

References and Suggested Readings

Bernstein, B., "Social Structure, Language and Learning." *Educational Research,* **3** (1961), 163–176. (This article has produced considerable controversy on the nature and differences between members of social classes and their use of language.)

[9] Note: Source information for many of the problems and topics may be found in the list of References and Suggested Readings.

Bloom, L., *Language Development: Form and Function in Emerging Grammars.* Cambridge: The M.I.T. Press, 1970. (A report on the acquisition of grammar by three children beginning at about 19 months of age. Interpretations of cognitive functioning are included.)

Bloom, L., and M. Lahey, *Language Development and Language Disorders.* New York: John Wiley & Sons, Inc., 1978.

Boehm, A. E., *Boehm Test of Basic Concepts.* New York: Psychological Corporation, 1971.

Bornstein, H., "Signed English." *Journal of Speech and Hearing Disorders,* **39** (1974), 330–343.

Braine, M. D. S., "The Ontonegeny of English Phrase Structure." *Language,* **39** (1963), 1–13.

Bronfenbrenner, U., "Toward an Experimental Ecology of Human Development." *American Psychologist,* **32** (1977), 513–531.

Brown, R., *A First Language: The Early Stages.* Cambridge: Harvard University Press, 1973.

———, "The Development of *Wh* questions in Child Speech." *Journal of Verbal Learning and Verbal Behavior,* **7** (1968), 279–290.

———, and U. Bellugi, "Three Processes in the Child's Acquisition of Syntax." *Harvard Educational Review,* **34,** 2 (Spring 1964), 133–151. (An exposition of a study of two children, "Adam" and "Eve," who were selected because they were both very talkative and very intelligible.)

Cazden, C. B., *Child Language and Education.* New York: Holt, Rinehart and Winston, Inc., 1972. (Basically deals with early language acquisition. However, Cazden also includes discussion of dialects and the role of language in cognition. A readable book for nonspecialists.)

Carroll, J. B., "Words, Meanings, and Concepts." *Harvard Educational Review,* **34,** 2 (Spring 1964), 178–202. (An exposition of how word meanings and concepts can be taught effectively by classroom teachers.)

Clark, H. H., and E. V. Clark, *Psychology and Language.* New York: Harcourt Brace Jovanovich, 1977.

Chomsky, C., *The Acquisition of Syntax in Children from Five to Ten.* Cambridge: The M.I.T. Press, 1969. (Describes the author's investigation of the acquisition of syntactic structures in children between five to ten years of age. Her findings indicate that the grammar of a five-year-old differs in a number of ways from adult grammar "and that the gradual disappearance of these discrepancies can be traced as children exhibit increased knowledge over the next four or five years of their development.")

Curtis, J. F., Ed., *Processes and Disorders of Human Communication,* New York: Harper & Row, Publishers, 1978.

Dale, P. S., *Language Development: Structure and Function.* New York: Holt, Rinehart and Winston, 1972. (Discusses language acquisition and evaluates language training approaches.)

Darley, F. L., Ed. *Evaluation of Appraisal Techniques in Speech and Language Pathology.* Reading, Mass.: Addison-Wesley Publishing Co., 1979. (Critical evaluations of published assessment procedures and tests in the fields of language, speech, and hearing.)

Davis, E. A., *The Development of Linguistic Skills in Twins, Singletons with Siblings and Only Children from Ages Five to Ten Years.* Minneapolis: University of Minnesota Press, 1937. (A classic and basic study of the language development of single and multiple-birth children.)

DeVilliers, P. A. and S. G. DeVilliers, *Early Language.* Cambridge, Mass.: Harvard University Press, 1979.

Donaldson, M., *Children's Minds.* Glasgow, Scotland: Fontana-Collins, Ltd. 1978.

Dunn, L. M. and Dunn, L. M., *Peabody Picture Vocabulary Test (PPVT), Revised.* Circle Pines, Minnesota: American Guidance Service, 1981.

Eimas, P. D., E. R. Siqueland, P. Jusczyk, and J. Vigorito, "Speech Perception in Infants." *Science,* **171** (1971), 303–306.

Ervin-Tripp, S., *Language Acquisition and Communicative Choice.* Stanford, Calif.: Stanford University Press, 1973.

———, "Discourse Agreement: How Children Answer Questions." In J. R. Hayes, Ed., *Cognition and the Development of Language.* New York: John Wiley & Sons, Inc., 1970. (The *comprehension* of questions develops sequentially from *yes-no* to *what, where, what-do, whose, who, why, where-from, how,* and *when.*)

Fry, D. B., "The Development of the Phonological System in the Normal and Deaf Child." In F. M. Smith and G. A. Miller, *The Genesis of Language.* Cambridge: The M.I.T. Press, 1966.

Gardner, M. F. *Expressive One-Word Picture Vocabulary Test,* Novato, California: Academic Therapy Publications, 1979.

Ginsburg, H. and S. Opper, *Piaget's Theory of Intellectual Development.* Englewood Cliffs, N.J.: Prentice-Hall, 1979.

Goldfarb, W., "Effects of Psychological Deprivation in Infancy and Subsequent Stimulation." *American Journal of Psychiatry,* **12** (August 1954), 102–129.

Gustason, G., D. Pfetzing, and E. Zawolkow, SEE: *Signing Exact English.* Rossmoor, Calif.: Modern Press, 1972.

Halliday, M. A. K., *Explorations in the Functions of Language.* New York: American Elsevier, Inc., 1977.

———, *Learning How to Mean.* New York: American Elsevier, Inc., 1977.

Hardy, J. C., "Neurologically Based Problems" In Curtis, H. F. *Processes and Disorders of Human Communication.* New York: Harper & Row, Publishers, 1978.

Ingram, D., *Procedures for the Phonological Analysis of Children's Language.* Baltimore: University Park Press, 1981, Chap. 7.

———, "Phonological Rules in Young Children." *Journal of Child Language,* **1** (1974), 49–64.

———, and Jon Eisenson, in Jon Eisenson, *Aphasia in Children.* New York: Harper & Row, Publishers, Inc., 1972.

Irwin, O. C., "Speech Development in the Young Child." *Journal of Speech and Hearing Disorders,* **17,** 3 (1952), 269–279.

Jakobson, R., *Child Language, Aphasia and Phonological Universals.* The Hague: Mouton & Company, 1968.

Kimura, D., "Functional Asymmetry of the Brain in Dichotic Listening." *Cortex*, **3** (1967), 163–178. (Dichotic listening, an approach to indicate ear preference, is explained in its relationship to cerebral dominance and language functions.)

Kirk, S. A., and W. D. Kirk, "Uses and Abuses of the ITPA." *Journal of Speech and Hearing Disorders* **43** (1978), 58–75.

Labov, W., *Language in the Inner City*. Philadelphia: University of Pennsylvania Press, 1972.

Lee, L. L., *Developmental Sentence Analysis*. Evanston, Ill.: Northwestern University Press, 1974. (Describes procedures for assessing a child's language status based on a taped language sample.)

———, "Developmental Sentence Types: A Method for Comparing Normal and Deviant Syntactic Development." *Journal of Speech and Hearing Disorders*, **31**, 4 (1966), 311–330. (An approach to the assessment of levels of syntactic development based on comparisons between a normally developing child and one with language delay.)

Lenneberg, E. H., *Biological Foundations of Language*. New York: John Wiley & Sons, Inc., 1967.

———, "Language Disorders in Childhood." *Harvard Educational Review*, **24** (Spring 1964), 152–177. (Devoted to language and learning; highly recommended for teachers and language clinicians.)

Lewis, M. M., *How Children Learn to Speak*. New York: Basic Books, Inc., 1959. (An English author's observations about speech development.)

Locke, J. L., "The Inference of Speech Perception in the Phonologically Disordered Child." *Journal of Speech and Hearing Disorders*, **45** (1980), Part I, 431–444; Part II, 445–468.

Macnamara, J., Ed., "Problems of Bilingualism." *The Journal of Social Issues*. **23** (1967). (The entire issue is concerned with problems of bilingualism. It includes articles by authorities from a variety of disciplines, each dealing with an important aspect or question related to bilingualism.)

McCarthy, D., "Language Development in Children." In L. Carmichael, Ed., *Manual of Child Psychology*, rev. ed. New York: John Wiley & Sons, Inc., 1954, 492–630. (Deserves reading as a classic report.)

McNeill, D., *The Acquisition of Language*. New York: Harper & Row, Publishers, Inc., 1970. (A fast-moving, technical discussion of language acquisition by children.)

———, "The Development of Language." In P. H. Mussen, Ed., *Carmichael's Manual of Child Psychology*, 3rd ed. New York: John Wiley & Sons, Inc., 1970, 1061–1161. (A survey of recent literature on language acquisition emphasizing the relationships among language development, intellect, and maturation in the child.)

Menyuk, P., *Sentences Children Use*. Cambridge, Massachusetts: M.I.T. Research Monograph Series, 1969.

Morehead, D. and D. Ingram, "The Development of Base Syntax in Normal and Linguistically Deviant Children." *Journal of Speech and Hearing Research*, **16** (1973), 330–352.

Muma, J. R., *Language Handbook: Concepts, Assessment, Intervention.* Englewood Cliffs, N.J.: Prentice-Hall, Inc., 1978.

Piaget, J., and B. Inhelder, *The Psychology of the Child.* New York: Basic Books, Inc., 1969. (Chap. 3 of this book is devoted to an exposition of the development/evolution/of language and thought in the child.)

Prather, E. M., D. L. Hedrick, and A. Kern, "Articulation Development in Children Aged Two to Four Years." *Journal of Speech and Hearing Disorders,* **40** (1975), 179–191.

Sander, E. K., "When Are Speech Sounds Learned?" *Journal of Speech and Hearing Disorders,* **37** (1972), 55–63.

Silverman, F. H., *Communication for the Speechless.* Englewood Cliffs, N.J.: Prentice-Hall, Inc., 1980. (Presents modes of communication that do not employ vocal and oral modalities for output. Several sign systems, not necessarily limited to use by the deaf, are described and evaluated.)

Slobin, D., Ed., *A Field Manual for Cross-Culture Study of the Acquisition of Communicative Competence.* Berkely, Calif.: University of California Press, 1967.

Smith, M. E., "Measurement of the Vocabularies of Young Bilingual Children in Both of the Languages Used." *Journal of Genetic Psychology,* **34** (1949), 305–310.

Templin, M. C., "The Study of Articulation and Language Development During the Early School Years." In F. M. Smith, and G. A. Miller, *The Genesis of Language,* Cambridge: The M.I.T. Press, 1966.

——, *Certain Language Skills in Children: Their Development and Interrelationships,* Minneapolis: University of Minnesota Press, 1957.

Tyack, D., and R. Gottsleben, *Language Sampling; Analysis and Training: A Handbook for Teachers and Clinicians.* Palo Alto, Calif.: Consulting Psychologists Press, 1974.

Van Riper, C., *Speech Correction,* 6th ed. Englewood Cliffs, N.J.: Prentice-Hall, Inc., 1978.

Weiss, C. E., and H. E. Lillywhite, *Communicative Disorders,* 2nd ed. St. Louis: The C. V. Mosby Company, 1981.

Winitz, H., *Articulatory Acquisition and Behavior.* New York: Appleton-Century-Crofts, 1969, chap. 1. (An excellent review of the research literature on prelingual stages of language development and theories about the onset of speech.)

——, "Sex Differences in Language of Kindergarten Children." *ASHA,* **1** (1959), 86.

Yasuko, N. and K. Owada, "Echoic Utterances of Children Between the Ages of One and Three." *Journal of Learning and Verbal Behavior,* **12** (1973), 658–665.

Zimmerman, I. L., V. G. Steiner, and R. L. Evatt, *Preschool Language Scale.* Columbus, Ohio, Charles E. Merrill, 1969.

8

Stimulating Language Development

As noted in Chapter 7, most children learn to speak well and quickly. Their competence and performance in all aspects of language—phonological, semantic, morphemic, syntactic and pragmatic are usually so readily apparent that we take them for granted. The following soliloquy by a kindergartner illustrates performance in language: After considerable, obvious deliberation, she called a Siamese cat a puppy cat. When asked why it was a puppy cat, she responded with: "He's small like a cat . . .He's on a leash like a dog. . . . Walks like a dog. . . . Looks half cat, half dog. . . . Sounds like a baby." With decided satisfaction and with assurance, she announced, "That's why he's a puppy cat."

For a five-year-old, this child's monologue displayed considerable facility with language. Her phonological system virtually equaled that of an adult with no observable substitutions or deletions of sounds. Although her sentences were mostly simple ones, she did use one with a dependent clause. Her vocabulary was adequate for her explanation. For her age, she displayed an unusual degree of language sophistication through her deductive powers. In her monologue, she used each remark, based on an analogy, as a cue for further extension and expansion of ideas. In this process, she presented a series of concepts. Finally, she arrived at her generalization, "That's why he's a puppy cat."

The next conversation is that of a three-and-one-half-year-old city boy. When *The Big City Book* by A. Ingle (New York: Platt & Munk, 1975) was shown to the child, Joey said, "I wanta read the book. You read the book." Whereupon the book was opened to its fly page, which includes pictures of a taxi, City Hall, a police car, a bus, and a grocery store—all items found in a large city. The adult said, "Joey, tell me about it." The boy enumerated items on the page including a policeman. As there was no policeman in the picture, the adult remarked, "I don't see a policeman." Joey said, "He's inside the car." Then he turned to pages 10 and 11 with buildings and a helicopter. Joey pointed to the helicopter and said *helicopter* very clearly. He responded to "Tell me about it" with "It opens." When this remark was followed by the adult's "Yes?", he added, "It makes a noise. . . . It flies." He turned to another page and named the animals such as giraffe [dræf], crocodile, duck, and hippopotamus [hɪpʰɑməˌmɪs]. Then he saw a car on top of a truck of melons and said, "The car is on the flowers." Then he noticed a pileup of cars on one side of the page and announced, "They got in an accident." When prodded with "Tell me about it," he responded with "They did." When he was prodded again with, "Why do you suppose there was an accident?", he responded again with, "They did." Joe's sound production is beginning to approximate that of an adult. Occasionally he uses /t/ and /d/ for /θ/ and [ð], consistently uses /t/ for /tʃ/ and /d/ for /dʒ/. He did particularly well in naming all of the objects and he spoke grammatically. When Joey was questioned about the policeman, he said that the policeman was in the police car. He used his own experience to call the melons *flowers,* but was accurate in placing the car on top of the flowers. He was not able to tell the "why" of the accident. Surely at this age, we cannot expect this explanation. This boy, too, is well on his way to using language with proficiency.

All children do not progress as rapidly in the receptive and expressive functions of language as these two children. Probably much of their learning has taken place in their homes with parents helping to motivate their language competence and production. Much of language learning takes place before the child enters school. The school's language arts programs are but extensions of the child's early language training with each individual child organizing his/her own language learning and advancing to another level when ready.

Both the teacher and the clinician are aware of differences in language abilities of children. The teacher makes an informal evaluation based on listening to the children's language. The teacher and clinician are equally interested in seeing that the development of language is at the level that is needed for academic achievement. When the level of a child's development appears to be decidedly below the level of his/her peers, the teacher suspects that the child is language delayed.

DEFINITION OF LANGUAGE DELAY

The simplest definition of language delay is a condition where the child's language development is significantly below his/her chronological age. Of course, children in the primary grades use new words in odd ways, skip from one subject to another, misuse pronouns, use the wrong tense—but even so they have a sound basic language competence. They just need more time to experiment with language in a variety of communicative situations. But children with delayed language do not have the abilities of their peers to use sounds, vocabulary, sentences, syntax, or pragmatics.

In other words, language-delayed children speak like much younger children, without the sentence-producing ability of their peers. They seem unable to use language purposefully. They lack concepts that their classmates have that are essential to classroom instruction. These children are not fluent, do not use language in an imaginative or original way, do not participate wholeheartedly in the discussion of problems. In some situations they may remain silent a large portion of the time, for they cannot meet the demands of communication in the classroom.

We are assuming that the delay is not caused by a hearing problem, mental retardation, emotional or behavioral problems, neurological impairment, peripheral oral motor deficits, or an oral-facial anomaly. The children's language use would be a year or more behind their chronological or mental age (as measured by tests described in an earlier chapter). The speech/language clinician makes an assessment of the delay after he/she has administered a language screening test or after the teacher's informal evaluation of the child's language.

The teacher may have collected a language sample from the child suspected of being language delayed. The teacher and the child look at pictures in a book together, talk about what they have seen, play with toys—conversing as they play, talking about what happens at home, or even playing a pretend game. No strong evidence exists as to what kind of situation brings forth the most useful language sample. For example, James and Button (1978) elicited samples in three clinical situations: (1) talk about toys from the clinic stack; (2) talk about toys brought from home, and (3) talk with no stimulus material. The use of the three samples showed no significant difference for the three groups in mean length of utterance, syntactic complexity, and the number of usable utterances in the first fifteen minutes of each situation. Individual variations did exist. Other factors such as the interests of the child, the child's intellectual ability, or the severity of the disorder may well play a role.

Volunteers or paraprofessionals often can give clues as to children's language development. The *New York Times* (March 25, 1981, page B-11) reports on a program in which 10,000 volunteers, mostly parents, help tutor New York City school children. In this article, one volunteer is quoted, "I have some kids in kindergarten who, if you point to their forehead, don't know what the word for *forehead* is." Many young children, of course, would not know the word *forehead*, but the volunteer goes on to say that these children are unaware of less sophisticated words for other parts of their bodies or for colors. Incidentally, some of these children may well have come from sterile, impoverished homes. Likely they have not had the language training, administered by parents, brothers, sisters, cousins, aunts, uncles, and neighbors, found in most homes.

Let us summarize some of the important observations cited earlier that are relevant to this chapter. First, language is used for a variety of purposes. The purposes are related to the conceptual, social, and physical contexts in which the talk occurs. Classroom talk usually revolves around the learning of academic content and acceptable social behavior.

We have indicated in the previous chapter that language grows out of a child's need or desire; this is true regardless of how we view competence and production of language. We have shown that the use of words gets people to do one's bidding or to satisfy one's needs physically and psychosocially. We explained that when the child says "up," he/she may be getting ready to be picked up—expecting this response from his/her adult mentor. Or when he/she utters "mama" with the proper intonation, he/she may mean, "I've had enough of you now." Through language, he/she successfully manipulates those around him/her.

Until recently we thought of language mainly in terms of its sets of systems: phonology, morphology, semantics, and syntax. The assumption was frequently made that learning to use language depended on the ability to manipulate these forms to make sentences. Today we believe that the intent resulting in the function of language is equally important—what the child is using language for and what he wants to accomplish through its usage. Bloom (1970) indicates that the form and function of language are intertwined.

Beyond the form and function of language, the kind of language used makes a difference in learning to mean. We have already discussed the use of varieties of pronunciations and syntax in Chapter 3 on "Intercultural and Intracultural Language Usage." A class or clinic group may contain students speaking many varieties of English, such as Standard English, English with a Spanish base (either Puerto Rican or Mexican), or Black English.

We have also stressed the importance of using the children's own experiences as a base for teaching language. These experiences include the cognitive concepts that they have come to possess. As indicated earlier, some concepts cannot be taught to first- and second-graders, for they are not yet ready to internalize some ideas.

Earlier, in Chapter 2, we pointed to the influence and importance of parents' communicative assets on children's ability to communicate. We noted, too, that parents are frequently very effective language stimulators and teachers for their children. Admittedly the parental influence does decline by the time the child enters school; then the child's peers, teachers, and other educational specialists take over.

PARENTS AS LANGUAGE TEACHERS

We should, therefore, like to call attention to principles of language training that obviously work for parents and other adult mentors in the early years of the child's life. The principles seem to us important whether they are inherent in a commercial program for language development or whether they are the language intervention programmed by the teacher or clinician.

The first principle followed by parents and other mentors is that there exists an inherent function of language in the communicative act: to entertain, to exchange objects, to comfort, to direct behavior, among many others. The communicative intent is uppermost in the minds of both the child and the mentor. Because the verbal interaction (intent and reaction) is what counts, the mentor rarely corrects a child's inappropriate form. A phrase like, "Wa baya" for I want the teddy bear is rewarded with the teddy bear. When the request is not clear or when the child's comments do not make sense, the mentor voices uncertainty. The child then attempts to change his/her language to clarify his/her intent.

As the child makes the intent clear and as the mentor responds appropriately (by providing the teddy bear, with relevant conversation, or with a smile), the child's particular communicative act is reinforced in a positive manner. Mentors tend to reinforce naturally. Further, they use modeling procedures. For example, as the child says, "The wed car aint no good" the mentor may respond with, "No, that red car isn't any good. What can we do?" The emphasis is not on semantic, syntactic, or phonological aspects but on content. This leads us then to the second principle.

Mentors do not attack phonemes one day, syntax another, semantic features another, and morphological aspects still another. Rather the child is bombarded with most of these systems at the same time; however, they are often simplified. One factor is obvious: mentors ask many questions of children. Admittedly some of the adult questions make little sense. A question such as, "Aren't you a pretty little girl?" does little to invite conversation. But others like, "Do you see that robin? What color is his breast? What did you do at play school today?" do make sense. The mentor noticeably uses quite short and simple sentences (see Snow, 1972). The language structure with its various aspects is the road that leads the way to communication and admittedly the road must be improved as the child matures. Mahoney (1975) indicates that in language development, the critical dimension of the set goal is precisely the social function of the human communication system, efficient communication. He goes on to note that the set goal is never a specific language structure, but that the linguistic structure is a way to achieve efficient communication within a variety of social environments.

Third, the communicative situation is one based on the child's experiences. It may involve toys, food, clothes, family. Or the child may be riding on a train, visiting his/her father's office, swinging on Grandma's porch, or being ridden around the block on his/her brother's bike. Talks needs experience as a base.

Fourth, effective interaction usually exists between the child and his parents or other adult mentors. The child hopefully is not "lectured to" or "talked at." Children carry their language learning to other situations. One five-year-old heard an adult use the word "ridiculous." Perhaps because she liked the sound and rhythm of the word, she wanted to know what it meant. After the adult explained its meaning through context, the child generalized and found her own synonym "silly." That night at the dinner table quite unobtrusively she used "ridiculous" appropriately. Probably she felt good about her use of the new word.

PRINCIPLES FOR LANGUAGE INTERVENTION

These observations on how parents and other adults motivate children to speak help to provide us with a set of principles that both teachers and clinicians could well follow in their language intervention sessions.

PRINCIPLE 1: INTERACTION. The clinicians or teachers interact with the child through language—often as individuals—so that they talk *with* the children and not *at* them. This interaction occurs within the framework of functions of language. The role of the adult is to listen, learn, question, be an active communicator in the group—in other words, to motivate communication involving its many aspects and functions. Unless language is functional, serving a useful purpose, unless the child feels the need to say something important, unless the intent of the message is appreciated by active listeners, language is occurring in a vacuum with no visible results.

The Bullock report (1975) suggests that the teacher in the intervention of language difficulties recognize the following uses of language:

> Reporting on present and recalled experiences.
> Projecting into the future; anticipating and predicting.
> Collaborating toward agreed ends.
> Projecting and comparing possible alternatives.
> Perceiving causal and dependent relationships.
> Giving explanations of how and why things happen.
> Expressing and recognizing tentativeness.
> Dealing with problems in the imagination and seeing possible solutions.
> Creating experiences through the use of imagination.
> Justifying behaviour.
> Reflecting on feelings, their own and other people's. (Bullock, 1975, p. 67.)

Both the clinician and the teacher should make sure that the language-delayed child has an opportunity for spontaneous speech. Clinicians seem to achieve their goals more successfully when they listen more and lead conversation less. On the basis of results of a study by Fey, Leonard and Wilcox (1981), this suggestion might well be carried further. They advise:

> It may be important to include as part of the therapy program some relatively unstructured periods during which the language-impaired children can interact freely with children of similar or lower ages and linguistic skills. Such interactions may serve two valuable purposes: By placing fewer constraints on conversational participation, they may assist the children in becoming more active communicators. Similarly, these less constraining situations may optimize the opportunities for language-impaired children to practice newly taught linguistic skills. (Fey, Leonard and Wilcox, 1981, p. 96)

The teacher also must make sure that the language-delayed children have opportunities for spontaneous speech. Sometimes classroom talk involves too many teacher's questions and commands. Verbal interaction that follows a child's play or conversation enhances language and cognitive development, for the child learns from his/her own language experience—particularly when the communication is given genuine feedback from the teacher and other children.

One teacher used as a base for talk *Ask Mr. Bear,*[1] the story of a boy trying to decide what to give his mother for her birthday. In the story, an egg, a pillow, cheese, a blanket are suggested. To each suggestion, Danny responds, "No, it isn't. . . ." The teacher then asked what Mr. Bear could suggest. All kinds of responses followed:

> Fur—it feels good.
> A big, big elephant. Protection against burglars.
> A bright, shiny kitchen clock.

This activity involves Searle's (1969) illocutionary act of posing a question where information is not readily available. The listeners to the question are providing possible bits of information. These children went on to Searle's act of "argue" wherein the speaker believes a proposition and wants his listeners to believe it. The children's responses included:

> "Fur's a good idea. All women like fur."
> "What protection could an elephant be against burglars? Need an alarm connected to the police station for that."
> "Costs a lot to feed an elephant."
> "Furs and elephants cost too much."

When the teacher suggested the answer in the book—"bear hug," almost all the children liked the idea although one child responded with, "Doesn't cost anything." Again the cognitive level was apparent: One child responded with, "Where'd you get a bear to hug? That's silly." He obviously did not know the connotation of the phrase *bear hug.* This remark leads us to the next principle.

PRINCIPLE 2: MATCHING LEARNING TO COGNITION. There should be a match between the concepts or learning experiences presented and the learner's cognitive readiness for these concepts and experiences. Parents tend to talk to their children about the here and now and about concrete experiences happening around them that the children readily understand. Both teachers and clinicians must be aware of the relationship between cognition and language comprehension. Saltz (1979) illustrates the need for this match with an examination of the use of proverbs and their meanings with children of different ages.

Saltz collected samples of typical responses of children at several different grade levels, using three proverbs, one of which was: *When the cat's away, the mice will play.* The children in kindergarten and grades two and three responded with completely literal concrete interpretations but in grades five and six the children began to respond

---

[1] Flack, M., *Ask Mr. Bear.* New York: Macmillan Publishing Co., Inc., 1932.

with interpretations not completely literal. Responding to "When the cat's away, the mice will play," a five-year-old said, "The people go looking after it;" a six-year-old, "When the cat goes, the mice stay;" a seven-year-old, "When the cat's away, the mice will get cheese and be happy;" a nine-year-old, "So, the mice won't get caught;" a ten-year-old, "The mice will play because the cat is not around to bother it"; but another ten-year-old said, "When parents are away, children will wreck the house." The younger children clearly were not cognitively ready to abstract a general meaning from the proverb. Even when the teacher attempted to teach the implicit meaning of proverbs to second-graders, she was not successful. Saltz (ibid.) concludes that children cannot be pushed in their use of understanding of language beyond their cognitive stage of development.

PRINCIPLE 3: REINFORCEMENTS. The child's contribution should be rewarded on the basis of its meaning. The reward is not offered because of correct phonology or syntax but because of the child's ability to get ideas across to listeners. For example, one clinician was working on language development with several children. She was using two puppets—a tall gangly man and a little boy. Said the clinician, "Where do you suppose they're going?" Answers varied: "home," "church," "a synagogue," "to the store to buy toys—that's his granpa." The children agreed on *to the store*. They then built a story based on the expedition to the store. The reinforcement came from the appreciation of each answer, from the actions of the puppets, from the interest inherent in the activity. These children were receiving feedback from the clinician and from their peers. Admittedly there were deletions such as "Daddy store," unusual use of language as "him walk; her ride." and "he wented fast" but these were immaterial to the success of this particular communicative act.

We emphasize that we believe in natural reinforcement, because automatically it rewards what happens in communicative situations. Tokens undoubtedly work simply and quickly but our question is, for how long? Muma (1978) suggests that extrinsic reinforcers may be little more than a numbers game for clinicians. The question is: Is the child who is reinforced by tokens for using a copulative verb appropriately, for combining two sentences into one, or for using *we* and *us* accurately, going to continue following the precepts that have been taught in another environment, at another time?

When, however, the training takes place within the bounds of accomplishing certain purposes of language, when the child feels success in the communicative act, the newly acquired form is, we believe, more likely to be permanent and to transfer to other situations—even to the playground. Bloom and Lahey (1978) note that merely a clinician's appropriate response to a child's utterance may be sufficient reinforcement.

Donaldson (1978, p. 115) says that there are dangers in the token awards: (1) Those who don't get stars may consider themselves failures, and (2) if the activity is rewarded by some extrinsic price token —something quite external to the activity itself—then the activity is less likely to be engaged in later in a free and voluntary manner when rewards are absent—and, too, less likely to be enjoyed.

We hope that some of the strategies we are about to describe will have reinforcement built into them. As we have watched children respond to activities with adults, such as listening to a story, reinforcement is obvious in terms of the pleasure of the activity, in the successes of children's responses, and in just plain "fun."

CAN LANGUAGE DEVELOPMENT BE STIMULATED?

Probably the two language development programs that are most frequently discussed are the "Sesame Street" television program and the Peabody Language Kit, both of which are linguistically based. Evidence points to the success of both of these programs.

Ball and Bogatz (1971) report on the success of "Sesame Street" with 943 subjects, many of whom have disadvantaged backgrounds. They reveal that:

1. Boys and girls who watched the programs showed greater gains than those who did not.
2. Watching time was positively correlated with learning.
3. Skills that were best learned were those that received the most time and attention on the program.
4. Regular watching by disadvantaged children produced gains superior to those of middle-class subjects who watched infrequently.
5. Greater gains were made by three-year-olds than by older children.
6. Children who watched the shows and then discussed them with their mothers showed the greatest gains.

Hamre (1972), noting the success of "Sesame Street," recommends that schools plan programs in language stimulation activities in a similar manner. He explains that "Sesame Street" provides a wealth of linguistic experiences some of which might be considered "controlled."

Milligan and Potter (1971) reviewed the studies of the Peabody Kit and concluded that it does accelerate growth in language development with both the advantaged and the disadvantaged. They also concluded that it appears to improve reading.

STRATEGIES FOR STIMULATING
LANGUAGE DEVELOPMENT

In planning strategies to stimulate language development, we believe that the principles we have just cited are important. We believe that language growth and meaningful experiences involving important concepts are intertwined. Young children, to be successful with language, should talk about persons, objects, and ideas with which they are familiar. The teacher or clinician then must take advantage of children's everyday experiences and, in addition, provide them with new, untried exciting ones. Bloom (1971) maintains that therapeutic language programs must give attention to content, for it appears that learning a linguistic code depends upon the child's learning to distinguish, understand, and express certain conceptual relations. Language learning can take place as a result of such experiential activities as trips, science experiments, creative drama, puppetry, and discussions.

In planning strategies for stimulating language development, we should like to stress the child's cognitive readiness for the concepts to be taught and the experiences containing these concepts. Just as there is a time for reading readiness, there is a time for readiness for certain language abilities. For example, Vasta and Lievert (1973) point to significant differences between first- and third-graders in the discrimination of unfamiliar syntactic constructions.

Similarly Lesser and Drouin (1975) found that they could not teach the two meanings of some "double function" terms such as *hard, soft, sweet,* and *sharp* to a group of first-, second-, and third-graders. The "double function" is represented by a *sweet pear* as opposed to a *sweet person.* They concluded that children cannot be pushed in their use of language much beyond their current cognitive level. They also found, however, that a teacher can move a child just a little beyond the original language understanding.

Evidence is accumulating that rarely if ever does a child have difficulty with only a single facet of language. The child who has difficulty with syntactic structures may well also have difficulty with phonology (see Menyuk and Looney 1972). Panagos (1974) points out that a phonological difficulty is often but one symptom of a more generalized language disorder, the cause of which may be tied to other deficits of cognitive and linguistic development. Some of the strategies that follow may appear to emphasize one facet of development more than others. Most of the strategies, however, are multifaceted.

Furthermore, while we are suggesting specific language activities, we should like to emphasize again that each activity should possess, if possible, an experiential base and that each activity should not be produced as an isolated exercise but as an integral, meaningful part of the school day's learning. For example, we might use the sentence: Ice cream tastes _____ than medicine. Children will not learn the concept of *better* from a repetition of this one sentence. When, however, they talk about: Smelling roses is better than _____; Petting a cat is better than petting a _____; Eating chocolate cake is better than eating _____, they are likely to acquire the meaning and concept of *better*. If, in addition, as they play the roles of two men, one good and one bad, the children talk about Jim's being *the better man* of the two, another dimension is added to the concept of *better*. With the reminders that meaning is important, that children must feel a need for an activity and find satisfaction in it, we list activities which can serve as examples of many others that stimulate language development.

Strategies for Stimulating Language Development in the Primary Grades

Understanding and Responding to Spoken Language

Some strategies for improving understanding and response to spoken language are:

1. Reading nursery rhymes and then answering questions about the content:

   Jack and Jill: Who went up the hill?
   What happened to Jack?
   What happened to Jill?

   Little Jack Horner: What was Jack eating?
   What did he say when he put his thumb in the pie?

2. Playing the game, "Simple Simon Says." For example, Simple Simon says, "Jump on one foot." If the leader omits *Simple Simon*, the children do nothing.

3. Following directions as given in a book:

   H. Rockwell, *I Did It* (New York: Macmillan Publishing Co., Inc., 1974). This book, intended for five- to seven-year-olds, gives simple directions that tell how to do such things as making a paper bag mask, a paper airplane, a secret message, or a mosaic picture.

4. Responding to: Could this happen? (Following an explanation such as: Some things can happen; some can't. "Can a little boy

really eat his desk?" "No." True—he might eat food on his desk but not the desk.)

> A little boy was eating his desk.
> He has fingers on his feet.
> She has a thumb on his foot.
> She has very dark hair.
> With his legs and feet, he can run.
> He puts food into his mouth.
> She drinks from a plate.
> She eats from a glass.
> He sometimes has bacon for breakfast.
> She sleeps in a bed.
> She sits on a chair.

5. Making changes of wording in some of the following sentences so that they make sense. (After an explanation such as: We have names for people who have particular jobs to do. For instance, what do we call the man who drives the school bus? What do we call the man who cleans up our classrooms?)

> The man who paints the house is a plumber.
> The man who fixes the electric lights is a carpenter.
> The man who drives the limousine for the rich lady is a chauffeur.
> The man who cooks the dinner is a cook.
> The lady who prescribes medicine for you is a doctor.
> The lady who goes to court to try cases is a policeman.
> The lady who plans the building of a bridge is an engineer.

6. Identifying objects inside the room from descriptions:

> I am thinking of something in this room. It is round; it is red. We can eat it. What is it?

7. Identifying objects outside the room from descriptions:

> I am thinking of something that goes high into the sky.
> The man in it gives us traffic reports in the morning.
> It can go from one airport to another. It can land on top of a building or in a field. What is it?

Categorization

Some strategies to improve the ability to categorize are:

1. Providing pictures of four green hats and one red hat. The children put those together that belong with each other.
2. Providing pictures of four hats and four caps. The children again sort these into the two proper categories.
3. A discussion after a visit to the supermarket. The first aisle we went

down had all the dairy products in it. What are some of the dairy products? The next aisle was the one with fresh fruit and vegetables. What did that have in it?

Remembering Language
Some strategies to stimulate and reinforce language memory are:

1. Using stories as a base:

> The teacher shows the pictures in such a book as A. Ingle, *The Big City Book* (New York: Platt & Munk, 1975). These pictures contain items that belong in schools, television stations, subways, parks, airports, and the like. The teacher enumerates the items, and the children talk about their functions. The children then recall the items in the various spots.

> The teacher reads *George and Martha: One Fine Day* by J. Marshall (Boston, Houghton Mifflin Company, 1978). George and Martha are two hippopottami; they take turns being nice to each other and then getting the best of each other. Martha walks a tightrope. Martha keeps George away from her diary. Martha improves George's table manners. George scares Martha. Martha turns the tables on George in an amusement park. Children usually enjoy this book. After reading it, the teacher might ask what Martha did, what George did, and what happened at the end of the book.

2. The teacher reads a story with a definite number of persons with different occupations. The children then enumerate the occupations.
3. Children repeat simple stories such as "The Three Bears."

Manual and Verbal Expression
PANTOMIMING ACTIVITIES:
1. Pantomiming nursery rhymes such as "Humpty Dumpty" and "Little Miss Muffet."
2. Pantomiming such activities as looking for a cat, bouncing a ball, catching a ball, vacuuming the floor, peeling potatoes, beating an egg, eating meat, eating spaghetti, drinking milk, picking flowers, playing a piano or violin.
3. Pantomiming in pairs: looking for a lost ring, rowing in a boat, walking on a very icy street, walking in mud, going through the woods at night when it is very dark, shopping in a store that is very crowded.
4. Pantomiming in groups:

> A fussy old lady, a bashful person, and a big bully being waited on by a brash waiter or waitress in a restaurant.

After a bomb has gone off at an airport, one relative is looking for two others. They all finally find each other and are very happy.

ADDING VERBALIZATION:

1. Pretending to represent certain occupations: cook, bus driver, lawyer, doctor, policeman, policewoman, painter, carpenter, schoolteacher.
2. Dramatizing nursery rhymes, such as "Mistress Mary" or "Wee Willie Winkie."
3. Dramatizing stories.
4. Making up stories based on some of the children's experiences such as a visit to the supermarket, to the firehouse, or to the post office, or going on a boat ride or a train ride. Or stories may be based on two words such as *ugly* and *beautiful,* or a set of objects.
5. Discussion based on such problems as:
   a. Let us suppose that you saw one of your classmates hide a barometer that you had been using in your science exhibition in his locker. He really loves that barometer. What would you do?
   b. Your cousin, from another town, arrives who is very, very bright and very, very beautiful. She draws attention to her high grades, her ability to write poetry, and her good looks. What would you do in this kind of situation?

Language for Fun

Sometimes children use language just for fun. Children in the middle grades begin to enjoy limericks—and often make them up. S. Brewton and J. E. Brewton's *Laughable Limericks* (New York, Thomas Y. Crowell Company, 1965) has one section on limericks according to topic and another on how to write limericks. Their limericks tend to amuse children. For children in the primary and intermediate grades William Cole's *The Square Bear and Other Riddle Rhymers* (New York, Scholastic Book Services, 1976) can bring laughter and, at the same time, provoke thought. The riddles are answered by two words that rhyme. Another book that entertains children is Leonard Kessler's *Ghosts and Crows and Things with O's* (New York, Scholastic Book Services, 1976). The child must find the letter O that is hidden in various pictures and find the use of O's in such games as tic-tac-toe. The book also lists words containing O's.

Limericks, riddles, jokes, and tongue twisters, while they often fascinate young children, sharpen their appreciation of the uses of language. Children frequently play with language by inventing jokes, riddles, or nonsense words. As a result, they begin to develop an ability to use language creatively.

PIAGET'S CONTRIBUTION TO OUR UNDERSTANDING OF COGNITIVE DEVELOPMENT

Many clinicians and language arts teachers recently have come to regard the contributions of Piaget as being helpful in planning for the cognitive development of children. Jean Piaget a Swiss developmental psychologist who was concerned with changes in cognitive functioning from birth through adolescence. Unlike Skinner, Piaget does not conceptualize behavior in terms of stimuli, responses, and reinforcement. Rather he describes children's behavior by asking them questions, noting their responses, and carefully and in detail observing their verbal behavior at different stages of their lives. Piaget designed his approach to discover the nature and level of development of the concepts that children use and not to produce developmental scales (Wadsworth 1973, p. 5). Because of the influence of his training in biology, Piaget views cognitive behavior as acts of organization and adaptation to the environment.

Piaget believes that the child controls the procuring and organizing of experiences in his own environment. For instance, babies follow with their eyes, explore with their hands, hold crackers and throw them. Such activities provide the base for absorbing and organizing experiences. This process, which Piaget calls *assimilation,* is fundamental to learning throughout life. It is, however, modified by *accommodation,* which steers children into adaptation to the world by resisting some patterns and by bringing in new results, which, in turn, enrich the patterns. A child's learning might be likened to a data-processing operation wherein the child feeds the data that is relevant into the machine and rejects that which is not relevant. The results of this operation represent learning. Piaget's hypothesis is that cognitive development is a coherent process of successive qualitative changes of cognitive structures with each structure and its concomitant changes deriving logically and inevitably from the preceding one (Wadsworth 1973, p. 25).

As regard the relation of age and stage, Piaget claims no more than that the ranges he cites represent his actual findings on the Geneva, Switzerland, schoolchildren whom he tested. His detailed figures plainly show a large overlap between the stages. In noting this, Isaacs (1974, page 46) says: "Thus some four-to-five-year-olds produce replies characteristic of the seven-to-eight average and some seven-to-eight's respond like average four-to-five's. Piaget has himself insisted that his age-ranges are no more than a useful framework of reference for the way in which the stages succeed one another; it is the order of succession that matters, and not any particular chronological age."

We should keep in mind Donaldson's (1978) admonitions in following Piaget: (1) Children are not as egocentric as Piaget has claimed; (2) They are not so limited in ability to reason deductively in their earlier stages, and (3) language learning skills are not isolated from the rest of the child's mental growth. (Donaldson, 1978, p. 58) These conclusions are the result of her findings as she manipulated some of the factors in Piaget's experiments. She found that three factors and their interactions made a difference in the outcomes of the experiments:

1. The child's knowledge of the language.
2. His assessment of what we intend.
3. The manner in which he would represent the physical situation to himself if he were not there at all. (Donaldson, 1978, p. 69)

She also notes that learning is bound up with the understanding of the intentions of the speaker. (Donaldson, 1978, p. 38).

PIAGET'S BUILDING STAGES

Stage 1. First Two Years: Sensorimotor Period

The earliest behavior shows no sense of persisting objects or of space or time concepts. But presently, the behavior changes and each month it takes into account more features of the world. At birth, children possess innate reflexes only, but gradually they begin to explore objects in their environment, watching the parts of the mobile move, holding a teddy bear, shaking the rattle. They discover, as a result of their interaction with their environment, that the world is a succession of objects with permanence in its surroundings. They discover tools for eating although they may try to use their rattles for this purpose. They find out that movements in specific direction carried out at specific times lead to the same results; for example, they hold out their arms and they are lifted. They learn to use words as symbols. By two years of age, the child invents new patterns of behavior, using words, actions, and symbolic play with and without words.

Stage 2. Two to Four Years: Preconceptual Thought

At this stage, children really explore their world—walking, touching, pulling, investigating everything they can reach. They climb on top of things, get below them, touch them, manipulate them. They imitate adults—running the vacuum cleaner like Mommy or hitting a nail like big brother. Words begin to symbolize images although a single symbol, in the early part of this stage, may carry many meanings: [bʊ] for book may mean, "Read to me," "Give it to me." or "Put it away." Slowly words not only accompany actions but represent something. At this stage the child is basically egocentric and he may play by himself, putting his dolly to bed and saying, "Put baby to bed." Recently when a ball (on a string) in the form of a music box was pulled down, and "Silent Night, Holy Night" was produced, the three-and-a-half-year-old said, "Christmas," and then "What is it?" (He had begun to classify.) Whereupon he pulled the ball down to hear the music. But the precocious five-and-a-half-year-old said, "It's a music box with a mechanism inside. The pull triggered the music." And then, "Can you get inside it?" This second child belonged in the next stage.

Stage 3. Four to Eight Years: Intuitive Thought

This boy related the sound heard to the sound in the music box in his own home. He would have liked to get inside it to see how it worked. At this stage, children are busy with what they see around them and what is happening around them. They really put things together—comparing and contrasting. The example given at the beginning of this chapter exemplifies this stage. The child listed a series of analogies until she arrived at "puppy cat." As children begin to categorize, they begin to think. Children at this age should be given opportunities to experiment with a variety of objects and should take part in many happenings such as trips, creative drama, puppet plays, and science experiments such as planting seeds and watching them grow.

Stage 4. Eight to Eleven Years: Concrete Operations

At this stage, children increase their logical thought processes. They think in concrete terms and must be given many opportunities to practice this concrete thinking. On reading about a fire in Chicago, they ask and answer, "What started the fire?" They answer the question, "How high is the Trade Center Building?" in terms of the number of stories, which answer is concrete and clear. They may talk about, if they live in Manhattan, "How far away is Times Square?" And then, "How far away is California?" They can understand concepts about lengths, numbers, speed, and sizes. At this stage, teachers give their students many opportunities to reason in concrete terms; *because, although,* and *if* are heard frequently.

Stage 5. Eleven Years On: Formal Operations

This stage is particularly important because here children attain the power of abstract thought. They operate freely with their own imagined possibilities and hypotheses. They can abstract, manipulate ideas about ideas, examine relationships. They set up miniature research studies and carry through their investigations.

Piaget did not intend that these stages represent norms; therefore, the ages given are approximate and can vary as much as two years or more. But Piaget's research does predict that each child develops through these sequential stages.

Teachers and speech/language clinicians in the schools can initiate language activities that facilitate and enhance the natural cognitive development in successive stages. For example, there follows illustrations of activities largely based on children's literature for various stages. We begin with stage 3, because this book is targeted on school years. We do this while recognizing the importance of stages 1 and 2. (See pages 250–261 for characteristics of delayed language acquisition.)

LANGUAGE ARTS ACTIVITIES FOR THE VARIOUS STAGES

Stage 3. Intuitive Thought

This stage should provide a wealth of experiences involving everyday happenings.

Concept—Numbers
Book—J. J. Reiss, *Numbers*, Scarsdale, N.Y.: Bradbury Press, 1971. This book helps children to count five arms on a starfish, seven segments on a horse chestnut leaf, and 100 legs on a centipede. It can be used to capture an interest in numbers and in counting.

Concept—Differences Between Winter and Summer
Books: E. Schick, *City in the Winter* (New York: Macmillan Publishing Co. Inc., 1970). E. Schick, *City in the Summer* (New York: Macmillan Publishing Co. Inc., 1960). These books can serve as a basis for a discussion on how the city in the winter differs from the city in the summer. For example, in *City in the Winter*, Jimmy wakes up to find the world is very white. He and his grandmother explore what the snow has caused—bootprints, buried sidewalks, and a closed store. The teacher may then say, "But suppose that Jimmy woke up on a very, very hot day in the summer. What would Jimmy and his grandmother have found then?" Clues can be found in *City in the Summer*. The teacher may go on to explore many differences between winter and summer: play activities, clothes worn, foods eaten, and trips taken.

Concept—Roles of Mothers
Books: W. Wiesner, *Turnabout* (New York: Seabury Press, 1972). J. Lasher, *Mothers Can Do Anything* (Racine, Wis.: Whitman Publishing Company, 1972). The Wiesner book is a Norwegian tale in which the farmer and his wife change roles for a day. While the wife calmly rakes the hay, the farmer

breaks the eggs, lets the cider run out of the keg, spoils the porridge, nearly kills the cow and gets stuck halfway up the chimney. The Lasher book contains a series of pictures showing mothers on jobs that are fundamentally different from the traditional women's jobs: policewoman, taxi driver, painter, judge, ditch digger, architect, dentist, plumber, cook, archeologist, and astronaut.

These books can serve as the base for a variety of activities: playing the role of mother as the children themselves see the role, playing the roles as suggested in either of the two books; discussing the roles of mothers in their own neighborhood; writing a poem about the roles of mothers.

Concept—The Five Senses

Books: Aliki, *My Five Senses* (New York: Thomas Y. Crowell Company, 1962). This book points to the functions of the five senses and shows that a combination of senses can be involved in any perception.

P. Showers, *The Listening Walk* (New York: Thomas Y. Crowell Company, 1961). This is the story of a boy who goes walking with his father; they don't talk but just listen to all the sounds around them.

Reading these two books can serve as the initial step in classroom work involving all the senses. From this vantage point, children can talk about the sounds they normally hear: the screeching of tires, the banging of doors, and the wind whistling. Or they may talk about kitchen sounds: the kettle whistling, the coffee pot going "ploppety plop, plop," the toaster going "zing," the dishes clattering, the pans banging, the bell going "brrrrr." Next they may consider smells: smells in the winter, in the summer, in the spring, what smells warn of danger; what smell is the best of all smells; what smell is the worst of all smells. And they can then attack the other senses. This work makes children aware of the world around them and, incidentally, increases their vocabulary. They may well learn new words such as *prickly, sticky, tangy,* or for some the difference between *hard* and *soft.*

Concept—Sibling Rivalry

Stegmaier (1974) in an article "Teaching Interpersonal Communication Through Children's Literature" shows how children's literature can provide a vehicle for teaching about conflict between siblings. She suggests two books for this purpose: Ezra Jack Keats's *Peter's Chair* (New York: Harper & Row, Publishers, Inc., 1967) and Russell Hoban's *A Baby Sister for Frances* (New York: Harper & Row, Publishers, Inc., 1964). Another more recent book is Eloise Greenfield's *She Came Bringing That Little Baby Girl* (Philadelphia: J. B. Lippincott Co., 1974). In this book Kevin wanted a baby brother but "she came bringing me that little girl wrapped all up in a pink blanket." Kevin is disappointed and annoyed as he sees relatives and neighbors fussing over a wee, wrinkled baby with tiny hands and feet. From a discussion of the concepts in these books, children recognize that natural rivalries do exist in such situations.

Concept—The Passing of Time; Size of Animals (For Some, the Futility of a Threat)

Book—E. Carle, *The Grouchy Ladybug* (New York: Thomas Y. Crowell Company, 1977). For a full twelve hours a grouchy ladybug looks for a fight, challenging everyone she meets with, "Hey you . . . Want to fight?" and then flies off with, "Oh, you're not big enough." The hours pass—the size of the animals increases. Finally the story ends with her and a friend ladybug eating aphids from a leaf.

Concept—The makeup of a Frog's Body

Book—J. Cole, *A Frog's Body*, New York, William Morrow & Co., Inc., 1980. This book explains the details of the frog's anatomy with exceptionally fine photographs. The text is well written—clear and succinct. The diagrams also are very clear.

Stage 4. Concrete Operations

This stage should involve many concrete problem-solving activities.

Concept: Analyzing a Personal Problem

Problem: Inability to cope with a new school environment with such problems as making new friends.

Genevieve Gray, *Sore Loser* (Boston: Houghton Mifflin Company, 1974). (This book tells about Loren who cannot seem to do anything right in his new sixth-grade class. He has trouble adjusting to the school and in making friends. The plot is revealed through letters written by Loren and by his mother, notes to the school principal from his teacher, school bulletins, and essays by students.)

A number of ways can be used to help solve this problem:

1. Playing the story as it is written and then replaying it as it could have been written, adding scenes and changing scenes.
2. Discussing Loren's problem and possible solutions to it.
3. Asking a counselor in the school to come in to give his viewpoints on the problem.

Concept—Numbers

Book: S. Shapman, *Numbers, How Many? How Much?* (Chicago: Follett Publishing Company, 1972).

This book contains 14 amusing arithmetic problems involving addition, subtraction, multiplication, and division. Objects in the problems include squishy grasshoppers, mud pies, basketballs, crocodiles, and kissing relatives.

This book can be used as reinforcement of many of the mathematical concepts and, at the same time, sections of it can be the basis for amusing creative drama.

Stage 5. Propositional or Formal Logic.

At this stage teachers should be encouraging abstractions, research abilities, and problems that involve either induction or deduction.

Two examples are given for this stage. The first involved a study of the Erie Canal undertaken by 13- and 14-year-olds. The second, involving a study of literature having to do with *pride*, was undertaken by 15- and 16-year-olds in a drama class in Jamaica High School, Jamaica, New York.

Teachers at both the elementary and high school levels frequently plan their work with their students. As the work of the unit progresses, many speech activities take place. Children give talks, report, discuss, debate, interview, read aloud, and dramatize.

For example, children in an eighth grade were studying the early history of New York State. While studying this era, one 12-year-old, reporting on his trip across New York State on the Thruway, compared the Thruway to the Erie Canal. The report of this trip motivated members of the class to study the building of the canal. The writer of their social studies text explained the reasons for the building of the canal and its values to the country, but the children wanted more information than their text contained. They discussed what more they would like to know about the Erie Canal. Specifically they wanted answers to the following:

- What were the factors that made a canal seem advisable?
- Who decided a canal was necessary?
- Why was Van Buren opposed to it?
- Why did Clinton approve the building of the canal?
- What were the times like in the early 1800s?
- What kind of clothes did people wear then?
- What did they do for entertainment?
- How did they live?
- What did they do for a living?
- How was the building of the canal planned?
- What was the route of the canal?
- What were some of the difficulties encountered in building the canal?
- Who built the canal?
- What was its opening like?
- What were the effects of its opening?

After they had listed these questions on the blackboard, they broke up into groups to decide how to do their research and how to report on their findings. The project demanded oral communication in its planning and in its execution.

Throughout this activity, groups frequently gave progress reports. As the children read, they found other items that they thought should be included. Finally, individuals and groups of individuals reported on what they had read. One boy gave an account of the way people talked in the 1800s. This item was not included originally, but he and the members of his group felt it added to their understanding of the period. "Oh, go sandpaper your nose" became one of the favorite expressions of the group. Another panel of students gave a very interesting discussion of the songs sung during this era. Through such activities children learn to participate in discussion.

The teacher helped these children in a number of ways to prepare and give reports. He reminded them of the necessity of gaining and holding the interest of their listeners. He suggested ways and means of collecting material and of organizing it. He stressed their having a thorough knowledge of their topic, a real interest in it themselves, and a desire to communicate this interest to their listeners.

The teacher also taught them to be more successful participants in a discussion group. He taught them how to state a problem, analyze it, and examine its solutions. The children learned that they must have a basis for the choice of a particular solution. Although these children had already learned to be fairly effective members of a discussion group, the teacher reinforced their learning. Frequently he stressed that they must have knowledge and background before speaking. Because the discussion sometimes went off on a tangent, he emphasized that they must keep it relevant. He helped the students to consider all points of view, participate well, and listen carefully. He encouraged each boy and girl to be a responsible member of the group.

In this work on the Erie Canal the students found it necessary to read aloud from various sources. One boy read the speech made by DeWitt Clinton at the opening of the canal. The teacher helped him to prepare this speech for reading aloud by making sure he understood the material both intellectually and emotionally. As the boy mentioned bringing together the waters of the Hudson River and Lake Erie, his classmates felt pride in his voice. Because he knew the background so well, he needed almost no help in preparing his material to read aloud.

Finally, as a culminating activity, the class wrote and produced a play that depicted the struggle to build the canal. The play included a chorus of singers who sang about the Erie Canal and a choral-speaking group who, dressed in overalls, carrying shovels, and pushing wheelbarrows, spoke, "We are digging the ditch through the mire." The play, quite elaborately staged and executed, ran for three nights.

A drama class taught by Mrs. Kirchman, formerly of Jamaica High School, Queens, studied the various concepts of *pride* as portrayed in a variety of plays. The following is the first page of a booklet that was the end result of the study.

Dear Students,

The word *pride* has been bandied about and used so loosely that we may have forgotten what we mean by it. I thought you would enjoy thinking about the layers of meaning covering the bare bones of the word. After discussing the connotations of the word, via dictionaries, quotations, and illustrations from drama, we were asked to dissect *pride* in a brief composition, poem, or sketch.

We selected fragments from your written work in an effort to explore the anatomy of *pride*. You may like having a copy of this class assignment, written by your classmates.

With proud shades of Antigone, Dr. Stockman, Masha, Kurt Muller, Annie Sullivan, Cyrano, St. Joan, and all the other people we've touched through plays,

Yours,
Rose Kirchman

People are isolated
By walls of their own making.
They cannot help each other
Or tell their problems honestly.
Shame and false pride
Lock the doors to understanding.
While trying to help a friend
They judge him, but say nothing;
Their opinions are shadowed in silence.
Guilt and fear combine and mix.
They will never remove their facades.
Being disapproved of is a large enough threat;
Crying comes later,
Behind a closed door.

—Patricia Truscelli

I sold out to the enemy at Berlin
I begged to go home in a box
But the punishment redeemed me—I died clear-conscienced and
    with pride
As I plunged head first to the rocks.
I no longer worry about the Proud
Who nurture the cancer in their mind.

I owe Pride nothing—I already gave.
I died for the false star,
My Pride.

—*Les Cohen*

The study of the Erie Canal involved many opportunities for reasoning. For example, the boys and girls talked about the evidence used to prove the feasibility of the canal. They discussed how leaders can put across even unpopular ideas. They were also able to look at progress over several decades—first, the stagecoach; then, the canal; then, the railroads; and finally, airplanes. They projected into the future. What could possibly be available in another 20 years—space ships? They analyzed the attitudes of reactionaries in Clinton's day and made analogies with the attitudes of today's reactionaries.

The high school drama group explored the concepts that can be attached to the word *pride*. They enlarged their horizons both from a cognitive and affective standpoint. They assumed a mental set for the abstractions of what pride can be. They shifted from one concept to another all within the rubric of *pride*. They grasped a variety of concepts having to do with *pride* and put these abstractions into writing.

Following the general philosophy of Piaget, we believe that the classroom teacher helps the child to develop thought processes and appropriate language for logical thinking. This development means that children use language to meet cognitive demands, to compare, to contrast, to draw inferences, to see cause and effect relationships, to take things apart and put them together, to talk about things and events that are present or absent. When the classroom teacher promotes such activities, boys and girls progress through the natural sequential way of cognitive development.

READING—A LANGUAGE ACTIVITY

Reading is probably the language activity most discussed by educators, parents, members of school boards, politicians. When the reading scores of children in a public school system increase, the fact commands front-page headlines even in the most prestigious newspapers. Probably all of us agree that reading involves a process of seeing print and converting the print to meaning. But differences arise when we attempt to allocate language skills to the reading program.

DeStefano (1981) gives broad descriptions of two interpretations of reading and its development:

Some reading experts maintain that in getting meaning from printed language, we apply strategies that are parallel to those we apply in understanding spoken language. They hold that we apply processing skills and strategies to sound in oral language which are applied to print in reading. Put another way, in reading we do not translate print into speech and then interpret that speech. In contrast to this position, some reading researchers argue that the ability to process and understand written text is dependent on oral language processing strategies. For them, decoding is crucial as we translate printed language into its phonological representation, applying skills used in the spoken language in the reading process. (DeStefano, 1981, p. 372)

Goodman (1979, p. 661) notes that literacy, reading and writing, is learned in the same way as oral language. If language learning is learning how to mean then literacy learning is learning how to mean through written language. Goodman goes on to note that children, from their experiences at home and at school, learn that print represents meaning. They learn general and specific meanings of print found in situational contexts: stop signs, cereal boxes, toothpaste cartons. At the same time, they develop some awareness of the form of print: directionality, letter names, key features. They distinguish print from pictures. From teachers and parents, they know the basic functions of books, letters, newspapers.

Teaching Reading

The teaching of reading must be language-centered to capitalize on the learners' existing language competence and performance as they learn to process language for meaning. Like Hall (1979), we prefer teaching reading through language experience. According to Hall, the premises on which language-centered reading are based include consideration of the language learning children bring to the reading situation, of the conditions that foster language and reading acquisition, of the use of relevant content and language for reading instruction, of the purpose of reading, and of the relationship between the reading and writing in the acquisition of literacy. Her recommendations for language-centered reading instruction include providing exposure to written language in prereading, using language experience in teaching reading, stressing comprehension, correlating reading and writing, and immersing children in a literate environment.

Prereading can be easily woven into classroom activities. Meaning must be present for real learning to take place. Janey, a language-delayed child, and her first-grade classmates had been to a plant that processed grape juice. The next day, the teacher produced a huge sheet of paper with a recipe for grape jelly; she also produced all the essentials for making grape jelly. Reading the recipe with the teacher, the children, step by step, made grape jelly. Later they ate the jelly with bread and peanut butter. The prereading situation was natural, was the result of a class experience, was interesting, and was rewarding. The written language held meaning for these children. When the speech/language clinician came to get Janey for clinical work, Janey went to the recipe and "read" parts of it to her. Incidentally the teacher had suggested that the clinician pick up Janey that particular day.

We also believe reading is successfully achieved when it is related to what the child already knows. The child must have a cognitive base from which to proceed. Sounding out words is not enough. The child must comprehend what is being sounded. Again meaning is all-important. Teachers must help children to build understandings, concepts, vocabulary—and they review whatever experiences and concepts are relevant before children read a particular printed text.

Durkin (1981) explains schema theory and defines schemata. (*Schema* is the singular, *schemata* the plural.)

In schema theory the basic assumption is that what is experienced (learned) is organized and stored in the brain not in static, unchanging form but in a way that permits modification through further development. Development occurs, the theorists say, when what is known (about an object, an event, a role, a process or whatever) interacts with what is new but related.

Durkin goes on to say that schemata may be thought of as networks of concepts. What is already known is called a schema, which is like a concept—and then some. Schemata, according to present beliefs, are arranged hierarchically. A person's schema for something like *sparrow*, for instance, is thought to be one part of the more encompassing schema for *bird*, which, in turn, is part of the still larger schema for *animal*, and so on. (Durkin, 1981, p. 25.)

The major thrust would seem to be that what is in a reader's head influences comprehension as much as what appears in print. But from the reading, new concepts may be learned and added to the schemata.

RELATIONSHIP BETWEEN SPEAKING AND READING

Investigators who have done research on children with reading disabilities point to the co-occurrence of language difficulties—usually in the areas of oral expression and listening comprehension. For example, Bruininks, Lockes, and Gropper (1970) in comparing the psycholinguistic abilities of good and poor readers found that the poor readers were inferior to good readers on ITPA subtests that required listening and oral expression. Incidentally, there were no differences on those subtests requiring skills involving visual and motor channels of expression. Kirby, Lyle, and Ambie (1972) found that problem readers did not do well on the auditory subtests of the ITPA. Wakefield (1973) found that normal readers did better than clinic readers on the digit span section of the WISC and the auditory sequential memory test of the ITPA. Flynn and Byrne (1970) reported that advanced readers did better on auditory discrimination tests and on two blending tests than did normal readers. Semel and Wiig (1975) discovered that elementary school learning-disabled children showed reductions in both the comprehension and expression of syntactic structures. These studies point to inabilities in competence and production of language in reading-disabled children.

Gibson (1972) points to the similarities between hearing-speaking and reading-writing. She notes that there exist similarities in the phonological system of hearing-speaking and the graphological system of reading-writing, in the semantic systems of both, and in the syntactic rule structure of both. Further relationships probably exist in the two areas in independence, transfer, and mapping rules.

Gibson draws a parallel between the phonological system and the graphological system: She notes that productive speech beings with babbling (although disagreement does exist as to the role of babbling in speech acquisition) and that graphic production begins with scribbling. In both instances, feedback (auditory in the first case, visual in the second) provides an opportunity to learn by self-regulation.

Discussing the semantic relationship, Gibson stresses that spoken words are symbols for real events, things, and ideas, and that written words are but symbols for spoken words. However, she stresses that reading for meaning does not always come easily.

Gibson believes that the syntactic aspects are easier to compare— that rules of grammar are the same for spoken and for written language. A knowledge of syntactic structure in both instances must be picked up to process units that communicate meaning. She notes that how the child does this for reading is not known and that the clues to syntax in both instances are comparable but not identical.

Mattingly (1972), comparing reading and listening, notes that the usual view is that the processes are parallel and summarizes this viewpoint: ". . . written text is input by eye and speech by ear, but at as early a stage as possible, consistent with this difference in modality, the two inputs have a common internal representation. From this stage onward, the two processes are identical." Mattingly further notes that even with the recent view of speech perception with a different model of linguistic processing wherein the process is active and similar to production, the assumption of a parallel between reading and listening remains.

Mattingly then points out differences between listening and reading: (1) Listening is a more natural way of perceiving language. Listening is easy and reading is hard, although listening is not a more efficient process in all respects. (2) Listening is slower. (3) The manner in which information is presented is basically different in reading and listening. The listener is processing a flow of complex acoustic signals and while listening has to separate the cues from irrelevant detail. Cues are not discrete events but tend to blend into one another. On the other hand, the reader is processing a series of symbols that are quite simply related to the physical medium that conveys them. Readers can see the letters if they want to, for, in writing a string of separate symbols is connected for practical convenience. Speech signals cannot be viewed in this way.

Mattingly concludes that reading is a language-based skill, that it is parasitic on language. Reading in the visual mode is not a parallel activity to speech perception in the auditory mode; differences cannot be explained by differences of modality. Reading is rather a deliberately acquired language-based skill that is dependent upon the speaker-hearer's awareness of certain aspects of primary linguistic activity.

It is clear that more research needs to be done to ascertain how speaking, listening, and reading are related. In the meantime, we develop strategies for both language competence and performance for both the speech communication specialist and the reading specialist.

Stark (1975) summarizes the role of the speech and language clinician in this area:

> . . . we believe that there is a significant amount of evidence to indicate that speech and language pathologists can make a very important contribution to the prevention and treatment of reading problems. Assisting parents, teachers, and other specialists by providing information about the nature of language acquisition and training children in linguistic processing may produce highly desirable results. At the least, speech and hearing clinicians may be able to modify currently used teaching techniques and materials so that teachers can more effectively understand the role that language development plays in reading. (Stark 1975, p. 834).

In summary, we subscribe to the theory that normal language acquisition involves a set of skills that develop in a more or less parallel fashion with each skill being possibly related to another, and possibly to some still undesignated language ability that increases with maturity. Sometimes a particular skill may be slow to develop but is still within normal range. In other cases, some of the skills do not develop, and these underdeveloped skills may well interfere with many of the other skills. The clinician intervenes to help the child develop particular language skills, whereas teachers plan to develop all the skills. As children mature, their thinking and their ability to attack more complex, cognitive problems develop. Reading is a language-based activity and, consequently, as language skills are built so is a basis for reading.

Problems

1. Visit a classroom in an elementary school or in a high school. List the activities that went on in the classroom that would stimulate language development. Describe each activity in one sentence.
2. Find five pieces of children's literature and indicate (a) how a clinician would use each piece for language intervention—that is, developing strategies for accelerating specific language abilities; and (b) how a classroom teacher would use each piece of literature for stimulating language development.
3. Visit a nursery school and a third-grade class. Indicate, in general, the differences in vocabulary, syntax, and articulation.
4. Watch "Sesame Street." Indicate the language abilities being stimulated and the strategies used to stimulate them.
5. Try any of the exercises listed for developing language abilities with two kindergarten children. Report on your progress.
6. List and describe one or two language activities for Piaget's stages 3, 4, and 5. Justify your choice.
7. Read Isaacs (1974, pp. 48–49) and Durkin (1981). Compare the concepts.
8. Observe children in a playground or in the back yard of a home. For what purposes are they using language? Could any of these activities be a base for either clinical or classroom intervention? Explain.
9. List some of the experiences of a four- to six-year-old child whom you know well that seemingly helped him/her develop language. Are any of these experiences pertinent in planning a language remediation program? Explain.
10. Read any section of a language arts book or article. Extract from it a particular strategy that might work well in helping a language-delayed child.
11. Work out a prereading experience that could be started in the classroom and implemented in the clinical setting, or vice versa.
12. Watch parents with preschool children in a supermarket. What kind of language are the parents using? How are the children responding? Watch parents with children from eight to ten years old in a similar situation. Again what kind of language are the parents using? How are the children responding? Indicate strategies for stimulating language.

References and Suggested Readings

Andrews, M. and C. Brabson, "Preparing the Language-Impaired Child for Classroom Mathematics: Suggestions for the Speech Pathologist." *Language, Speech, and Hearing Services in Schools,* **8** (1977), 46–53. (Suggests ways of teaching mathematical concepts)

Applebee, A. N., "Environments for Learning: ERIC Resources in the Language Experience Approach." *Language Arts,* **55** (Sept. 1978), 756–760. (Contains references on relationship of reading to oral communication and on Language Experience Approach to Reading.)

Aram, D. M., and J. E. Nation, "Patterns of Language Behavior in Children with Developmental Language Disorders." *Journal of Speech and Hearing Research,* **18** (June 1975), 229–240. (Classifies children with similar patterns of language based on their ability to comprehend, formulate, and repeat specified phonologic, syntactic, and semantic aspects of language.)

Ball, S., and G. A. Bogatz, "The First Year of Sesame Street: An Evaluation." *Today's Education* (National Education Association Journal), **60** (March 1971), 72.

Baratz, J. C., "A Bi-Dialectal Task for Determining Language Proficiency in Economically Disadvantaged Negro Children." *Child Development,* **40** (September 1969), 889–901. (Compares the language behavior of standard and nonstandard speakers when repeating standard or nonstandard sentences. Concludes that the major difficulty for black children is one of "code-switching" rather than language deficiency.)

Biederman, S., "Integrating Language Exercises into Academic Curricula in a Self-Contained Language Disabilities Class." *Language, Speech, and Hearing Services in Schools,* **7** (1976), 41–47. (Gives examples of language activities based on the ITPA Model—based on an Eskimo unit.)

Bloom, L., "Why Not Pivot Grammar?" *Journal of Speech and Hearing Disorders,* **36** (February 1971), 40–50.

——, *Language Development: Form and Function in Emerging Grammars.* Cambridge, Massachusetts: MIT Press, 1970.

—— and M. Lahey, *Language Development and Language Disorders.* New York: John Wiley & Sons, Inc., 1978.

Boehnlein, M. M., and J. M. Ritty, "Integration of the Communication Arts Curriculum: A Review." *Language Arts,* **54** (April 1977), 372–377. (Shows the interrelationships of spelling, reading, listening and written and oral composition.)

Boynton, K. R., and L. L. Henke, "Conversational Expansion in Young Children." *Communication Education,* **27** (1978), 202–211.

Bruininks, R. H., W. G. Lockes, and R. L. Gropper, "Psycholinguistic Abilities of Good and Poor Reading Disadvantaged First-Graders," *The Elementary School Journal,* **70** (April 1970), 378–388.

Buckley, M. H., "A Guide for Developing an Oral Language Curriculum." *Language Arts,* **53** (September 1976), 621–627. (Includes material on basic elements, interactive patterns, content, role of teacher and of students, and evaluation.)

Bullock, Sir Alan, Chairman, *A Language for Life*. Report of the Committee of Inquiry appointed by the Secretary of State for Education and Science. London: H. M. Stationery Office, 1975.

Burns, P. C., *Assessment and Correction of Language Arts Difficulties*. Columbus, Ohio: Charles E. Merrill Publishing Company, 1980. (Contains teaching strategies for listening and oral composition.)

Bush, C. S., "Creative Drama and Language Experiences: Effective Clinical Techniques." *Language, Speech, and Hearing Services in Schools*, 9 (October 1978), 254–258. (Tells how to use creative language experiences with the language-disabled.)

Cahir, S. R., and R. W. Shuy, "Classroom Language Learning: What do Researchers know?" *Language Arts*, 58 (March 1981), 369–374.

Carter, T., "Creative Dramatics for Learning-Disabled Children." *Academic Therapy*, 9 (Summer 1974), 411–417.

Chappell, G. E., "A Cognitive-Linguistic Intervention Program: Basic Concept Formation Level," *Language, Speech, and Hearing Services in Schools*, 8 (1977), 23–32. (Explains a strategy wherein "test-teach" can be used to help children develop basic concepts.)

———, "Language Disabilities and the Language Clinician," *Journal of Learning Disabilities*, 5 (December 1972), 611–619. (Indicates where the language performance may break down.)

———, "Oral Language Performance of Upper Elementary School Students Obtained Via Story Reformulation." *Language, Speech, and Hearing Services in Schools*, 11 (October 1980), 236–250. (Presents data on the mean length of utterance, use of five syntactical structures and use of five features of story content that characterize the oral language of children in grades four through seven.)

Chenfield, M. B., *Teaching Language Arts Creatively*. New York: Harcourt Brace Jovanovich, Inc., 1978.

Cholewinski, M., and S. Holliday, "Learning to Read: What's Right at Home is Right at School." *Language Arts*, 56 (September 1979), 671–674.

Chomsky, C., *The Acquisition of Syntax in Children from Five to Ten*. Cambridge, Mass.: The M.I.T. Press, 1969. (Ascertains children's competence in four grammatical structures.)

Coleman, R. O., and D. E. Anderson, "Enhancement of Language Comprehension in Developmentally Delayed Children," *Language, Speech, and Hearing Services in Schools*, 9 (October 1978), 241–253. (Describes the use of receptive language tasks presented in a cognitive, problem-solving context as a method for enhancing language comprehension in developmentally delayed children.)

Dally, A., "Language Remediation with Primary School-Age Children." *Language, Speech, and Hearing Services in Schools*, 9 (April 1978), 85–90. (Gives the advantage of exposing the language-disabled child to visual symbols—particularly in terms of later class placement.)

Davis, F. R. A. and R. P. Parker, Jr., *Teaching for Literacy: Reflections on the Bullock Report*. New York: Agathon Press, Inc. 1978.

DeStefano, J. S., *Language, the Learner, and the Schools*. New York: John Wiley & Sons, Inc., 1978.

————, "Classroom Language Learning: What Do the Researchers Know?—S. R. Cahir and R. W. Shuy." *Language Arts*, **58** (March 1981, 369–374.)

Donaldson, M., *Children's Minds*. Glasgow, Scotland: Fontana/Collins, Ltd., 1978.

Doughty, G. Thornton, and A. Doughty, *Language Study: The School and the Community*. New York, American Elsevier, Inc., 1977. (Focuses upon a meeting point between the insights of linguistic science often in conjunction with the other social sciences, and the linguistic questions raised by the study of a particular aspect of individual behavior or human society.)

Dunn, L. M., and J. O. Smith, *Peabody Language Development Kit*. Circle Pines, Minn.,: American Guidance Service

Durkin, D., "What is the Value of the New Interest in Reading Comprehension?" *Language Arts*, **58** (January 1981), 23–43.

Edelsky, C., "'Teaching' Oral Language." *Language Arts*, **55** (March 1978), 291–296. (Gives classroom implications based on findings from adult-child reaction studies.)

————, and T. J. Rosegrant, "Language Development for Mainstreamed Severely Handicapped Non-Verbal Children." *Language Arts*, **58** (January 1981), 68–78. (Shows the impact of Public Law 94–142 and the resultant mainstreaming.)

Engler, L. F., E. P. Hannah, and T. M. Longhurst, "Linguistic Analysis of Speech Samples." *Journal of Speech and Hearing Disorders*, **38** (May 1973), 192–204. (Shows the way to contrast a child's speech with that of an adult or other children his own age or development. Tells how to elicit and record the sample.)

Fennimore, F., "Choral Reading as a Spontaneous Experience." *Elementary English*, **48** (November 1971), 870–885. (Describes an informal approach to choral speaking based on the children's own language.)

Fey, M. E., L. B. Leonard, and K. A. Wilcox, "Speech Style Modification of Language-Impaired Children." *Journal of Speech and Hearing Disorders*, **46** (February 1981), 91–96. (Gives results of language interaction of normal children of same age, normal children of younger age, and language-impaired children.)

Flynn, P. T., and M. C. Byrne, "Relationship Between Reading and Selected Auditory Abilities of Third-Grade Children." *Journal of Speech and Hearing Research*, **13** (December 1970), 731–740. (Tests for significant differences between advanced and retarded readers on auditory tasks.)

Foulke, P. N., "How Early Should Language Development and Pre-Reading Experience be Started?" *Elementary English*, **51** (1974), 310–315.

Gans, R., *Guiding Children's Reading Through Experiences*, 2nd ed. New York: Teachers College Press, Columbia University, 1979.

Gibson, E. J., "Reading for Some Purpose." In J. J. Kavanagh and I. G. Mattingly, *Language by Ear and by Eye*, Cambridge, Mass.: The M.I.T. Press, 1972, 3–17.

Ginsburg, H. and S. Opper, *Piaget's Theory of Intellectual Development*, 2nd ed. Englewood Cliffs, New Jersey: Prentice-Hall, Inc., 1979. (Introduces Piaget's basic ideas and findings concerning children's intellectual development.)

Goodman, K. S., "The Know-More and the Know-Nothing Movements in Reading: A Personal Response." *Language Arts,* **56** (September 1979), 657–663.

Gruenewald, L. J., and S. A. Pollak, "The Speech Clinician's Role in Auditory Learning: Reading Readiness." *Language Speech and Hearing Services in Schools,* 4 (July 1973), 120–126. (Lists auditory activities associated with reading. Shows how the speech clinician is involved with the auditory-vocal language of children.)

Hacker, C. J., "From Schema Theory to Classroom Practice." *Language Arts,* **57** (Nov./Dec. 1980), 866–871.

Hall, M. A., "Language-Centered Reading: Premises and Recommendations." *Language Arts,* **56** (September 1979), 664–670.

——, *Teaching Reading as a Language Experience;* 2nd ed. Columbus, Ohio: Charles E. Merrill Publishing Company, 1976. (Gives the theoretical basis for the language experience approach and suggests how to proceed with this theory in the classroom.)

Halliday, M. A. K., *Explorations in the Functions of Language.* New York: American Elsevier, Inc., 1973. (Learning language is learning how to mean. Emphasizes the concept of linguistic focus as contributing to an understanding of language in socially significant contexts.)

——, *Learning How to Mean: Explorations in the Development of Language.* New York: American Elsevier, Inc., (1977). (Focuses on the functions that communication serves the child. Emphasizes the role of language in teaching and learning.)

Hammill, D. E., and S. C. Larsen, "The Relationship of Selected Auditory Perceptual Skills and Reading Ability." *Journal of Learning Disabilities,* **7** (August-September 1974), 429–435.

Hamre, C. E., "The Sesame Street Challenge." *Journal of Learning Disabilities,* **3** (April 1972), 207–209.

Haniff, M. H. and G. M. Siegel, "The Effect of Context on Verbal Elicited Imitations." *Journal of Speech and Hearing Disorders,* **46** (February 1981), 27–30. (Indicates that for most children performance on imitation tasks was significantly improved with picture context.)

Hegde, M. N., "An Experimental-Clinical Analysis of Grammatical and Behavior Distinction Between Auxiliary and Copula." *Journal of Speech and Hearing Research,* **23** (December 1980), 864–877. (Investigated whether auxiliary and copula belong to a single response class. Found that training in either generates production in both.)

Hendricks, B. L., "Beyond Dramatic Play." *Communication Education,* **26** (September 1977), 197–200. (Explains a semi-structured playing of a narrative thread by a child or group of children and an adult to provide opportunities for problem-solving.)

Hildebrand, V., *Guiding Young Children,* 2nd ed. New York: Macmillan Publishing Co., Inc., 1980. (Includes materials on mainstreaming of exceptional children, communicating with parents, and understanding behavior of children.)

Hutton, B. A., "Moving Language Around: Helping Students Become Aware of Language Structure." *Language Arts,* **57** (September 1980), 614–620.

(Includes material on: a rationale for developing concepts about language structure and some suggestions for developing concepts about language structure.)

Isaacs, N., *A Brief Introduction to Piaget.* New York: Schocken Books, Inc., 1974.

James, S. L., and M. Button, "Choosing Stimulus Materials for Eliciting Language Samples from Children with Language Disorders." *Language, Speech, and Hearing Services in Schools,* **9** (April 1978), 91–97.

Kaliski, L., R. Tankersley, and R. Iogha, *Structured Dramatics for Children with Learning Disabilities.* San Rafael, Calif., Academic Therapy Publishing Company, 1971.

Kirby, E. A., W. Lyle, and B. Ambie, "Reading and Psycholinguistic Processes of Innate Problem Readers," *Journal of Learning Disabilities,* **5** (May 1972), 295–298.

Klein, M., *Talk in the Language Arts Classroom.* Urbana, Ill.: National Council of Teachers of English, 1977. (Explains oral language, its pragmatism and factors influencing its application and development in children.

Kramer, C. A., S. L. James and J. H. Saxman, "A Comparison of Language Samples Elicited at Home and in the Clinic." *Journal of Speech and Hearing Disorders,* **44** (August 1979), 321–330.

Lasky, E. Z. and A. M. Chapandy, "Factors Affecting Language Comprehension." *Language, Speech, and Hearing Services in Schools,* **7** (1976), 159–168. (Shows the effects of syntactic complexity, semantic familiarity, interaction between the semantic and syntactic complexity, contextual clues, and rate of presentation in messages presented to listeners by a clinician or a teacher.)

Leonard, L. B., "A Preliminary View of Generalization in Language Training." *Journal of Speech and Hearing Disorders,* **39** (November 1974), 429–436.

———, "What is Deviant Language?" *Journal of Speech and Hearing Disorders,* **37** (November 1972), 427–446. (Suggests the way to determine clinically significant aspects of syntactical deviations and to distinguish between the slow language developer and the deviant language developer.)

——— and L. Reid, "Children's Judgments of Utterance Appropriateness." *Journal of Speech and Hearing Research,* **22** (September 1979), 500–515.

Lesser, H. and D. Drouin, "Training in the Use of Double Function Terms." *Journal of Psycholinguistic Research,* **4** (1975), 285–303.

Levenstein, P. "Cognitive Growth in Pre-Schoolers Through Verbal Interaction with Mothers." *American Journal of Orthopsychiatry,* **40** (April 1970), 426–432.

Liles, B. J., and M. D. Shulman, "The Grammaticality Task: A Tool for Language Assessment and Language Intervention." *Language, Speech and Hearing Services in Schools,* **11** (October 1980), 260–265. (Tells how to obtain a language sample. Describes gramaticality task.)

Lindfors, J. W., *Children's Language and Learning.* Englewood Cliffs, New Jersey: Prentice-Hall, Inc., 1980. (Synthesizes research in language. Includes material on language—structure, acquisition, cognition, in social contexts, and linguistic variations.)

Lodge, D. M., and E. A. Leach, "Children's Acquisition of Idioms in the English Language." *Journal of Speech and Hearing Research,* **18** (September 1975), 521–529. (Shows strong preference for literal meaning in younger children.)

Mahoney, G. J., "Approach to Delayed Language Acquisition." *American Journal of Mental Deficiency,* **80** (1975), 139–145.

Mattingly, I. G., "Reading for Linguistic Process and Linguistic Awareness." In J. J. Kavanagh and I. G. Mattingly, Eds., *Language by Ear and Eye,* Cambridge, Mass.: The M.I.T. Press, 1972, 133–147.

Mecham, M. J., "Enhancing Environments for Children with Cultural-Linguistic Differences." *Language, Speech, and Hearing Services in the Schools,* **6** (July 1975), 156–160. (Proposes the thesis that attitudinal tensions affect relationships between different socioeconomic classes and that such differences may be recognized in dialectal or linguistic characteristics.)

———, "Measurement of Verbal Listening Accuracy in Children," *Journal of Learning Disabilities,* **4** (May 1971), 257–272.

Meline, T. J., "The Application of Reinforcement in Language Intervention." *Language, Speech, and Hearing Services in Schools,* **11** (April 1980), 95–101. (Talks about natural reinforcements versus token reinforcements.)

Menyuk, P., and P. L. Looney, "Relationships among Components of the Grammar." *Journal of Speech and Hearing Research,* **15** (June 1972), 395–406. (Examines the relationship between the accuracy of repetition of syntactic structures and phonological sequences by language-disordered children and the effect of meaning on the phonological sequence repetition accuracy of a group of language-disordered and normal speaking children.)

Meyer, W. J., and J. Shane, "The Form and Function of Children's Questions." *Journal of Genetic Psychology,* **123** (December 1973), 285–296. (Compares the question-asking behavior between two groups of children separated by a span of some three years. In general, the data support Piaget's conceptualizations concerning question-asking behavior.)

Milligan, J. L., and R. E. Potter, "The Peabody Language Development Kit and Its Function in a Language Development and Pre-Reading Program." *Reading World,* **2** (December 1971), 130–136. (Review the studies of the values of the Peabody Kit.)

Mog, C., "A Language Experience Bibliography." *Language Arts,* **55** (November-December 1978), 979–980.

Moran, M. R., and M. C. Byrne, "Mastery of Verb Tense Markers by Normal and Learning Disabled Children," *Journal of Speech and Hearing Research,* **20** (1977), 529–542.

Muma, J. R., *Language Handbook: Concepts, Assessment, Intervention.* Englewood Cliffs, New Jersey: Prentice-Hall, Inc., 1978. "The Communication Game: Dump and Play." *Journal of Speech and Hearing Disorders,* **40** (August 1975), 296–309. (Explains the dump and play operations and the social enterprise of the speaker-listener situation. Dump operations refer to mental processes in preparing and giving a message. Play operations refer to adapting the message (such as changes in semantic or syntactic structure) so that the listener is able to respond to the message.)

————, "Language Assessment: Some Underlying Assumptions." *ASHA*, **15** (July 1973), 331–337. (Contains an excellent bibliography.)

Musselwhite, C. R. and S. Barrie-Blackley, "Three Variations of the Imperative Format of Language Sample Elicitation." *Language, Speech, and Hearing Services in School*, **11** (January 1980), 56–67. (Elicited samples on basis of noun task, procedure task, and action task. The variations are noted.)

Navratil, K., and M. Petrasek, "An Approach to Mainstreaming Language-Disabled Children in the Elementary School." *Language, Speech, and Hearing Services in Schools*, **9** (January 1978), 17–23. (Describes a program which provides daily resource remediation to elementary school children with language handicaps.)

Nelson, L. K., and M. Weber-Olsen, "The Elicited Language Inventory and the Influence of Contextual Clues." *Journal of Speech and Hearing Disorders*, **45** (November 1980), 549–563. (Indicates the importance of contextual clues in obtaining language samples.)

Panagos, J. M., "Persistence of the Open Syllable Reinterpreted as a Symptom of Language Disorder," *Journal of Speech and Hearing Disorders*. **39** (February 1974), 23–31.

Piaget, J., (trans. by M. Gabain), *The Language and Thought of the Child*. New York: New American Library, Meridian, 1974.

————, (trans. by Helen Weaver), *Psychology of the Child*. New York: Basic Books, Inc., 1969.

Rees, N. S., "Imitative and Language Development Issues and Clinical Implications." *Journal of Speech and Hearing Disorders*, **40** (August 1975), 339–350.

————, "The Speech Pathologist and the Reading Process," *ASHA*, **16** (May 1974), 255–257. (Talks about the contribution that the speech pathologist can make to the process of reading acquisition both in normal and learning-disabled children.)

————, "Auditory Processing Factors in Language Disorders: The View from Procrustes' Bed." *Journal of Speech and Hearing Disorders*, **38** (August 1973), 304–315. (Cites the evidence and the lack of it for an auditory perceptual factor in language learning and disorders.)

————, "Bases of Decision in Language Training." *Journal of Speech and Hearing Disorders*, **37** (August 1972), 283–304. (Discusses six theoretical bases for selecting grammatical structures in training language-disordered children.

Robinson, H. A., "Psycholinguistics, Sociolinguistics, Reading, and the Classroom Teacher." *International Reading Association Conference Papers*, **17** (1972).

Saltz, R. "Children's Interpretations of Proverbs." *Language Arts*, **56** (May 1979), 508–513.

Sawyer, D. J., "The Relationship Between Selected Auditory Abilities and Beginning Reading Achievement." *Language, Speech, and Hearing Services in the Schools*, **12** (April 1981), 95–99.

Schiefelbusch, R. L. (Ed.), *Bases of Language Intervention*, Baltimore, MD: University Park Press, 1978.

Schiefelbusch, R. L., and L. L. Lloyds, Eds., *Language Perspectives: Acquisition Retardation, and Intervention.* Baltimore: University Park Press, 1973.

Schwartz, E. R., and C. B. Solot, "Response Patterns Characteristic of Verbal Expressive Disorders." *Language, Speech, and Hearing Services in the Schools,* 11 (July 1980), 139–144. (Examines the need to analyze free expression as part of assessment of language in school age children. Lists linguistic symptoms of language delay.)

Schwartz, J. I., "Implication of Early Linguistic and Cognitive Development for Teaching Reading." *Language Arts,* 56 (September 1979), 675–680. (Notes that language experience is essential.)

Scofield, S. J., "The Language-Delayed Child in the Mainstreamed Primary Classroom." *Language Arts,* 55 (September 1978), 719–723. (Includes strategies for working with language-delayed children.)

Searle, J., *Speech Arts.* London: Cambridge University Press, 1969.

Semel, E. M., and E. H. Wiig, "Comprehension of Syntactic Structures and Critical Verbal Elements by Children with Learning Disabilities." *Journal of Learning Disabilities,* 8 (January 1975), 46–53.

Shewan, C. M., "The Language Disordered Child in Relation to Muma's Communication Game," *Journal of Speech and Hearing Disorders,* 40 (August 1975), 310–314. (Indicates that the concept of communicative competence is clinically relevant and important.)

Shipley, K. G., and S. C. McFarlane, "Facilitating Reading Development with Speech and Language Impaired Children." *Language , Speech, and Hearing Services in Schools,* 12 (April 1981), 100–106. (Suggests ways in which the speech/language clinician can help in developing reading abilities.)

Shuy, R. W. and P. Griffin, Eds., *The Study of Children's Functional Language and Education in the Early Years.* Washington, D.C., The Center for Applied Linguistics, 1978.

Silvestri, S. and R. Silvestri, "A Developmental Analysis of the Acquisition of Compound Words." *Language, Speech, and Hearing Services in Schools,* 8 (1977), 217–221. (Examines the acquisition of compound words in relation to receptive vocabulary and grade level.)

Simon, C. S., "Cooperative Communication Programming: A Partnership Between the Learning Disabilities Teacher and the Speech-Language Pathologist." *Language, Speech, and Hearing Services in Schools,* 8 (1977), 188–200. (Lists how speech-language clinicians and learning disabilities specialist can cooperate.)

Snow, C., "The Development of Conversation between Mothers and Babies." *Journal of Child Language,* 4 (1977), 1–22.

———, "Mothers' Speech to Children Learning Language." *Child Development,* 43 (1972), 549–565.

Snyder-McClean, L. K., and J. E. McClean, "Verbal Information Gathering Strategies: The Child's Use of Language to Acquire Language." *Journal of Speech and Hearing Disorders,* 43 (August 1978), 306–325. (Views language development delay as a process rather than product deficit. Suggests that selective imitation partnership is functional at specific stages of language development.)

Stark, J., "Reading Failure: A Language Based Problem." *ASHA*, **17** (December 1975), 832–834.

———, R. L. Rosenbaum, D. Schwartz, and A. Wisan, "The Nonverbal Child: Some Clinical Guidelines." *Journal of Speech and Hearing Disorders*, **38** (February 1973), 59–72. (Describes principles and procedures related to language training for nonverbal children.)

Stauffer, R., *The Language Experience Approach to the Teaching of Reading*, 2nd Ed., New York: Harper & Row, Publishers, 1980.

Stegmaier, N. K., "Teaching Interpersonal Communication Through Children's Literature." *Elementary English*, **51** (October 1974), 927–932. (Explains how children's literature can be a vehicle for communicative activities that further honest, wholesome, and sound interpersonal relationships.)

Tyack, D. L., "Teaching Complex Sentences." *Language, Speech, and Hearing Services in Schools*, **12** (January 1981), 49–56.

——— and R. H. Gottsleben, "Constructing Reading Material to Match a Child's Oral Language Patterns." *Journal of Learning Disabilities*, **10** (December 1977), 12–16.

Vasta, R., and R. M. Lievert, "Auditory Discrimination—Syntactic Structure." *Developmental Psychology*, **9** (1973), 79–82.

Veatch, J. et al., *Key Words to Reading: The Language Experience Approach Begins*. Columbus, Ohio: Charles E. Merrill Publishing Company, 1979. (Tells how to develop. organize, and implement a reading/language arts program based on a child's own language experiences.)

Wadsworth, B. J., *Piaget's Theory of Cognitive Development*. New York: David McKay Co., Inc., 1973.

Wakefield, M. W., "Sequential Memory Responses of Normal and Clinic Readers." *Elementary English*, **50** (September 1973), 930–939.

———, and N. J. Silvaroli, "A Study of Oral Language Patterns of Low Socioeconomic Groups." *The Reading Teacher*, **22** (April 1969), 622–624. (Attempts to discover whether differences in speech patterns were influenced more by the ethnic or socioeconomic background of the children. Results indicated that economic background was a stronger influence on language than ethnic background.)

Westby, C. E., "Assessment of Cognitive and Language Abilities Through Play." *Language, Speech, and Hearing Services in Schools*, **11** (July 1980), 154–168. (Describes ten stages in development of symbolic play abilities and relates language concepts and structures at various levels.)

White, D. E., "Language Experience." *Language Arts*, **57** (November-December 1980), 888–889. (Contains a bibliography with emphasis on reading through language experience.)

Wilcox, M. J. and L. B. Leonard, "Experimental Acquisition of Wh-Questions in Language-Disordered Children." *Journal of Speech and Hearing Research*, **21** (June 1978), 220–239.

9

Delayed or Retarded Language Acquisition and Development

The speech/language clinician and the classroom teacher who are concerned with a linguistically retarded child are faced, among other things, with the effects of delayed intervention. The attitude of "Don't worry, Johnny (or Mary) is likely to grow out of it," however well intentioned, is not supported by recent evidence, which indicates that there is a primary need to identify the "it" that the child is likely to outgrow. There is a critically important difference between the child who understands language and has begun to show such understanding before one year of age but is not yet speaking intelligibly at eighteen months and one who neither understands nor produces language. The first child may catch up; the second probably will not. Bricker and Carlson (1981, p. 479), based on the results of studies on early cognitive development and language acquisition, argue for the usefulness of (1) early (preschool age) intervention, (2) viewing language as interactive with and dependent upon other behavioral systems, and (3) the importance of environmental context.

We may not be able to undo the total effects of tardy intervention for a linguistically delayed child. There is, fortunately, much that can be done to minimize if not to overcome the developmental implications of what, at best, is benign neglect. To avoid any possibility of misunderstanding, when we use the terms *linguistic delay* or *linguistic retardation* or *delayed language development,* we are not referring to a child who lisps, or substitutes a *w* or *y*[j] sound for *l* or *r*. We are referring to children who, if they have such errors, have other deficiencies as well. These deficiencies or improficiencies include overall

231

slow development of articulation, sparse vocabularies, and slow acquisition of syntactic (grammatical) constructions. Perhaps even more important than these productive-expressive and therefore communicative limitations are those for language comprehension.

The most severe linguistic retardates may not be in school, or if they are, in special classes as part of mainstreaming programs. Some who have auditory perceptual problems may be in classes for aphasic or dysphasic children. Those with hearing impairments so severe as to render them deaf usually require special educational approaches, and may divide their time between instructional settings in keeping with their needs and regular classrooms. Identifications and approaches for these linguistically retarded children are considered in separate chapters.

The term *delayed language development* as it is usually applied to school-age children refers to a range of problems. If we except the most severely delayed for the reasons stated above, we have children who seem to comprehend and can engage in social conversations but have difficulty in understanding instructional language, who fail to appreciate subtleties that do not escape their age peers, and who have a vocabulary that limits them in communicative efforts. Others may have numerous articulatory defects, speak in comparatively short and simple sentences, and have difficulty in understanding complex sentences that are readily decoded by their age peers. Their deficiencies may become more apparent in their reading comprehension and their written language. Some children seem to persevere in their infantile articulation. Assessment of such children may reveal that they are also delayed in their syntactic and semantic acquisitions.

There are exceptions to these generalizations. There are some "late starters" who do catch up by school age or by the time they are six or seven years of age. These children are likely to come from families that include other "late starters." However, as we suggested earlier, though some children may be slow in producing language, in the absence of sensory, emotional, central auditory, or severe intellectual involvements, those "late starters" in active language use who "catch up" are not *late* in their capacity for comprehending spoken language.

IDENTIFYING LANGUAGE DELAY

Many children who enter school with delayed language development may be identified as requiring help for articulatory defects by the time they reach the second or third grade. These children do not suddenly or belatedly develop their articulatory difficulties. For the most part, their articulatory proficiency was delayed as one aspect of their overall language development. By the time the children began to establish a working vocabulary and a fair degree of syntactic ability, the defective articulatory component of their language acquisition became more obvious.

Menyuk (1964) compared 10 children diagnosed as using infantile speech with 10 matched children, ages 3.0 years to 5.10 years. The I.Q.s of the two groups were approximately 126, based on the Ammons Full-Range Picture Vocabulary Test. Menyuk concluded from her data that the term *infantile*, in regard to articulation, appears to be an incorrect designation because "at no age level did the grammatical production of a child with deviant speech match or closely match the grammatical production of a child with normal speech from two years on." Our own observations support those of Menyuk, with even greater differences found for children who are within the normal or below-average range of intelligence. Along the same line, and perhaps even more emphatically, Ingram (1977, p. 122) asserts that ". . . deviant phonology may be not just a phonemic disorder, but a more global linguistic one. . . . this added dimension provides some important implications for therapy."

Children with serious delay in language (verbal production) per se are not likely to progress normally in the primary grades. There are, of course, occasional and important exceptions. We sometimes find children with severe oral linguistic impairments who nevertheless learn to read and write and so evidence their educational achievement. More often, however, children with serious delays in language development also have difficulties in learning to read and to write and are generally retarded in educational achievement.

For the most part, the classroom teacher of the nonexceptional child may have one or two children who have the residuals of delayed language. These children often need the help of the speech/language clinician to improve their articulatory proficiency. They are likely also to need help with other aspects of language development.

MENTAL RETARDATION AND LANGUAGE DELAY

Despite recent criticism of intelligence tests as instruments for assessing mental capacity and intellectual potential, the relationship between functional mental retardation and language delay continues to be evident. We are still able to observe that the chief cause of prolonged language (speech) delay is mental retardation. This is so for the onset of speech as well as for the development of speech after onset. There is, however, considerable recent evidence that with direct teaching and training, many severely mentally retarded children are able to learn to speak even though they could not acquire speech by a "normal" amount of exposure in an essentially normal language environment.

In an experiment at the Institute for Childhood Aphasia at San Francisco State University, a group of severely retarded children (IQ's below 50) who had no functional oral language were directly taught language with a program primarily used for aphasic children. After a five-month, four-hour-per-week training period most of the children learned to understand and use a considerable amount of functional language. Emphasis in training was on vocabulary building, language concepts, and basic syntactic structures. Most of the children reached a level equivalent to a two-to-three-word mean length of utterance. This is roughly comparable to the acquisition of mean length of utterance in children between 15 and 18 months of age. All of the children learned some socially useful language.

With due reservation for and about intelligence testing and testers of intelligence, we present some studies that indicate the relationship between mental retardation and language delay. However, we again emphasize that *findings may be reversible* and are, often, happily, influenced by therapy.[1]

Lillywhite and Bradley (1969, p. 11) report that in a survey of communication impairment among the educably mentally retarded in the Portland, Oregon, public schools, 12 per cent were found to have speech and/or language defects, as compared with 4.5 per cent among the nonretarded. Generally, in their survey, Lillywhite and Bradley observed that the most severely retarded, those with IQ's ranging from 40 to 70, presented a variety of defects, including articulatory, functional, and organic voice quality disturbances such as excessive nasality, huskiness, and language delay. "All of the children showed speech and language functioning in one way or another significantly inferior to expectation based upon mental age." They were, of course, considerably more inferior in terms of actual age expectations. Contributing causes of speech defects are hearing losses, found in greater incidence among retardates than among nonretardates, as well as sluggish control of palatal and pharyngeal structures.

---

[1] P. W. Drash in "Habilitation of the Retarded Child: A Remedial Program," *The Journal of Special Education,* **6** (1972) reports on a delayed language child who tested at age four in the mid-50 to mid-60 I.Q. range on standardized tests of intelligence. After two years of speech and language training, the child tested well within the normal range of intelligence. Academic acheivement in two years of elementary school was also well within the average range.

Luchsinger and Arnold (1967, pp. 513–544) report that 52 per cent (69 of 134 cases) diagnosed as having delayed language development in a large New York City clinic tested on intake as having Intelligence Quotients below 75. Another 16 tested at the borderline level (I.Q. 80). As in the Lillywhite and Bradley survey, contributing or associated causes were also present. These included Down's syndrome, childhood schizophrenia, and endocrine disturbances.

Let us accept the notion of mental retardation as representing present capacity related to past experience and innate but not necessarily realized potential. On this basis we will find correlations between mental retardation and language proficiency along the following lines: the most severely mentally retarded may never acquire functional speech; moderately retarded children usually do acquire speech, but often with numerous defects in articulation, impoverished vocabularies, and very limited syntax; mildly retarded children acquire speech, but are likely to have limited vocabularies and use relatively simple sentence constructions. In general, moderate and mildly retarded children parallel and "shadow" normal children in all aspects of language development. Naremore and Dever (1975) studied the language performance of educable mentally retarded and normal children in the six-to-ten years age range. They found that the retarded children tended to use simpler grammatical constructions than the normal children. Specifically in regard to ten-year-olds, the investigators observed that the retarded children used few subordinate clauses and more "and" or "and then" constructions to relate parts of sentences. However, "The development . . . appears to be in the same direction as that of the normal child, although the same levels are not attained."

We sometimes find children with moderate mental retardation who seem to have as many words as their age peers. A discerning listener may be able to note, however, that these children use the words less meaningfully and that the words lack depth and richness of concept. It is our observation that some mentally retarded children who are well trained and well taught are able to acquire appropriate words on a low level of meaning for many situations and events.

Some mentally retarded children who "know the words but not too many of the meanings" may manage to get through the primary grades without too much trouble. These children, by virtue of the "halo effect" of their apparent linguistic ability, may not seem to be mentally retarded until they reach a level in school where the teacher begins to note their difficulty in dealing with concepts or ideas that cannot readily be objectified.

It is also important to recognize that there are some children whose difficulty with oral language makes them appear to be mentally retarded when they are not. Some children who are suspected of being mentally retarded because of their delayed development may, upon examination with nonlanguage tests of intelligence, turn out to be normal, or even above average, in intelligence. Other causes, such as slow general physiologic development, emotional disturbances, or hearing loss, may account for the language delay. The possibility of error in arriving at a causal diagnosis of mental retardation for language delay points to the need for a competent clinical psychologist or school psychologist to examine the suspected child and make an evaluation. If this cannot be done, both the speech/language clinician and the classroom teacher may entertain hypotheses about the child concerned, but judgments should be withheld until justified. They should be especially careful to reserve judgment about possible mental retardation for the child with uneven school achievement. If the child does average or better work when oral language is not required, but does poorly in areas that require speech competency, we should seek the cause for the disparity rather than conclude that we are dealing with a "nontypical" but nevertheless mentally retarded child.

Figure 10, taken from Lenneberg (1967, p. 169) presents a graphic comparison of the language development of retardates and normal children in relation to milestones for sitting and walking.

The classroom teacher is most likely to have contact with moderately (educable) retarded children. In general, these children tend to "shadow" normal children in their language acquisitions, developing language, articulatory proficiencies, and communication skills at a delayed rate. Weiss and Lillywhite (1981, p. 185) observe that

> . . . it is a mistake to assume that the delay is the only problem with communicative skills. Many other factors are involved, such as poor physical coordination, faulty or absent early stimulation, and the fact that the retardation creates a different environment for the child, which adds errors to speech, language, and often to behavior. These factors are likely to cause more delay than the mental age of the child would lead one to anticipate, as well as speech and language distortions beyond expectations for the intellectual and physical status of the child.

With individual exceptions, the most likely and apparent speech deficiencies of the moderately retarded child are in articulation. Some of the errors may be an expression of developmental lag and may include the simplification of sound blends (e.g., *poon* for *spoon, tand* for *stand, ty* for *try*), sound substitutions, omissions of final consonants, and distortions. At the risk of overgeneralizations, these errors may be regarded as the maintenance of normal infantilisms. Those sounds that are normally last to be controlled—the sounds *r, s, z, n, sh, ch, th*

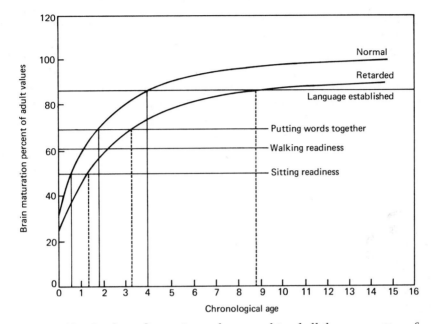

FIGURE 10. On the ordinate, Lenneberg combined all the parameters of brain maturation into a single factor. "Retarded children presumably attain the maturational values later in life than normal children. Attainment of brain maturation is correlated with behavioral achievements shown here as 'horizons.' A comparison of the growth curves of normal and retarded children explains why the relative distances among the various milestones become greater with advancing age. Normally, a child begins to join words together about 15 months after he is ready to sit up; in a retarded child it may take 24 months to achieve this. It takes about two years to acquire the general basis for language establishment once a normal child has begun to put words together. In a retarded child it may take five years or more to acquire the same facility in language." (From E. H. Lenneberg, *Biological Foundations of Language*, New York: John Wiley & Sons, Inc., 1967, p. 169.)

and *l*—are likely candidates for distortions (see tables on pp. 164 and 168–9 in Chapter 7).

Language deficiencies include a limited vocabulary and slow grammatical acquisition. These limitations tend, of course, to mirror receptive inadequacies. However, it is not always clear whether and when the overall language deficiencies are not a reflection of their cognitive development. It may well be that many if not most retarded children are really no more limited in their ability to say what they think and feel than are most normal children. Verbal facility varies greatly with the normal. We should expect such facility to be variable among the retarded.

Yoder and Miller (1972), based on their own observations and a review of the literature, found a positive correlation between level of intelligence and such linguistic factors as sentence length, sentence complexity, sentence completeness, and tense and structural variety. The lowest correlation was for the most severe retardates; the highest, but below that for children with normal I.Qs, was for the mild retardates. For an excellent review of the relationship of mental retardation to speech and language development we recommend Chapter 12 by McLean and Synder-McLean in R. J. Van Hattum, Ed. *Communicative Disorders*, Macmillan (1980).

As indicated earlier, problems of speech (voice or articulation), as well as of language, increase in severity and incidence and are more severe among retardates. These deficiencies are often associated with physical conditions that include organic anomalies and hearing loss. In their survey Lillywhite and Bradley (1969, pp. 13–14) report that educably retarded school age children have two to three times more hearing loss than the nonretarded population. The percentage and *severity* of loss increase with the more severely retarded.

Therapeutic Intervention for the Mentally Retarded

Treatment for the mentally retarded, whether we are dealing with "biological types" or with those whose development may be functionally delayed, should take the form of education and training geared to the cognitive and sensorimotor capacities of the individual child. Our emphasis would be on vocabulary building, language concepts, and syntax (grammar) associated with semantics (meanings) with intelligible communication as the goal. For low level retardates, socially functional language may be both the immediate and ultimate goal. However, an effort for more advanced language should be tried, even for children regarded as among the most severely mentally retarded.

Stimulation and improvement of the home environment, if this is possible, should help to bring the retardate to a level where potential for language usage and articulatory proficiency become highly and positively correlated. Specific training for the correction of specific articulatory and vocal defects is indicated for the higher grade retardates. Such children may be members of slow progress or "special" classes. For most children, a reasonable achievement objective is to strive for the proficiency level of a normal child whose chronological age is equal to that of the mental age of the retardate. In the absence of sensory, motor, or personality involvements, this level of achievement may be reached for most higher level retardates. (Miller, 1981, p. 335) Little progress, however, may be expected beyond age 14 (Goda and Griffith 1962 and Lenneberg 1967, pp. 154–155).

Language, regardless of the specific system or modality for intake and output, has one dominating purpose, to enable the speaker to communicate. Whatever the immediate therapeutic goal may be, the ultimate objective should always be to help the child to establish the basic skills that make communication possible. Unrealistic goals will frustrate this achievement.

Although voice and articulatory defects occur in a higher incidence in retardates than in children of normal intelligence, the chief factor in the mentally retarded child's communicative difficulties are to be found in limited and inadequate language. As already suggested, a lack of early stimulation and often a continued lack of parent-child interaction are high among the nonorganic causes.

What in language, in form (structure) and content, do we teach (stimulate and motivate) to retarded children who are slow in language development? By *slow* we imply even slower than we may have a right to expect based upon their degree of retardation. Miller and Yoder (1972) provide an answer. Based upon a review of the literature completed in 1970, they concluded that mentally retarded children who do have language develop their language code in a manner similar to that of normal children *but at a slower rate*. The implication of this finding is that what we know about normal language acquisition provides a basis for the language training of retarded children. The sample syntactic structures presented in Chapter 7 on "The Development of Language" constitute a body of information based upon normal language acquisition. Beyond this, we can endorse Miller and Yoder's (1974, pp. 507–508) principles and criteria for the individual retarded child. With some modification to reflect our own position, we have incorporated the Miller and Yoder criteria as follows.[2]

1. A language training program should begin by looking at where each child is linguistically (stage or level of development as ascertained by standardized testing or the analysis of a representative language sample). The program should project increments as to where the child should be helped to advance.
2. A program should be based on a realistic set of goals or behaviors in regard to language, both for the communication of ideas and the expression of feelings. The latter, admittedly, may come more easily and spontaneously as acquisitions by exposure to older speakers in

[2] Although these criteria are presented as specific to mentally retarded children, we believe that they pertain to all children who are retarded in language development.

the environment. A program should include intermediate and tentative terminal behaviors. These should be related and relevant to the child's home, social, and educational environment as well as to individual development capacities.

3. A program should be founded on what we now know about normal language acquisition.
4. A program should anticipate the variety of circumstances and situations that involve children and older speakers in their environments.[3]
5. Overall communicative competence, both verbal and nonverbal, should be aspects of the social goals.
6. A program should have a systematic approach to help the child achieve appropriate and proficient language. The systematic approach may employ operant procedures and techniques, or other approaches compatible with the speech/language clinician and the child. Seldom does inspiration of the moment suffice. However, a sensitive speech/language clinician will follow a child's lead if unexpected circumstances or unexpected language behaviors are presented.

It has become increasingly clear that language training to be meaningful requires interaction rather than drill. Interaction-communicative interchanges on a level consonant with the cognitive capacity of the child, based on assumptions and guidelines recommended by Bricker and Carlson (1981, p. 498), follow:

1. Early developmental processes are intimately related and virtually inseparable from educational or therapeutic objectives.
2. Children are constantly engaging in activities that involve other persons and so should normally instigate reciprocal behavior, including intervention efforts.
3. Behavior, including language learning, generally changes from the simple to the complex, thus providing behavioral goals (language included) for therapeutic intervention.
4. Disequilibrium (increasing and changing environmental demands) is required for the child to learn and establish new adaptive responses.

These objectives are, of course, not exclusively intended for the mentally retarded. They hold as well for all children with speech or language handicaps.

[3] Approaches for linguistic retardates that are directed toward the family, to teach the family intervention strategies, are described by MacDonald (1978).

Non-oral Communicative Approaches

Severe mental retardates, children who at best are considered to be trainable but not educable, are likely to have little functional oral language. Several recent studies indicate that a non-oral system may be taught with enough success in a sufficient number of cases to encourage the use of signing as an alternate mode of communication. Silverman (1980, Chap. 2) reviewed recently published and unpublished studies on the use of signing with mental retardates and other non-oral persons—the autistic and the orally apraxic (children who may hear and understand speech but who cannot control their organs of articulation to produce intelligible speech). We will restate some of Silverman's tentative conclusions:

1. Teaching a non-oral person to employ a nonspeech mode of communication does not have a negative effect on his or her motivation for eventually acquiring speech for communication.
2. Learning to use a nonspeech mode of communication may have a positive impact on verbal output. That is, a non-oral mode of communication may actually increase verbal output in some children.

It is not presently possible to assess all of the positive or possibly negative effects of the use of signing systems with severely retarded children. The studies reported by Silverman vary as to the kind of sign system taught and include American Sign Language (ASL), the American Indian Sign Language, Signing Exact English, and Signed English. The ages of the children studied and the degree of severity also varied. However, based on nine of the studies reported by Silverman that comprised 105 cases, 37 (35 per cent) are reported to have shown positive effect as judged by increased attempts at speech, compared with 68 (65 per cent) who, though they may have acquired some signing ability, did not increase in their attempts at oral speech. Important by-products even among the children who did not increase their attempts at oral language were observed. "13 of the children were reported to have noticeable changes in behavior,—i.e., reduction in frustration behavior such as temper tantrums and being more willing to participate in language activities" (Duncan and Silverman, 1977) and "increased willingness to interact with others; increased attention span" (Kimble, 1975).

Kahn (1981) is generally optimistic about the implications of the results of a study with hearing, nonverbal retarded children who were taught signing. The subjects, 12 children, ranged in age from 53 to 101 months, all diagnosed as profoundly retarded. Eight of the children were taught signing, four with accompanying oral language and four without; four children (the placebo group) were instructed in areas that did not include communication. Kahn notes that most of the children who were taught signing, with or without accompanying oral language (total communication), also began to produce oral language up to three- and four-word utterances. The placebo children did not. Kahn concluded that "In general, the teaching of sign language appears to be a useful procedure for some children." Further, Kahn observes "Future research should be directed toward comparing different sign training approaches . . . and toward investigating ways in which the transfer of signing to speech may be enhanced."

HEARING LOSS: THE DEAF[4]

Deaf children have insufficient hearing, at the time when speech normally is learned, to enable them to acquire oral language ability through the sense of hearing. Children with a hearing loss that is severe enough for them to be diagnosed as deaf do not learn to speak orally unless they are specially trained to do so through the use of devices and techniques that are not necessary for children with normal hearing. Virtually all children with severe hearing loss are likely to have significant defects of articulation, voice, and almost always of language development (vocabulary and syntax). However, as we observed in our discussion of the prelingual stages in language development, up to six months of age the vocalizations of deaf children are not ordinarily different from those of hearing children. Between six and eight months of age, differences in vocalizations and utterances between the deaf and the hearing tend to be quantitative rather than qualitative (Lenneberg 1964, p. 153). The deaf infant has a reduced inventory of sounds and spends less time in sound play than does the hearing child. This observation has an important therapeutic implication. If the child is recognized early as having a severe hearing loss every effort should be made by the parents to encourage vocalization and sound play. The parents should, for example, make certain that the child sees the parent who is talking, especially in direct parent-child interchange. Simple repeated statements should be directed to the child. A mirror, strategically placed above the child, may stimulate talking to the mirror image. Such activities will encourage the deaf child not to become a silent child. The child may respond to the low-pitched vocalization of the adult, that is, to the voice per se, and then

---

[4] The problems of the deaf and hard-of-hearing children are considered in some detail in Chapter 14.

learn to look and see, and perhaps begin to face-read some of the speech of the adult. Appropriate gestures accompanying the speech of the adult may well enhance the deaf child's understanding of the adult's speech.

The problems of the deaf child for language learning are sometimes complicated by some degree of associated mental retardation or by slower mental maturation. However, Lenneberg (1964, p. 156), after reviewing the literature on cognitive, nonverbal investigations of deaf children, observes: "On strictly cognitive tasks it has been experimentally shown that even pre-school and thus 'pre-language' deaf children perform no worse than hearing children."

Signing and the Deaf Child

The extent of delay in language development for many, if not for most, deaf children may be appreciated when we realize that the normal hearing child at primary school age has a *speaking* vocabulary of 2,000 or more words—and several times that number for comprehension. In sharp contrast, the deaf child who enters a school for the deaf at age five may have no working vocabulary at all. The deaf child who has not acquired either an oral or a gesture (sign) system that can be used with at least one other person to communicate and express thoughts and feelings is without functional language.

This is the basis of the position taken by Furth (1966, pp. 226–228) on the need to establish an early visual language (gesture) system for congenitally deaf children. Learning to talk, and so to think, without recourse to oral language enhances the deaf child's cognitive and intellectual development. Waiting to establish an oral language system may impair such development. So, Furth argues, "as a direct result of linguistic incompetence, the deaf fail or are poor in all tasks which are specifically verbal or on a few non-verbal tasks in which linguistic habits afford a direct advantage." As an indirect result, the deaf lack information and exhibit a minimal amount of intellectual curiosity. Moreover, "they have less opportunity and training to think." Based on these observations, Furth proposes that the deficiences associated with the linguistic incompetence of the deaf "would be avoidable if non-verbal methods of instruction and communication were encouraged both at home in the earliest years and in formal school education." He suggests that at home "parents must have recourse to distinguishable signs and use these together with speech. Practically all deaf children, instead of the present 10 per cent, could then be expected to reach a basic competence in English, just as all hearing children in any society learn the language to which they are exposed."

Furth may be overoptimistic in his projection of the training of deaf children through nonverbal (we believe he means nonoral) means. However, we accept his position that the intellectual potentials of most deaf children, as well as their linguistic limitations, could be improved if the implications of his suggestions are followed.

In recent years there is evidence of increased interest in the early introduction of a signing system for children who are identified as deaf. Educators of the deaf who recommend teaching a sign system find support for their position in studies that report advantages in language comprehension, academic achievement, and social skills in children who are exposed to signing early in life (Moores, 1970). Many educators who advocate signing also recommend that deaf children be simultaneously exposed to oral language (speech) as they respond to signs. This approach—simultaneous exposure to a signing system and oral speech—is referred to as *total* communication. Some advocates of an oral/aural approach for teaching deaf children continue to resist signing or the total (signing and speaking) approach. Their opposition is based on the assumption that children who sign have a limited social and vocational future. Further, children who sign are likely to resist learning oral language, a much more difficult achievement than signing. Certainly the final word has not been said on the controversy between the "oralists" and the "manualists." More long-term studies will be needed to enable us to predict for which deaf children oral language is a possible accomplishment, and for which a likely achievement—as well as for whom the results are likely to be only frustration born of failure. Further, we need more studies that will assess whether the long-term social, educational, and vocational outlooks favor children who have been exposed only to signing over those exposed to total communication or those educated with an oral approach.

Sanders (1980, 235–237) reviews the difference in position between the "oralists" and the "manualists" and makes some cogent observations.

> What is clear is that the issue should not be approached in the political terms of proving one method to be correct, or even superior. To do so is to make the a priori assumption that all children will learn best by one method. The task must be to determine the criteria for selecting a method most appropriate for a given child.

The Deaf Child in the Classroom

There are some exceptions among deaf children in regard to language development. Most of the exceptions are found among bright deaf children, especially among those whose parents were aware of the hearing impairment and initiated early training along the lines suggested. Other exceptions may be found among deaf children with sufficient residual hearing who are able to make use of their limited hearing. These children have learned to attend to speakers and to read their faces and their articulatory and accompanying manual gestures. Some children, though deaf, may have their residual hearing enhanced by a properly fitted hearing aid and so learn considerably more about speech and speakers than if they relied on vision alone. Still other exceptions are found among children who became deaf (adventitious deafness) after they had acquired speech. In general, however, the incidence of speech defects and of language retardation is almost universal among preschool deaf children.

Most deaf children of school age have a slower rate of academic achievement than do their hearing peers. However, unless mental retardation is an associated problem, most deaf children learn to read and to write, and to progress in other school subjects.

Silverman (1971, p. 411), sums up his position as well as a consensus of the literature as follows:

> The deaf child does not learn at the same rate as the hearing child. With the need to master new vocabulary and language, it takes about two or more years to achieve second grade school level and an additional one and a half to two years to complete the third grade.

Silverman, in common with other authorities on the deaf, believes that most deaf children do not achieve academically up to their intellectual potential. "The gap between mental ability and academic achievment can be reduced but is seldom eliminated." Improved instructional methods may, we hope, reduce the gap for some children and eliminate it for the most fortunate of the deaf. However, a survey by Lane (1976, p. 101) on the academic achievement of severely hearing-impaired children over a period of 50 years generated the conclusion that "there has been some slight improvement in educational achievement of the deaf, but the educational retardation is still one of the greatest barriers to academic and vocational success of the deaf."

Deaf-Aphasic Children

Before leaving the subject of the deaf child, we must briefly discuss a small subgroup: the congenitally (developmentally) aphasic-deaf.[5]

---

[5] For a survey of the literature of the evolving concept of developmental aphasia and the auditory and perceptual impairments of aphasic children, see H. Myklebust, in L. E. Travis, ed., *Handbook of Speech Pathology and Audiology* (New York: Appleton-Century-Crofts (Prentice-Hall, Inc.), 1972), Chaps. 46–47.

See also Wyke, M. A., Ed., *Developmental Dysphasia*, New York, Academic Press, 1978.

Our own position on developmental aphasia will be presented in Chapter 16.

Such children, who are also referred to as having *central deafness,* are not able to perceive and assign meanings even to sounds which, when reinforced by amplification, are physically received. We assume that such children, in addition to peripheral hearing loss, also have incurred damage or have severe maturational delay of an area, or areas, of the cerebral cortex that normally serves for the analysis of speech sounds. A child who is both peripherally and centrally deaf (aphasic), is likely to ignore and reject even very loud speech, and may be disturbed by and refuse to use hearing aids. The child is probably wise in doing so. If the youngster is unable to make sense out of any received human speech sounds, confusion and frustration may result from mere reception without perception. Such a child may be trained initially through a straight visual approach, with signing and finger spelling and later through graphic media alone for reading and writing. We need to emphasize, however, that the deaf-aphasic child constitutes a very small subgroup of the deaf. Nondeaf congenitally aphasic children, also a small group, are considered in Chapter 16.

HEARING LOSS: THE HARD-OF-HEARING

Language retardation and voice and articulation defects are prevalent in children who have sufficient hearing to learn to speak through the auditory modality, but whose hearing is sufficiently impaired to create problems in the easy and comfortable reception of oral language signals.

Silverman et al. (1978, p. 434) consider a hard-of-hearing person to be one who "generally with the use of a hearing aid, has residual hearing sufficient to enable successful processing of linguistic information through audition." Usually, not only auditory reception but perception (deriving meaning) is improved with appropriate amplification.

With important exceptions, the incidence of speech (voice and articulation) and language defects are positively related to the severity of hearing loss and to the time in the child's life at which the loss began. The child who develops a hearing loss at age three or four, when his/her speech is well established, is likely to have much less impairment for language, and possibly also for voice and articulation, than is the congenitally hard-of-hearing child, or one whose hearing loss was acquired before he/she spoke in sentences. Some children whose pure-tone audiometric results might lead us to expect severe speech difficulties may do better than those whose hearing impairment might be considered relatively mild judging by their audiograms. "Just as there are gradations in the usefulness of hearing, so there are gradations in the quality and intelligibility of the speech of the hard-of-hearing. Many hard-of-hearing children speak so well that the lay observer notices no abnormality, whereas the severely impaired may be almost unintelligible to those who are not accustomed to this type of speech" (Silverman 1971, p. 431).

We need to appreciate that both the quality and the quantity of the language of the hard-of-hearing child depend on many individual factors. These include the intelligence of the child, the early recognition of the hearing loss, and the motivation of both parents and child toward speech learning. A bright child who is well motivated and who has well-informed parents may achieve normal speech through combining lip (speech) reading and the maximum use of hearing. Amplified sound and the use of a hearing aid, if possible and appropriate, are usually of considerable help.

Speech Defects Associated with Hearing Loss

Almost all children who are more than mildly hard of hearing have some degree of difficulty in articulation and appropriate vocalization. Depending in part on the type and degree of hearing loss, distortions and omissions of consonants, and especially fricative sounds, are common. There is also likely to be some difficulty in distinguishing between voiced and voiceless cognates such as *b* and *p*, *d* and *t*, *v* and *f*, and the *th* sounds. Vowels and diphthongs may be distorted.

The improvement of the speech of the child with a recognized and appreciable hearing loss is the task of the professional speech/language clinician rather than the classroom teacher who specializes in "normal" children. The nonspecialist classroom teacher has an important auxiliary role in cooperating with the speech/language clinician and special educator. In this instance, the special educator is one whose responsibilities are specific to children who have significant hearing impairment.

Intermittent or Occasional Hearing Difficulty

Many teachers have had children who on occasion seem to have some difficulty in hearing. It is possible that some of these children have relatively slight though chronic difficulty with hearing, but are usually able to make up for the loss by good attentive effort. However, if such a child has a head cold, or suffers from enlarged adenoids because of a temporary inflammation, the hearing problem may be temporarily increased. Fatigue or ill-health may produce comparable results. There are, of course, other children who, for reasons related to their emotional problems in or out of the classroom, on occasion seem not to be able to hear. Perhaps these children block out spoken language because of difficulties that arise when they do hear, understand, and respond to speech. If the teacher suspects the latter to be the case, an understanding of what may be the basis for the "nonhearing" rather than a penalizing response is in order.

Whenever hearing loss is suspected, an audiological evaluation, which should include speech perception, is recommended. If hearing loss is found, its cause and possible treatment should be determined by a physician. Fortunately, in some instances, medical treatment can minimize or entirely clear up temporary difficulty in hearing resulting from pathology.

The Hard-of-Hearing Child in the Classroom[6]

The teacher can be of appreciable help in the classroom for a child believed to have a hearing loss. Among the things that can be done to be of direct help to the particular child are

1. Make certain that the teacher is constantly in direct view of the child during instructional periods.
2. Permit changing of seats to keep the teacher's face in direct view of the child.
3. Speak louder and somewhat more slowly when an activity is anticipated that will involve a specific response from the child suspected of having a hearing loss.

EMOTIONAL PROBLEMS AND LANGUAGE DELAY

The history of many children with language delay includes an item indicating that they began to speak at an age within normal limits but then seemed to give up speaking. On questioning, one or both parents may reveal that the cessation of speaking seemed to be associated with an unhappy familial situation. In some instances, it becomes apparent that the parents were disturbed about their own relationship, and frequently spoke harshly to each other in the presence of the young child. Occasionally, an admission is obtained that when the parents spoke to each other at all, it was in emotional outbursts. The young child apparently became afraid of the consequences of speech and retired into the relative safety and security of not speaking, at least not to the parents at home. Such a child may continue to be ap-

---

[6] See Chapters 1 and 4 for a more detailed discussion of the teacher's role.

prehensive about the consequences of speaking in other situations, including in school where the teacher may be perceived as a parent away from home. If the child meets any penalty resulting from speech behavior during the early school experiences, his/her apprehensions are confirmed. This kind of child may prefer to be ignorant or "dumb" or accept a scolding for apparent inattention or negativism rather than risk the greater penalty of saying the wrong or unacceptable thing. The child may decide that it is safer to be the "quiet one" than the one who becomes involved in difficulties for speaking thoughts or feelings.

Another situation associated with regression or cessation of speech and occurring frequently enough to be worthy of note is the birth of a new child. The two- or three-year-old may look upon the crying, non-speaking infant as a usurper of attention and affection. With what seems fair logic, the older sibling may decide that the only way to compete with the usurper is to imitate the newcomer's behavior. So speech, at least for a while, may regress to prelingual stages or come to a halt.

Childhood Schizophrenia

There are other children, more severely involved in their emotional relationships and human identifications, whose early history may begin with comparatively normal onset and development of speech. These children appear to be normal, at least as far as speech is concerned, until they are about two years of age. Then they regress or cease to talk or become fixed at the one-word labeling stage. These children also show other withdrawal behavior of sufficient degree as to be identified as childhood schizophrenics. Goldfarb (1961) presents a psychiatrist's view of the nature and treatment of children with childhood schizophrenia. Other psychiatric, psychological, and psycholinguistic viewpoints are included in the writings of Pronovost and Wakstein (1966), Rimland (1964), Rutter (1971), and Wing (1966). A behavior modification approach that is realistic both as to objectives and achievements is presented by Lovaas, Schreibman, and Koegel (1974).

Ross (1980, Chap. 11) reviews theories and behavioral educational approaches for children identified as suffering from childhood schizophrenia. Ross gives considerable emphasis to the role of language for both diagnosing and providing therapy to schizophrenic children.

> . . . the more severe the disorder, the greater the language impairment and the less favorable the prognosis. From this one might also conclude

that the earlier one intervenes and gives the child systematic language training and other treatment aimed at enhancing the socialization process, the more likely one will be to promote adaptive development. (Ross, 1980, p. 196)

Parental Expectations and Delayed Language

In Chapter 7 on "The Development of Language" we presented four basic assumptions relative to the parents and the home environment that were considered conducive to a child's normal acquisition of speech (see pp. 175–6). Some parents, perhaps in their effort to provide normal stimulation and have a normal speaking child, become anxious in their expectations. Perhaps they fail to understand that child language is not adult language in miniature form. A child speaks as a child, not only in thoughts but in phonology, vocabulary, pronunciation, and syntax. Perhaps it is well for us to remember that "When I was a child, I spoke as a child . . . When I became a man, I put away childish things" (Corinthians 13:11).

Chess and Rosenberg (1974) report on referrals made to them in a clinical psychiatric practice limited to children. Children with speech problems, they observe, are brought in earlier (peak ages four to five) than are children without speech problems (peak ages eight to nine). Out of a population of 563 children, 139 (24 per cent) had some type of language difficulty at the time of referral. Of this group, 81 had delayed onset of speech (fewer than 15 words by two years of age) and 51 immature speech (speech usage significantly below age expectation).

Chess and Rosenberg make two important clinical observations. "In the cognitively normal child with speech usage below age there may be a tendency to inhibit speech in situations where rebuff or misunderstanding are anticipated." The second observation is related to the higher incidence of boys to girls (three boys to one girl) in the clinical population. "Whether this is a function of the high language expectations of middle-class parents has not been determined."

Kleffner (1973, pp. 11–12), on the basis of rich clinical experience, observes that three factors are common in parental reactions to young children who have disorders of speech. Kleffner's observations are particularly relevant to the child who appears to be delayed in speech development.

1. Parental anxiety tends to produce "an insidious and pervasive pressure for the child to talk. Paradoxically, this pressure can coexist . . . with a reduction in the parent's efforts to engage in functional communicative interactions with the child."

2. Parents tend to intensify their efforts to evoke what little language their children have acquired rather than to help them to acquire new language or to broaden their concepts about language. Parents encourage labeling by asking children to name pictures or objects ("What's this?") rather than presenting a situation and themselves talking about the picture, for example, "The bird's wings are spread open when it flies."
3. Parents seem to have difficulty in determining the level of language usage and language stimulation that will result in an optimum verbal interchange. "Sometimes they talk far above the child's head; at other times reverting to rudimentary or even nonverbal communication well below the child's ability levels."

Perhaps the basic problem relative to parental expectations is that despite all possible good intentions, most parents do not know what to expect. Until the 1960s, parents were offered advice and opinions, much of which seemed to be logical but was in fact *not fact.* Since the 1960s we have been the beneficiaries of a wealth of sophisticated objective observations about normal language acquisition and the possible role of parents in the language development of their children. One of the authors (Eisenson, 1976) wrote a book addressed to parents to answer the question *Is Your Child's Speech Normal?* and to advise them as to what they as parents can do to enhance the likelihood of normality.

We shall offer some advice for parents, and for teachers and speech/language clinicians who are professionally concerned with delayed language children, advice that is the product of parent-to-preschool-child language interchanges. The advice is implied in the following observation from de Villiers and de Villiers (1979, p. 99).

Parents usually talk to their preschool children about what is present and concrete, about the here and now that can be seen, touched, and directly experienced. So referents and meanings are likely to be clear. Further, de Villiers and de Villiers note:

> Mothers and fathers . . . tailor the length and complexity of their utterances to the linguistic ability of their children. Mother's speech to one-and two-year olds consists of simple, grammatically correct, short sentences that refer to concrete objects and events. There are few references to the past and the future.

Caretaker speech—the speech of parents, older siblings, or some important "other"—should be syntactically simple, spoken more slowly than to older children or adults, with distinct pauses between the phrases and the *short sentences.* Moskowitz (1978, p. 94) observes that the speech of caretakers to young children may be describable by a grammar six months in advance of their own. We would characterize caretaker language to a child who is developing normally in language acquisition as having structure and content not so far above him or her as to be out of reach, yet far enough (or close enough) to make the reaching worth the effort.

Feeling of apprehension may continue to characterize the behavior of children who once were delayed in speech. The classroom teacher in the first or second grade would do well to be permissive in attitude and to avoid correcting the articulation or pronunciation of children who have a delayed-speech history. These children need the security of acceptance of themselves as they are, so that their speech efforts will not be conducive to disapproval or fear. Remedial speech work of specific speech faults may well wait until the third or fourth grade for these children. Of course, indirect efforts at correction take place whenever the child is exposed to a kind and permissive environment that stimulates good but not unrealistically perfectionistic speech. An attitude of permissiveness, incidentally, should be consistent and should not vary from day to day according to the whims of the adult.

Faulty Motivation

Human beings, we have emphasized, are expected to speak. The drive to speak is so strong in almost all children that we need to do little more than provide a decent environment for a child to have a child who will speak. However, the quantity of the child's speech and, to some degree, the quality of speech may well be modified by an unfavorable environment. In the preceding pages we considered the possible effects of parental anxiety and unrealistic expectation, perhaps a result of a lack of knowledge of what is normal. Now we turn our attention to what may well be the other side of the coin, the overprotected child.

The child who suffers—and suffers is really the word—from overprotection is a comparatively rare child. The overprotected child does start to talk and most likely will continue to acquire speech that is at least normal in form unless the child is completely overwhelmed by parents. But for the rare child who had adequate intellectual, sensory, and motor equipment, who does make a start but does not seem motivated to continue in language acquisition, what is presented in the next few paragraphs is relevant.

Children are not likely to develop many new skills, language acquisition included, unless such skills provide them with a sense of satisfaction and accomplishment that they cannot otherwise obtain.

Though almost every child is born to speak, and will have a normal age for onset of speech, the members of the family may either nurture or retard later language development. Children whose wants are regularly anticipated may be denied the opportunity for expressing their wants, thereby frustrating their need to do so. The magic of speech is the right of each child who is capable of exercising such potency. Parents who are overprotective, because of past or present injuries or illness of their children, and who hover over them when they first attempt to stand alone or to walk, do nothing to encourage standing or walking. Parents who cannot wait until their child completes a gesture without overwhelming the youngster with a number of things the gesture might signify produce a state of "what's the use" and confusion in the child. Children have the need and right to speak for themselves *just as soon as they are able.* Some overprotected children may be fortunate in having other less anxiety-ridden and overprotective adults or older siblings with whom they can identify. Speech may then be selectively produced. But the less fortunate of the overprotected children may begin to speak at the expected age but not make the expected acquisitions after onset. Among the immediate improvements and modifications sought for these children are the following:

1. An understanding on the part of parents, and any other overanxious, overzealous members of the child's environment, that the child is deserving of the right to entertain a want or a need, even if it is necessary to cry about it.
2. When an attempt at speaking is made, the attempt is to be heard out before the adults jump to do something about it.

For children who have not begun to speak, or who have not gone beyond "mama" and "dada" in their early naming, the following suggestions are in order:

1. A repeated vocalization, especially if it accompanies a repeated gesture in association with a given situation, may be the beginning of word usage. The adult should imitate the vocalization in the recurring situation before responding to the act of gesture-vocalization. In this way, attention is directed to the oral activity rather than to the pantomine.
2. Once repeated vocalization is established, the parent should take the initiative and give a simple monosyllabic name to a toy or object frequently used and desired by the child. This name should include sounds the child has successfully made and repeated in his sound-play activity. For example, if "da" is frequently uttered by the child, the name *da* can be given to a doll or some other play-

thing enjoyed by the child. The sound should be spoken by the parent each time the object is given to the child, and each time the adult, when present, observes the child reaching for the object. After one or two days of this practice, the object should be withheld, but not with a look of apprehension or threat, until the child makes some attempt to utter the sound-name for it. If the child is reasonably successful in making a sound that closely resembles, if not directly reproduces the sound-name, quick approval for the effort is in order. This, however, does not mean that the child is to be rewarded by another toy or overwhelmed with a flow of words too numerous and too rapid for assimilation or understanding. Easy is the mode for early parent-child interchanges. The longer this mode is maintained, the better are the interchanges.

THE INFLUENCE OF BILINGUALISM

In Chapter 7 on "The Development of Language," we discussed bilingualism and bidialectism. These subjects, however related, should not be confused. Neither should we fail to be aware of the sociopolitics involved in considerations of bilingualism. It is beyond the scope of this book to become involved in the questions and issues of bilingual or bidialectal education. (For an objective review of these matters, the reader is referred to Cazden 1972, pp. 143–181). Our concern in this chapter is to consider the influence of bilingualism relative to the acquisition and development of language in children who have no choice as to whether they might prefer a bilingual or monolingual environment or which of two languages they are to be exposed to first.

As suggested in Chapter 7, the group who come from a bilingual environment include a higher proportion of children with delayed language development than children exposed to a simple language from birth. The research data, unfortunately, are sparse as to the specific effects of bilingualism on onset of speech, lexical, phonological, and syntactic acquisitions. Even more rare are studies on the effect of conceptualization and verbal meaning for bilingual children. The bilingual children we see in a clinical setting are found frequently to have been delayed in onset of speech and even more delayed in their language acquisitions after onset. But this is a selected population of children referred for diagnosis or treatment because of their evident difficulties. We know very little about bilingual children who have no difficulties. An exception is a study by Smith (1949) who investigated the effect of bilingualism (Chinese and English) among children in

Hawaii. Smith found that even when the vocabularies of the two languages were combined, only two-fifths of the children exceeded the expected norms for monolingual children. On the strength of her data Smith concluded that "only the superior bilingual child is capable of attaining the vocabulary norms of monoglots . . ."

In a more recent study Carrow (1972) compared a group of monolingual preschool children in the age range 3.10 to 5.9 years with a bilingual group who lived in low socioeconomic areas in Houston, Texas. The groups were compared on aspects of auditory comprehension. Carrow found that the bilingual children scored significantly lower than the monoglots on comprehension of certain nouns, pronouns, plural forms of nouns, and noun phrases that included two-adjective modifiers. It is possible that the Carrow study, like the earlier one of Smith, may be measuring the related effects of low socioeconomic status and bilingualism rather than bilingualism per se on early language acquistions.

A significantly different conclusion was reached by Lambert, Just, and Segalowitz (1970, p. 233). However, these investigators—sociolinguists—were involved with the results of teaching a second language (French) to children brought up in monolingual (English) homes. The teaching was carried on in Montreal schools in the kindergarten. The authors consider that this age and school level are critical to the results. The teachers were French-speaking and described as highly skilled. Moreover, in addition to vocabulary building and listening comprehension, the children were taught art and music and played games in French. So, learning French became both fun and status achievement. Lambert *et al.*, say that the children in this ideal school situation "demonstrate a very high level of skill in both receptive and productive aspects of French, the major language of instruction; a generally excellent command of all aspects of English, the home language of the children; and a high level of skill in a nonlanguage subject matter, mathematics, taught through the foreign language only."

On the basis of these two references of studies made over a considerable distance in time and difference in social cultures, we are not ready to come to any conclusions. However, for children who are simultaneously exposed to two languages, and who do present indications of delayed or disordered speech, we can suggest the following:

On the whole, it would seem much safer for a child to have one language well established before being exposed to a second. If multiple language exposure cannot be avoided, as is the case in many homes and many cultures, the use of a given language should be identified consistently with a person or a situation. Some children seem to find it necessary to fit themselves and the speaking situation into a linguistic "groove" and to maintain that groove in a consistent manner. For example, if the parents spoke only English, and the grandparents, nurse, or housekeeper spoke a second language, the child would learn to associate a language pattern—a way of speaking—with a person or persons and so have less conflict than if the parents spoke English on some occasions and a second language on others. When the other times are unpredictable, or when the other times are reserved for admonishments, difficulty with the second language may intensify. So, also, unfortunately, may the child's attitude toward language behavior in general.

The observations we have made in regard to bilingual exposure hold true also for children who appear to have difficulty in language development. Many children present no such difficulty. Such children are often found in middle- and upper-socioeconomic-class homes. Penfield and Roberts (1959, pp. 251–255) recommend that children who live in bilingual environments, as, for instance, in Montreal, Canada, should intentionally be taught two languages by the direct method—that is, by having the children exposed to both languages in their home, but each in a systematic way—during the early preschool years. The argument for this natural and direct approach is that the child's brain before school age has a maximum plasticity and capacity for acquiring more than one language. A young child may respond "reflexively" to whatever language is spoken. The children will not, of course, realize that they may be speaking French on one occasion and to one person, and English to another person or on different occasions.

If, however, a child who has been exposed to more than one language appears to have difficulty in learning to speak, we strongly recommend that the parents decide which language is to be essential for the child and that the youngster be exposed to only one language until the child's speech behavior has become established. This frequently calls for control and modification of the home environment as well as of aspects of the environment outside of the home. Although such control and modification may not always be easy to achieve, it is important that it be done.

Bilingualism may present a variety of problems relative to language proficiency as well as to psychological and social development. These problems are discussed in a monograph edited by Macnamara (1967).

To avoid any possibility that our position will be misunderstood, we will re-emphasize that in the absence of evidence or indication that we are dealing with a child who is at high risk for language acquisition, on balance, bilingualism is beneficial. We agree with the view of Smith, Goodman, and Meredith (1976, p. 49) that a knowledge of a second language provides opportunities for cultural enrichment. "Bilingualism can be developed in varying degrees from elementary awareness of alternate ways of saying things and naming objects to full fluency in a second language; at any level it is beneficial and broadening."

Bidialectism: Black English

We have already indicated the need to distinguish between delayed and defective speech and the use of a dialect in which there are differences in phonology, vocabulary, and syntax with another dialect of the same language. Thus, children who speak Black English, or any other dialect of English for that matter, should be evaluated for how well they are doing in the particular dialect before decisions are made as to whether their linguistic proficiencies are normal, delayed, or defective.

The matter of whether a child's dialect should be changed involves educational and sociolinguistic considerations. We earnestly hope that it is not solely a political consideration. If the decision is made to encourage the child to change from Black English to another dialect of English that is more representative of a majority of speakers in the country or area in which the child lives, then necessary procedures can be undertaken. Another decision may be to establish bidialectism. In any event, it is essential that the clinician or teacher who is responsible for motivating and bringing about changes, *or teaching* a "standard" dialect, understands the child's first dialect.

Because the issues of bidialectism are so involved, we can make no definitive statements. We do suggest, as educators as well as clinicians, that if one dialect interferes with a second because of numerous overlapping features, a choice will need to be made as to whether a minority or majority dialect should be taught. Again we hope that the interests of the child rather than sociopolitical influences will determine the choice.

Before closing this necessarily brief consideration of bidialectism and its implications for children whose first English dialect is Black English, an observation of caution is in order. We previously advised to keep separate dialectical differences and delayed language development or defective speech. It is equally important that we do not attribute to a dialect actual delay in language development or indications of defective speech. In fairness to the children involved, we should keep in mind that developmental problems may be expected for any group within a culture that for reasons of its own or because of imposed causes has children who are at high risk. By *high risk* we mean children who are prematurely born, whose mothers were not well nourished, or who are themselves malnourished in their early years. The incidence of children who are delayed in language and often in intellectual and cognitive development as well is higher among Black English speakers than in the general population. The term *the language of poverty,* used for Black English, should not be confused with the effects of impoverishment on some of the children brought up in poverty.[7] The effects of poverty are by no means limited to blacks.

MULTIPLE BIRTHS

To what extent may we accept the observation that twins are double trouble? And if we double the potentialities for trouble with twins, is there a progressive likelihood of difficulty as the number of children per birth increases? Although most of our data are on twins, the answer in general is "Yes." With awareness that as individual children, children born as twins range in their intelligence, motor development, language development, and the like from retarded to precocious, we nevertheless find more delay and more problems in speech among twins than among single-born children. When the twins are identical, the liabilities, and happily some of the assets, are also likely to be amazingly similar.

After reviewing the literature on twins, Lenneberg (1967, p. 253) concludes:

> The developmental history of identical twins tends to be much more synchronous than that of fraternal twins. Among the former, motor milestones, menarche, change of voice, and growth rate are more likely to occur at the same time than among the latter. The same is reflected in the onset of speech (that is, the age at which the first few words appear, words are joined into phrases, and grammatical mistakes become minimal). It is only among the fraternal twins that difference in onset occurs, whereas identical twins seem to progress simultaneously. It is the general consensus of the investigators that these divergences cannot be simply explained on the grounds of imitation or differential treatment by parents.

[7] We strongly recommend the book *Language and Poverty,* edited by F. Williams (Chicago: Markham Publishing Co., 1970), for an excellent series of essays on dialects and their implications for attitudes on social change and education. We also recommend *Black English: Its History and Usage in the United States* by J. L. Dillard (New York: Random House, Inc. 1972). Dillard claims that 80 per cent of American blacks speak Black English as one of their dialects of American English.

Lenneberg (p. 252) summarizes the findings on delayed language and twins with the observation that 65 per cent of identical twins were delayed in onset of speech compared with 60 per cent of fraternal twins. Identical twins showed considerably more similarity in the features of their delay than did fraternal twins.

Onset of speech is delayed in twins, and twins are retarded in language acquisition up to about age four. The evidence suggests that most twins do catch up with single-born children by the time they enter the elementary school grades. Early language retardation among twins may be attributed both to organic causes and to an atypical social environment—the influence of each twin upon the other.

According to Nelson (1959, p. 305), most twins are prematurely born. Prematurity of birth is associated in many instances with vascular defects and with brain damage. Even when there is no clear evidence of damage to the brain, there is considerable evidence of a lag in overall physical maturation, which continues at least until the time the child is of age to enter school. Lags in psychological and social development parallel those for physical development. These disadvantages, we should emphasize, are associated with the combination of twinning and premature birth. Though there is evidence that some prematurely born children "may never catch up" (Silvern, 1961), we are more inclined to accept the older point of view of the geneticist Newman (1940), who maintains that if twins survive the hazards of being born and the consequences of prematurity, by the time they are well along in school they are as capable as their single-born peers.

Twins provide an atypical environment for one another. As they grow up they seem to be satisfied with their mutual social situation and so are less demanding of the attentions of older persons. Even if attention is demanded, it must be divided. Unfortunately, twins are not well qualified as language stimulators. The result is that they are exposed less to adults than are single children, and more to poor language stimulation. An interesting linguistic phenomenon among twins is their development of a special code for expression and communication—an idioglossia—which seems to serve the twins adequately but baffles all other members of the family. Because of the evident satisfaction twins derive from their idioglossia, they may not be motivated to learn the language of their homes or their more extended environment.

Evidence that most twins tend to catch up with single-born children comes from a study by Mittler (1970) on a middle-class population of twins in England. Mittler compared a population of 200 four-year-old twins with 100 singletons of the same age. All the children had just entered nursery school. The *Illinois Test of Psycholinguistic*

Abilities—ITPA (Kirk and McCarthy 1968) was used as the assessment measure. Mittler found that the twins' scores on all of the ITPA subtests paralleled those of the singleton children. Mittler concludes

> thus, twins do not appear to show any characteristic pattern of linguistic organization, and their performance can best be described as a more or less uniform retardation or immaturity.

The retardation in this study amounted to approximately six months.

Another finding that is worthy of note is that coming from a middle-class home was not as strongly a favorable factor for twins as for single children. Mittler speculates that by virtue of being a twin, each child is less receptive to the usual positive language values that are attributed to being a member of middle socioeconomic family.

> . . . It might be argued that the middle-class twin remains a "restricted" code user by virtue of the "twin situation" which renders him less receptive to the "elaborated" linguistic code used by his parents, whereas working-class twins, who are mainly exposed to restricted codes in any case, are relatively less handicapped (p. 755).

Though most twins do catch up by school age, there is a higher incidence of those who are retarded in language than in the population at large. A school-age population may not include many children who cannot be accepted or who are not accepted in schools by virtue of their language and associated retardations.

If twins arrive at school age still using their special language, they should, if at all possible, be put in separate classes. If this is not possible they should be put in separate groups so that they may associate with children using more conventional language.

THE ROLE OF THE CLASSROOM TEACHER WITH DELAYED-LANGUAGE CHILDREN

As indicated earlier, regular classroom teachers are not likely to have many children with seriously retarded language development among their pupils. By the time children of normal intellect, who began by being delayed in language, reach school age, they are likely to be speaking well enough to be accepted in the regular class. However, some residual signs of the problem may remain. Some of the children who were formerly delayed in language and speech may still be apprehensive about speaking and show anxiety when responsibility for communication is fixed upon them. These children are likely to be freer when responding as members of a group than when they are required to recite alone or to speak with, rather than in front of, their classmates. Others may have limited vocabularies or more than a normal number of speech faults. If teachers can determine which of the causes of retarded language development were present for any of the children, they can be of great help in controlling or preventing the pressure associated with the original cause for language retardation. These children need to learn that speaking is enjoyable before they become aware that with the acquisition of oral language there is an assumption of communicative responsibility. When pleasure replaces apprehension, goals for increased speech/language proficiency can be set. The children should be directed gently toward these goals and not goaded toward their attainment. Incidentally, we strongly urge that children who have just started their school careers be given no cause to become self-conscious about their lack of proficiency. Teachers must provide motivation, stimulation, and good and attainable models, as well as reinforcement for improvement. However, teachers should avoid any negative indications that might lead children to hold back on talking, or worse still, cause self-interruptions of what they, however improficiently, might be trying to say.

The current practice for "mainstreaming" to include as many children as possible in regular classes at least for part of their academic day may alter the situation in regard to serious language-delay problems. Regular classroom teachers may have to add another specialty to their broad array of general practice "specialties." We hope that at a minimum regular classroom teachers will have the assistance of language clinicians in their work with children who are seriously delayed in their language development.

Problems

1. What are the chief causes of delayed language acquisition? What is *the* chief cause?
2. What is the relationship between emotional upheavals in the family and possible language delay? Can you recall such a case?
3. Check with the parents of five children as to the ages when their children began to speak. Average the ages for the boys and for the girls. Which group had an older average age? Are there any present language differences?
4. Twins have been found to begin to speak at a later age than single children. How do you account for this? Are there any differences between fraternal and identical twins?
5. Read two of the references mentioned on childhood schizophrenia and childhood autism. Compare the early clinical histories of these two

"types" of children with emotional problems. Are all autistic children schizophrenic? Are all schizophrenic children autistic?

6. Read the article by J. Stark, J. J. Giddan, and J. Meisel, "Increasing Verbal Behavior in an Autistic Child," *Journal of Speech and Hearing Disorders*, **33** (1968), 42–47. What methods were used to get the child to speak? Did the child generate any new utterances based on the vocabulary and syntax he was taught?

7. Compare the approaches in the Stark *et al.* article with those described by E. G. Wolf and B. A. Ruttenberg, "A Communication Therapy for the Autistic Child," *Journal of Speech and Hearing Disorders*, **32** (1967), 331–36, and those in Lovaas et al., referred to in this chapter, and those of Seibert and Oller (*Journal of Autism and Developmental Disorders*, (**11**, 1, 1981, 75–81).

8. There is considerable evidence that children who have difficulty in learning to read include more than a "normal" number of children with delayed-language onset. Can you account for this?

9. Compare a three-year-old child's motor and speech development with the motor and language milestones of the table adapted from Lenneberg. (See Chapter 7 on "The Development of Language.") Make the same comparisons for a three- or four-year-old who has been designated as being delayed in speech. Where are the greater disparities?

10. In the light of the present move to "mainstream" as many children as possible in regular classes in the public schools, are there any additional responsibilities and roles the classroom teacher has that were not suggested in this chapter?

11. What is a language dialect? Define bidialectism. What are the major features of Black English compared with "Standard" American English?

12. There are several kinds of bilingualism. What are they and what determines the designation?

13. Under what circumstances might you recommend that a preschool child or a primary-school-age child be exposed, if possible, to a single language?

References and Suggested Readings

American Speech-Language-Hearing Association, "Position Statement on Nonspeech Communication." *ASHA*, **23**, 8 (1981), 577–581.

Bricker, D. D., and L. Carlson, "Issues in Early Language Intervention." In R. L. Schiefelbusch D. D. Bricker, Editors, *Early Language, Acquisition and Intervention*. Baltimore: University Park Press, 1981.

Carrow, E., "Auditory Comprehension of English by Monolingual and Bilingual Preschool Children." *Journal of Speech and Hearing Research*, **15** (1972) 407–412.

Cazden, C., *Child Language and Education*. New York: Holt, Rinehart and Winston, Inc., 1972. (A down-to-earth treatment of language development in the child. Reviews theories, facts, and their educational implications.)

Chess, S., and M. Rosenberg, "Clinical Differentiation Among Children with

Initial Language Complaints." *Journal of Autism and Childhood Schizo-phrenia,* **4** (1974), 99–109.

Day, E. J., "The Development of Language in Twins." *Child Development,* **3** (1932), 179–199. (A classic study.)

de Villiers, P. A. and J. G. de Villiers, *Early Language.* Cambridge, Mass.: Harvard University Press, 1979.

Dillard, J. L., *Black English: Its History and Usage in the United States.* New York: Random House, Inc., 1972. (As the title indicates, the book reviews the history of the origins of Black English in the United States. A readable and authoritative book.)

Drash, P. W., "Habilitation of the Retarded Child: A Remedial Program." *The Journal of Special Education,* **6** (1972), 149–159.

Duncan, J. L. and F. H. Silverman, "Impacts of Learning American Indian Sign Language on Mentally Retarded Children." *Perceptual and Motor Skills,* **44,** (1977), 1138.

Eisenson, J., *Is Your Child's Speech Normal?* Reading, Mass.: Addison-Wesley Publishing Co., 1976. (A book addressed primarily to parents to answer the questions implied in the title).

Furth, H. G., *Thinking Without Language.* New York: The Free Press, 1966. (An important book that emphasizes the need to teach deaf children cognition even before they begin to learn a language system.)

Giradeau, F. L., and J. E. Spradlin, Eds., *A Functional Analysis Approach to Speech and Language.* ASHA Monograph No. 14, Washington, D.C.: American Speech and Hearing Association, 1970.

Goda, S., and B. G. Griffith, "Spoken Language of Adolescent Retardates and Its Relation to Intelligence, Age, and Anxiety." *Child Development,* **32** (September 1962), 489–498.

Goldfarb, W., *Childhood Schizophrenia,* Cambridge, Mass.: Harvard University Press, 1961.

Ingram, D., *Phonological Disability in Children.* New York: American Elsevier, Inc., 1977.

Journal of Autism and Developmental Disorders, **11,** 1 (1981). (The entire issue, edited by Paula Menyuk, is devoted to the language and cognitive functioning of autistic children.)

Kahn, J. V., "A Comparison of Sign and Verbal Language Training with Non-verbal Retarded Children." *Journal of Speech and Hearing Research,* **24,** 1 (1981), 113–119.

Kimble, S. L., "A Language Technique with Totally Nonverbal, Severely Mentally Retarded Adolescents." Paper presented to the 50th Annual Meeting of the American Speech and Hearing Association, Washington, D.C., 1975.

Kirk, S., and J. McCarthy, *The Illinois Test of Psycholinguistic Abilities,* Urbana, Ill.: University of Illinois Press, 1968.

Kleffner, F. R., *Language Disorders in Children,* New York: The Bobbs-Merrill Co., Inc., 1973. (A brief and highly personal, clinical exposition of the nature of language disorders in young children.)

Lambert, W. E., M. Just, and N. Segalowitz, "Some Cognitive Consequences of Following the Curricula of the Early School Grades in a Foreign Language." In J. E. Alatis, Ed., *Twenty-first Round Table Bilingualism and Language Contact*, Washington, D.C.: Georgetown University Press, 1970.

Lane, H. S., "Academic Achievement." In Bolton, B., Ed., *Psychology of Deafness for Rehabilitation Counselors*. Baltimore: University Park Press, 1976.

Lenneberg, E. H., *Biological Foundations of Language*, New York: John Wiley & Sons, Inc., 1967.

———, "Language Disorders in Childhood," *Harvard Educational Review*, **34**, 4 (Spring 1964), 152–177. (A review of causes, prognoses, and therapeutic procedures for children with moderate and severe language disorders.)

Lillywhite, H. S., and D. P. Bradley, *Communication Problems in Mental Retardation*. New York: Harper & Row, Publishers, Inc., 1969. (Includes discussions of background, causes, and management of communication problems of mentally retarded children.)

Lovaas, O. I., L. Schreibman, and R. L. Koegel, "A Behavior Modification Approach to the Treatment of Autistic Children." *Journal of Autism and Childhood Schrizophrenia*, **4** (1974), 111–129.

Luchsinger, R., and G. E. Arnold, *Voice-Speech-Language*, Belmont, Calif.: Wadsworth Publishing Company, 1967.

MacDonald, J., *Environmental Language Inventory: A Semantic-Based Assessment and Treatment Model for Generalized Communication*. Columbus, Ohio: Charles E. Merrill Publishing Company, 1978.

Macnamara, J., Ed., "Problems of Bilingualism." *The Journal of Social Issues*, **23**, 2 (April 1967).

McLean, J. E., and L. Synder-McLean, "Communicative Disorders Associated with Mental and Behavioral Deviations." In R. J. Van Hattum, Ed., *Communication Disorders*, New York: Macmillan Publishing Co., Inc., 1980.

McReynolds, L. V., ed., *Developing Systematic Procedures for Training Children's Language*, ASHA Monograph No. 18. Washington, D.C.: 1974.

Menyuk, P., "Comparison of Grammar of Children with Functionally Deviant Articulation." *Journal of Speech and Hearing Research*, **7**, 2 (June 1964), 109–121.

Miller, J. F., "Early Psychololinguistic Acquisition." In R. L. Schiefelbusch, and D. B. Bricker, Ed., *Early Language Acquisition and Intervention*. Baltimore: University Park Press, 1981. (A multiple authored book with a strong psycholinguistic orientation. Includes good reviews of the current literature on early language, parental influence, and therapeutic procedures for children with language problems.)

Miller, J. F., and D. E. Yoder, "An Ontogenetic Language Teaching Strategy for Retarded Children." in R. L. Schiefelbusch, and L. L. Lloyd, Eds., *Language Perspectives- Acquisition, Retardation, and Intervention*, Baltimore: University Park Press, 1974, pp. 505–528.

———. "On Developing a Content for a Language Teaching Program." *Mental Retardation* (April 1972), 9–11.

Mittler, P., "Biological and Social Aspects of Language Development in Twins." *Developmental Medicine and Child Neurology*, **12** (1970), 741–757.

Moores, D. F., *Education of the Deaf in the United States, Research Report.* Minneapolis, Minnesota: University of Minnesota Research, Development, and Demonstration Center in Education of Handicapped Children, 1970.

Moskowitz, B. A., "Acquisition of Language." *Scientific American,* **239** (1978), 92–108.

Myklebust, H., "Childhood Aphasia: An Evolving Concept" In L. E. Travis, Ed., *Handbook of Speech Pathology and Audiology,* New York: Appleton-Century-Crofts (Prentice-Hall), 1972, chaps. 46–47.

Naremore, R. C., and R. B. Dever, "Language Performance of Educable Mentally Retarded and Normal Children at Five Age Levels." *Journal of Speech and Hearing Research,* **18** (March 1975), 89–95.

Nelson, W. E., *Textbook of Pediatrics,* 7th ed. Philadelphia: W. B. Saunders Company, 1959.

Newman, H. H., *Multiple Human Births.* New York: Doubleday & Co., Inc., 1940.

Penfield, W., and L. Roberts, *Speech and Brain Mechanisms.* Princeton. N.J.: Princeton University Press, 1959, pp. 251–255.

Pronovost, W., and M. P. Wakstein, "A Longitudinal Study of the Speech Behavior and Language Comprehension of Fourteen Children Diagnosed Atypical or Autistic." *Exceptional Children,* **33** (1966), 19–26.

Rimland, B., *Infantile Autism.* New York: Appleton-Century-Crofts, 1964. (An extensive report on theories as to the cause of autism in children. Excellent research on information available up to the date of the publication of the book.)

Ross, A. O., *Psychological Disorders of Children,* 2nd ed. New York: McGraw-Hill Book Company, 1980.

Rutter, M., Ed., *Infantile Autism: Concepts, Characteristics, and Treatment.* London: Churchill Publishers Ltd., 1971. (A multiple authored book that includes pertinent information on aspects of autism, as implied in the title.)

———— "Diagnosis and Definition." In M. Rutter and E. Schopler, Ed., *Autism: A Review of Concepts and Treatment.* New York: Plenum Press, 1978.

Sanders, D. A., "Psychological Implications of Hearing Impairment." in W. M. Cruickshank, Ed., *Psychology of Exceptional Children and Youth,* 4th ed. Englewood Cliffs, N.J.: Prentice-Hall, Inc., 1980.

Silverman, F. H., *Communication for the Speechless.* Englewood Cliffs, N.J., Prentice-Hall, Inc., 1980.

Silverman, S. R., "The Education of Deaf Children." In L. E. Travis, Ed., *Handbook of Speech Pathology and Audiology.* New York: Appleton-Century-Crofts (Prentice-Hall), 1971, 398–430.

Silverman, S. R., H. S. Lane, and D. R. Calvert "Deaf Children." In H. Davis and S. R. Silverman, *Hearing and Deafness.* New York: Holt, Rinehart and Winston, 1978.

Silvern, W. A., *Dunham's Premature Infants,* 3rd ed. New York: Paul Hoeber, 1961, pp. 76–83.

Smith, E. B., K. S. Goodman, and R. Meredith, *Language and Thinking,* 2nd ed. New York: Holt, Rinehart and Winston, 1976.

Smith, M. E., "Measurement of Vocabularies of Young Bilingual Children in Both of the Languages Used." *Journal of Genetic Psychology*, **74**, (June 1949), 305–310.

Van Riper, C., *Speech Correction*, 6th ed. Englewood Cliffs, N.J.: Prentice-Hall Inc., 1978, Chap. 5. (The chapter surveys the causes and treatment of delayed speech and contains suggestions for stimulating language in reluctant speakers.)

Weiss, C. E. and H. S. Lillywhite. *Communicative Disorders*, 2nd ed. St Louis: The C. V. Mosby Company, 1981. (Considers the prevention, identification, and treatment of communicative disorders.)

Williams, F. Ed., *Language and Poverty*. Chicago: Markham Publishing Co., 1970. (A series of essays on dialects, especially of persons who are economically disadvantaged. Attitudes of dialect speakers and the educational and social implications of "substandard" dialect speakers are considered.)

Williams, F., and R. Naremore, "Social Class Differences in Children's Syntactic Performances." *Journal of Speech and Hearing Research*, 12 (1969), 777–793.

Wing, L. Ed., *Early Childhood Autism*. Oxford, England: Pergamon Press, 1976.

Wyke, M. A., Ed., *Developmental Dysphasia*. New York: Academic Press, 1978. (A multiple authored book with essays by leading authorities on aspects of identification and treatment of developmental [congenital] dysphasia.)

Yoder, D. E., and J. F. Miller, "What We Know and What We Can Do." In J. E. McLean, D. E. Yoder, and R. L., Schiefelbusch, Eds., *Language Intervention with the Retarded: Developing Strategies*. Baltimore: University Park Press, 1972.

10

Articulation Disorders
(I) Theory

In the chapter on normal language development, we have indicated that some children become quite phonologically proficient by the age of three or four and many have adult level articulatory proficiency by the age of five. We note, however, that children usually do not level off in phonemic control until about the age of six or seven. This chapter also contains the characteristics of early phonemic development, the pattern of phonemic development and norms for speech sound proficiency.

Many children, therefore, by the time they enter first grade have developed articulatory proficiency. Arlt and Goodban (1976) studied the age at which children acquire proficiency in articulatory skills. By five years of age, 75 per cent of the males and females produce all sounds correctly. This study, incidentally, points to a somewhat earlier acquisition of sounds than do the studies mentioned earlier.

Although most children do acquire articulatory proficiency by at least the fifth grade, there are some who do not. Bradley and Stoudt (1977) report the results of a five-year longitudinal study of the spontaneous development of articulatory proficiency in 60 elementary-school children who misarticulated at least one phoneme in the first grade. Out of the 60, 47 developed adequate articulation during the five years of schooling with no speech intervention. This study suggests that a significant amount of phonological maturation occurs without interventive speech services. That some fifth-graders, however, did continue to demonstrate articulatory errors is significant, for obviously these children needed the services of a speech/language clinician.

ORIGINS OF ARTICULATORY DEFICIENCIES

Organic Articulatory Deficiency

Some errors of articulation are obviously due to anatomical irregularities of the vocal mechanism. Facial clefts, cleft lip, and cleft palate may involve such parts of the articulatory mechanism as the alveolar process, upper lips, one or both of the nares, and the hard and soft palate (see Chapter 15). Dental irregularities may also prevent accurate articulation. Or various malformations of the tongue may cause articulatory deficits. Or there may exist a neuromotor disturbance which interferes with the fine motor skills needed for articulation (see Chapter 16). Or there may exist an auditory dysfunction (see Chapter 14). Some articulatory errors are clearly based on organic or neurological malformation or malfunction.

Non-organic Articulatory Deficiency

When there is no obvious organic difficulty, the question that arises is: Is the articulatory pattern that emerges similar to that of the language of a younger child or instead is it unique and deviant? That some phonological processes tend to persist longer than others is clear—but do some of these processes differ from one articulatory defective child to another and can these differences be classified? The deviant-articulatory child may use unique or uncommon processes in a general fashion. Certain processes do not drop out as the child matures.

For example, Ingram (1976) notes that such processes as reducing clusters—[tɪk] for [stɪk], making fricatives into stops—/f/→/p/ as [pæt] for [fæt], gliding—/r/→/w/ as [wɛd] for [rɛd], fronting—/k/→/t/, voicing—/t/→/d/ as [bæd] for [bæt] are frequently found in the language of articulatory-delayed children. Other processes, however, are unusual, as where /s/ is substituted for /θ/ or /t/ for /f/. Similarly Pollack and Rees (1972) point to the unusual nasalization of /w/ wherein /w/ becomes /m/. Pollack and Rees (1972) note that phonemic inability reflects the child's inadequate or deviant phonological system rather than inability to execute certain articulatory movements.

Through phonological process analysis, we discover that children use phonological processes to simplify the forms used by adults. These children who exhibit inappropriate processes in articulation for their age have *phonological disorders*.

Hodson and Paden (1981) analyzed and compared the phonological systems of sixty children between the ages of three and eight years who were essentially unintelligible and of sixty children who were four-year-olds who were normally developing intelligible youngsters. Hodson and Paden's phonological analysis of the two groups showed that all of the unintelligible subjects used cluster reduction, stridency deletion and stopping whereas fewer than five of the intelligible four-year-olds gave any evidence of these processes. In addition about two-thirds of the unintelligible speakers used one or more of the following processes: final consonant deletion, fronting of velars, backing, syllable reduction, prevocalic voicing, and glottal replacement; these same processes were virtually non-existent in the speech samples of the normally developing four-year-olds. This study suggests that there are specific processes which are symptoms in terms of kinds of patterns of the unintelligible speakers and not of the normally developing children.

PHONETIC AND PHONEMIC ARTICULATION DISORDERS

Pollack and Rees, then, are pointing to *phonemic errors,* which include what are sometimes called *functional articulatory errors* or *defects.* No neurological or physiological basis seems to exist to account for such disorders, which usually consist in the substitution of one sound for another. On the other hand, *phonetic errors* result from clearly indicated problems, such as muscular or neuromuscular disorders and structural abnormalities and deviations. Children with phonetic errors may possess adult phonological competence but may still be unable to demonstrate the competence because of the problems just mentioned. In this instance the speech/language clinician trains these children by helping them initiate and develop compensatory movements to disguise the physical and/or neurological impairment.

Johnson (1980) indicates that phonetic and phonemic articulatory errors may manifest themselves in the same client and that deficits underlying phonetic mastery often interfere with normal phonemic development. Johnson's table, indicating the distinctions between phonetic and phonemic errors appears on page 270.

Perception of Listeners

Listeners assess sounds usually by: (1) whether or not the incorrect production of a phoneme is obvious and (2) what the perceived symptoms of the incorrect production are. Judgments by speech/language clinicians as to whether a phoneme is uttered correctly or incorrectly are not unanimous. Norris, Harden and Bell (1980), using graduate

Major Distinctions Between Phonetic and Phonemic Articulatory Disorders*

Phonemic Disorders	Phonetic Disorders
1. Predominantly substitution errors.	1. Predominantly distortion and omission errors.
2. Misarticulations related to specific feature errors.	2. Misarticulations may be related to specific structural or neurologic deficit or motoric complexity.
3. Errors may be inconsistent.	3. Errors typically consistent.
4. Difficulty with auditory discrimination of errors.	4. Frequently normal ability to discriminate errors.
5. Client may be stimulable on some errors.	5. Error stimulability is frequently low.
6. Structurally intact speech mechanism.	6. Structural defect may be present.
7. Diadochokinesis[1] within normal limits.	7. Diadochokinesis may be slow and labored.
8. Oral sensation and perception normal.	8. Oral asterognosis[2] may be present.

* Johnson 1980, p. 122.
[1] Diadochokinesis: ability to alternately start and stop the rapid movement of the articulators, as in repetition of syllables [tʌt], [tʌt].
[2] Asterognosis: inability to determine the shape of an object through feeling or touching it. In this instance, a child might not be able to tell that the sourball in his mouth is spherical.

students in speech pathology as assessors, found that agreements on judgment of correct and incorrect sounds varied from 77 to 89 per cent. Differences in the judgments of assessors may be due to such factors as the acceptance or nonacceptance of a particular phoneme and to different standards for correct articulatory performance. Norris, Harden and Bell found that the disagreement increases when the error is classified.

CATEGORIES OF ARTICULATION DISORDERS

Articulatory disorders are usually categorized on the basis of the listener's perception of sounds. As a result of this perception, clinicians may categorize articulatory difficulties as:

1. The omission of sounds.
2. Substitution of one sound for another.
3. The distortion of sounds.

Every child who has an articulatory disorder possesses one or all of these symptoms.

Substitution of One Sound for Another

The substitution of one sound for another is the type of articulatory error that children in the primary grades make most frequently. In a detailed study, Snow (1963) reports on the sounds most frequently substituted for other sounds. She found these substitutions most frequent: /ʃ/, [ts], and /s/ for [tʃ]; /θ/ and /f/ for /s/; /f/, /s/, /t/ for [θ]; /s/ and /tʃ/ for /ʃ/; /d/ and /v/ for /ð/; [dz] and [tʃ] for [dʒ]; [dz] and /s/ for /z/; /z/, [dʒ], [dz] for /ʒ/; /w/ for /r/; /w/ for /l/; /w/ for /ʍ/, and /l/ for /j/. An examination of these data reveals that the substitutions have many of the same phonetic features as does the incorrect sound. For example, in comparing /θ/ and /s/, both are fricatives and both are unvoiced; the difference lies in the parts of the articulatory mechanism involved. /θ/ involves the tip of the tongue and the cutting edges of the teeth, whereas /s/ involves the tip of the tongue and the alveolar ridge or the ridge behind the lower teeth. In comparing the sounds in the substitution /w/ for /r/, both are glides and both are voiced. The difference again lies in the involvement of particular articulatory agents. In comparing /d/ with /ð/, both are voiced but the manner of articulation is different, for /d/ is a stop whereas /ð/ is a fricative. Furthermore, the articulatory agents involved are different, for /d/ is made with the tip of the tongue on the teeth ridge and /ð/ is made with the tip of the tongue against the cutting edges of the teeth. All in all, the features of the substitutions and the correct sounds share many characteristics; despite their differences, there are many basic similarities.

The following are substitutions made by a seven-year-old boy and by a six-year-old girl. Indicate the substitutions, as /s/ for /θ/, and, according to the system just described, identify the changes as:

	/s/	/θ/
Place of Articulation	Tip of tongue and alveolar ridge.	Tip of tongue on cutting edges of teeth.

Then, using the one of the systems of distinctive features as noted in Chapter 6, list the changes in features as:

	/s/	/θ/
	/+ strident/	/− strident/

Substitutions made by Mary, a six-year-old girl in a large school system:

[sʌm]	for *thumb*
[tusbrʌʃ]	for *toothbrush*
[tæt]	for *cat*
[stos]	for *stove*

[naɪs]   for *knife*
[tɪkɪ]   for *chicken*

Substitutions made by Jimmy, a seven-year-old boy:

[stɝəl]   for *squirrel*
[prʌʃ]   for *brush*
[trʌm]   for *drum*
[lɛlo]   for *yellow*
[fɛdɚ]   for *feather*

Most children seemingly are not consistent in their substitutions. They may substitute /f/ for /θ/ in one word and not in another. They may substitute /f/ for /θ/ but also substitute /θ/ for /s/. Consistent patterns of substitution may seem to occur infrequently. But when the substitutions are analyzed carefully, a pattern usually emerges (see Oller 1973, Ingram, 1976, and McReynolds et al., 1974). The child devises a set of rules that translates the usual sounds heard in adult speech into a different but particular phonetic forms. Usually, as noted later, the substitutions maintain many of the features of the target sound and are easier to produce. In general, children are more likely to make substitutions when the sound occurs in the middle or at the end of a word than when it occurs at the beginning of a word.

The Role of Distinctive Features in Substitutions

Research by Menyuk (1968) points to the importance of the distinctive features of consonants. She studied the mastery of consonantal sounds in terms of gravity and diffuseness (aspects of place of articulation); stridency, nasality, and continuancy (aspects of manner of articulation); and the vocal component (presence or absence of voice) for two groups: (1) children with normal speech development for whom data were obtained by transcribing phonetically the substitutions made as the children were spontaneously generating sentences, and (2) children with articulatory difficulties, for whom data were obtained by giving the Templin-Darley Articulation Test and analyzing the results.

The data for the group with normal speech development were analyzed by determining the percentage of sounds containing a feature that was used correctly at various ages in the developmental period of two and a half to five years of age. The rank order of use of features in correctly uttered phonemes was (1) nasal, (2) grave, (3) voice, (4) diffuse, (5) continuant, (6) strident. In other words, the feature first mastered in terms of percentage of correct usage was nasality (the presence of nasal resonance as in /m/ and /n/; the second, grave (being produced at the outer boundaries of the speech mechanism as /p/, /b/,

/k/, and /g/); the third, the voicing or unvoicing feature; the fourth, the diffuse feature (involved in anterior sounds such as /t/, /d/, and /θ/; the fifth, the continuant feature; and the sixth, the strident feature, where interference is high as in the /tʃ/ and /s/.

Prather, Hedrick, and Kern (1975) in a study of 147 children using the same set of distinctive features, found a similar progression in learning. As Menyuk analyzed phonological developmental data, she found the rank order for Japanese children to be identical with that for American children. From this, one can hypothesize that the ability of children to perceive and to produce distinctive linguistic features of sounds is universal. The features dominating the acquisition of phonemes in the early stages of morphemic structure are two aspects of manner of production—use of nasality and use of voice—and one aspect of place of articulation, grave—placement periphery of the mechanism.

In her analysis of distinctive features of phonology of children with articulatory defects, Menyuk makes the point that children in learning to utter a phoneme must perceive several features. She notes that distinction between sounds that differ in the feature of place of articulation causes the greatest difficulty. In *tate* for *cake*, /t/ and /d/ are alike except that /t/ is an alveolar sound and /k/ is a palatal sound. The other feature she mentions is continuancy in manner of production, as *tink* for *think*. She observes that when two features are disturbed, as *date* for *cake*, where the substitution involves both the place of articulation and voicing, the speech becomes less intelligible.

It is obvious that considerable phonetic likenesses exist between the substituted sound and the target sound. Usually the change involves no more than two features and often only one. Much of the change seems to be related to ease of production. For example, in the substitutions of /f/ for /θ/ and /w/ for /l/, the only distinctive feature change is from /+coronal/ to /−coronal/ (a feature involving raising the front of the tongue from a neutral position). When we think in terms of articulatory phonetics, the only change is in the place of production in both substitutions (see Cairns and Williams (1972); and McReynolds, Engmann, and Dimmitt 1974). Winitz (1972) notes that the phonetic similarity of the sound to be learned and the sound that is substituted may be an important variable governing phonetic acquisition.

Leonard (1973) found that the feature errors of the children in the Cairns and Williams (1972) study were precisely those used most frequently by children he studied who were receiving therapy in a public school setting. Both groups of children used errors characterized by distinctive feature sets that required only the addition of one or two features to achieve the target sound. He notes that children who exhibit such errors as substituting /w/ for /r/, /d/ for /ð/, and /f/ for /θ/ eventually will develop standard articulation. Maturity will help these children to reach adult articulatory proficiency.

Leonard points out, however, that another group of children acquire articulation in a deviant manner. He bases this conclusion partly on the Menyuk study (1968) just cited. He notes that children who follow the Menyuk schedule but who are acquiring sounds later than their peers are simply using a less mature phonological system. Other children, however, are following a deviant pattern wherein the features /+strident/, /−anterior/, and /+continuant/ are seldom maintained in their substitutions. Leonard found that out of 200 children with articulatory difficulties not caused by known organic or intellectual factors, 70 per cent showed deviant errors.

Some writers point out that the existing distinctive feature systems are not always practical for the speech clinician. They believe that a particular distinctive feature may be overgeneralized and may encompass too great a phonetic space. Walsh (1974) contrasts the Jakobsonian theory of distinctive features with one of language-specific articulation features, which he believes helps the clinician to see the sort of articulatory problems involved in certain cases. He illustrates with the use of the substitution of /j/ for /l/, noting that this would be described in (Jakobsonian) theory as a change in such features as vocalic, consonantal, and coronal, all of which are used to differentiate large classes of sounds. Walsh describes his preference as follows:

	/l/	/r/
Lower articulator	+ tongue tip	− tongue tip
	− tongue blade	+ tongue blade
Upper articulator	+ tooth ridge	− tooth ridge
	− prepalate	+ prepalate

Walsh notes that when the substitution is described in this way, the misarticulation can be seen either as a retracted articulation rendering a lateral release impossible or as a motor failure requiring compensatory articulation in a retracted position.

Such lack of precision in the distinctive feature analysis of phonetic events, as illustrated, leads to questions concerning the theory's potential as a model of speech production. For example, Gallagher and Shriner (1975) found that /s/ and /z/ were more likely to be produced correctly when followed by /t/ and /d/ than when followed by other sounds. Distinctive feature theory would classify /s/ and /z/ as having more features in common with /θ/ and /ð/ than with /t/ and /d/. Gallagher and Shriner explain that their results may be influenced by the similarity between /θ/ and /ð/ and their children's incorrect productions of /s/ and /z/. In this area, the need for more research and phonological analysis is evident.

To meet some of these objections and to provide a basis for computer analysis, Telage (1980), as noted in Chapter 6, compiled a set of features considered as a production matrix divorced from phonemic theory. For this purpose, articulatory attributes replace distinctive features. After reviewing the Chomsky and Halle features, Telage eliminated those features that relate to vowels: *rounded, tense,* and *low. Consonantal* was also eliminated since no attention was to be given to vowels. *Vocalic, nasal, continuant, voicing,* and *strident* remained. He changed *vocalic* to *glide* to indicate minimal constriction in the oral cavity for consonants. Because these attributes still did not appear to delineate enough information, he further differentiated by adding the features *stop, fricative,* and *lateral.* Telage excluded *low,* leaving four place features: *coronal* and *high* were retained; *back velar* and *glottal* were substituted for *back. Anterior* was considered too general a feature. In reviewing the consonants, he found that /k/, /g/, /ŋ/, and /h/ occur posteriorly but that the remaining twenty include a considerable degree of differential activity involving the lips, alveolar process, and different aspects of the tongue and palate. He therefore increased the number of features by eight: *bilabial, labio-dental, tip alveolar, tip dental, blade alveolar, blade prepalatal, front-palatal,* and *central palatal.* His place features include *bilabial, labiodental, tip-alveolar, tip-dental, blade-alveolar, blade prepalatal, front-palatal, central-palatal, back velar, glottal, high* and *coronal.* His features involving manner include: *stop, continuant, fricative, strident, nasal, lateral, glide,* and *voicing.* See page 129 for Telage's chart of the features.

Omission of Sounds

A sound may be omitted. The following are examples of omissions of sounds by David, a ten-year-old boy:

[bɛd]	for *bread*
[dɛs]	for *dress*
[taɪ]	for *try*
[ten]	for *train*

Most youngsters will not be as consistent as this child in omitting sounds. Their omissions may be more like those of Susie, a five-year-old, whose examples follow:

Air you dowin? [er ju doɪn]	for *Where are you going?*
Me ante o too. [mi antə o tu]	for *I want to go too.*
I or? [aɪ or]	for *Why for?*

Obviously, omissions occur much more freqeuntly in the young child's speech than they do in the older child's speech. As noted earlier, children omit final consonants more often than the initial consonant and they commonly omit one of the sounds in clusters of two consonants, such as *tr*[tr], *pr*[pr], *st*[st], or *sl*[sl]. But as children grow older, their *pide* becomes *pride*. Omissions then are not particularly common and tend to decrease after the age of three.

The clinician needs to be aware of the many factors that affect perception of a child's omission of sounds. He/she must be cognizant of the assimilative processes. A speech/language clinician may hear clearly a child's *old bat* as [oʊl bæ]. But when the clinician is aware that both /l/ and /d/ are voiced sounds and that the /d/ may well have been assimilated, is there an omission of a sound? Perhaps one speech/language clinician heard a faint /t/ at the end of [bæt]; another, nothing. Is then /t/ omitted, is there some kind of substitution, or is /t/ distorted? Only a spectographic analysis can tell for sure. Furthermore, the clinician also must make sure that the omission is not the result of a dialectal difference. For example, a child may be perfectly capable of making a final /t/ but say, *Yesterday I walk home* rather than *I walked home.* Or he may not be aware of some process such as pluralization. He may say *I have five pencil* not because he cannot make the final /s/ but because he does not understand the process of pluralization.

Distortion of Speech Sounds

A sound may be distorted. The listener recognizes the sound but is distracted by it. Again perception plays a role. One speech/language clinician perceived a child's /s/ as distorted. A second pathologist asked, "How?" The first responded with, "I saw Jane's tongue protrude." But was the result distorted enough to be noticeable? Did it differ from most adult speakers? Or was it largely the result of the observation of the tongue's protruding? In another situation, two clinicians and a teacher unanimously judged an /s/ to be lateral. Even the children noticed this quality with such remarks as: "He sounds like he's telling us to be quiet." "Gary makes an /s/ like he's getting ready to spit."

Winitz (1975, p. 2) defines *distortion* as a substitution of an uncommon English sound for the target sound. He describes a lateral lisp as a sound that is voiceless, made with more frication than the normal /s/, and lateralized. He uses the symbol /ɫ/ for the lateral lisp. The /l/ indicates the lateral quality (both sides of the tongue are lowered); the /-/ indicates the dark quality of the /l/; and // indicates the voiceless quality.

Both omissions and distortions can be considered substitutions. In omissions there is a substitution, for a time gap replaces the target phoneme. Distortions involve the substitution of an unacceptable English sound for a target phoneme. In distortions, the child recognizes and selects the correct phoneme but doesn't achieve an accurate sound. The result begins to approximate the sound but is not perceived as the actual sound by listeners.

PHONETIC CONTEXT

The phonetic context makes a difference in the speaker's rendition of phonemes. We have already pointed to assimilative processes—the effect of one speech sound on another. As phonetic context and position of a sound in a syllable differ, allophones of a single phoneme occur. For example, consider a variety of *t*'s. When you place /s/ before *tab*, making the word *stab*, the *t* in *stab* is different from the *t* in *tab*, for the *t* in *tab* is fully aspirated. When you say *tat*, the initial and final /t/ differ in that the initial /t/ is fully aspirated while the final /t/ is not. Again when you say *bat the ball*, the /t/ is made differently with the tip of the tongue not on the alveolar ridge but against the teeth.

Seldom are words spoken alone; rather they are in a phrase or sentence. Therefore, the final consonant in a word may not really be a final consonant, as in "Won't you do it?" which frequently becomes ['wonₜt∫ə'duₜɪt]. Obviously no final /t/ exists in *wont*, for the process of assimilation is at work. Articulatory movements continue throughout the phrase. When you add to the question *either now or later, Won't you do it now or later* may all be spoken on one exhalation. The syllables within the phrases take various forms as:

oh	V	tried	CCVC
day	CV*	strayed	CCCVC
aid	VC	baste	CVCC
tray	CCV		

*C=consonant; V=vowel

The diagnosis of the errors, then, cannot be readily assigned in terms of initial, medial, and final consonants. And a phoneme may be correct in one phonetic context and not in another. A speech sound, however, that is an inaccurate acoustic representation of the intended sound represents an articulatory error. Because the movements of the articulating mechanism do not produce the intended speech sound, these movements are also symptoms. The competent clinician will assess the inaccuracy of the speech sounds and will account for them in terms of the producing mechanism. Telage (1980), as noted earlier, presents such a system based on articulatory (see p. 129) attributes. Ingram's (1976 and 1981) terminology for articulation errors is useful in that it describes clearly what is happening to the intended sound— at least on the surface level.

Ingram (1981) explains how to analyze a child's phonological processes and how to record them. His summary sheet includes a way of reaching an articulation score, syllable types, an analysis of homonyms (where the child produces the same phonetic form for two or more adult words that normally are not homonymous as [bat] for both *bath* and *blanket*), which sounds are substituted for other sounds, and finally a phonological process analysis. We are including an example of this last item, based on a sample of one child's misarticulations.

- **FINAL CONSONANT DELETION**: [me] for *made;* [bu] for *broom*
- **REDUCTION OF CONSONANT CLUSTERS**: [tɪ] for *stick* and [bu] for *broom.*
- **SYLLABLE DELETION AND REDUPLICATION**: [te] for *table;* [bɛbɛ] for *bell* [bɛll].
- **FRONTING OF PALATALS AND VELARS**: [tʌm] for *come;* [do] for *go;* and [su] for *shoe.*
- **STOPPING OF FRICATIVES AND AFFRICATES**: [paɪ] for *five;* [pouə] for four; [ti] for *see.*
- **SIMPLIFICATION OF LIQUIDS AND NASALS**: [daɪs] for *nice.* [padɪ] for *Polly;* [wɛd] for *red.*
- **OTHER PROCESSES:**Backing [kæp] for *tap*
  Nasalization [mɛmo] for *yellow.*
  Voicing [bæd] for *bat*
  Lisping [θe] for *say*
  Glottal replacement [paʔɪ] for *Polly;* [taʔɪ] for *stocking.*

Ingram (1981, pp. 78–79) also gives a more detailed form of analysis. We have included the first two sections of this form to illustrate his method:

Examples of Phonological Processes as Listed on the Phonological Sheet

---

Syllable Structure Processes

DELETION OF FINAL CONSONANTS (The deletion of any single consonant that occurs at the end of a syllable)

1. Nasals: /m, −n, −ŋ/ Example: [kʌ] for come; [kɪ] for *king*
2. Voiced stops: /b, −d, −g/ Example: [ro] for *robe*
3. Voiceless stops: /p, −t, −k/ Example: /ʌ/ for *up*

Examples of Phonological Processes as Listed on the
Phonological Sheet (*continued*)

Syllable Structure Processes

4. Voiced fricatives: [v, −z, −ʒ, −dʒ] Example: [mu] for *move*
5. Voiceless fricatives: [f, −θ, −s, −ʃ, −tʃ] Example: [li] for *leaf*

REDUCTION OF CONSONANT CLUSTERS (The deletion of one or more consonants that occur together within the same syllable)

6. Liquids

reduced to consonant	clock [kak]	cry [kaɪ]	queen [kin]
consonant deleted	[lak]	[raɪ]	[win]
cluster deleted	[ak]	[aɪ]	[in]

7. Nasals
8. *s* Clusters

Ingram goes on to include three aspects of syllable deletion and reduplication (9, 10, and 11), five aspects of substitution processes including fronting and stopping, three aspects of simplification of liquids and nasals (17, 18, and 19), four of other substitution processes (20, 21, 22, and 23) and four of assimilative processes, (24, 25, 26, and 27). Clearly this program could define the surface phonological processes in a child's substitutions accurately.

PERSISTENCE OF SOUND PREFERENCES

Ingram (1976) discusses the persistence of sound preference as a characteristic of children with phonological disabilities. He gives examples of children preferring nasal or fricative sounds over others; in other words, some children tend to make excessive use of certain articulatory features. Weiner (1981) investigated and analyzed the articulatory deficiencies of eight children who exemplified the sound preference system. For example, one of the children substituted /h/ for nonlabial voiceless stops; [tɛnt] became [hɛnt], [kom] became [hom]. Of course, many other substitutions also occurred. The process of substituting /h/ obviously did not apply to the labial, voiceless sound /p/.

Weiner (1981) notes that sound preference is different from phonological processes like stopping of fricatives or fronting of velar stops in that the latter processes involve feature changes, as *fricative→stop*. Sound preference is not a feature changing process per se; rather it is more appropriately termed a *collapsing process*, where a group of sounds having certain features in common are represented by a restricted feature arrangement. For instance, where all voiceless fricatives are replaced by /t/, there is the substitution of a specific feature complex (e.g. +stop, −voice and +alveolar for +fricative, −voice.)

Weiner emphasizes that making the distinction between feature-changing processes and the sound preference process is important both in terms of accuracy of description and in planning speech intervention programs. In the sound preference situation, the preference sound needs to be contrasted with each member of the general class of sounds that were collapsed. Such analysis can lead to efficient therapy.

POSITION OF SOUND IN A WORD.   Children exhibit superior performance across all features for the initial position as compared with the medial and final phenomenon. Features in the initial position are less constrained by contextual conditions than are those in medial or final positions (Ingram 1976), and thus lend themselves to more distinct perceptual contrasts. Singh, Hayden and Toombs' (1981) research supports the thesis that the initial position carries a higher information load and this increased importance enhances the role of distinctive features.

ARTICULATORY DISORDERS AND COMMUNICATION

There are social consequences to articulatory disorders. Children frequently tease the child with articulatory disorders, calling him/her "baby" or mimicking some pronunciations. Such evaluations on the part of listeners affect the child's concept of self. A negative concept of self can, in turn, affect ability to communicate. The classroom teacher is of inestimable worth in fostering acceptance of the handicapped on the part of other students. The teacher's contribution of reinforcing the clinician's therapy is equally valuable.

Lisping seems to be particularly detrimental to effective communication. Mowrer et al. (1978), studying the effects of lisping on listeners, found that lisping negatively influences the first impression judgments of an adult audience as to the speaking ability, intelligence, education, masculinity, and friendship (social appeal) of the speaker. Interestingly, a speaker with a mild lisp is rated more favorably than one with a moderate lisp. Similarly Silverman (1976) found that on an initial encounter an adult with a lateral lisp is likely to be evaluated by peers as handicapped. Such disorders obviously need remediation— and the remediation needs reinforcement by the teacher.

The atmosphere of the communicative situation itself can have an affect on articulation. Most of us when we find we are not understood speak more slowly, rephrase, or give greater detail to help clarify our communicative intent (Longhurst and Siegel, 1973). Different communicative atmospheres may bring about different results of articulation testing. Weiner and Ostrowski (1979) set out to determine the effects of uncertainty on the part of the listener on articulatory inconsistency on the part of the speaker. In this instance, phonetic context was held constant; the only difference was in the attitude of the listener. When the listener pretended to be uncertain of what the speaker said, the number of sound errors decreased significantly. More significance should be attached to the interaction of the speaker and listener as a factor in the variations in speech sound production.

CONCOMITANT DIFFICULTIES

Other speech problems may be associated with articulatory difficulties. For example, the child with a denasal voice has three defective sounds: *m* /m/, *n* /n/, and *ng* /ŋ/. The child with a muffled voice keeps his/her mouth almost clenched shut; the quality is in part the result of the lack of clear-cut articulation of sounds. These two difficulties are labeled *voice disorders*.

The term *retarded speech development* includes many articulatory defects—omissions, substitutions, and distortions; in fact, some writers include their discussion of the articulatory defects of the primary-grade children under retarded speech development. Retarded speech development, however, does connote, in addition to articulatory difficulties, meager vocabulary, overly simple structure, and, in general, retarded language development.

Cleft-palate speech and defective speech caused by impaired hearing are also characterized by articulatory difficulties. Even in cluttering, because of its rapid rate, the child noticeably slurs over and distorts the consonantal sounds. Thus, defective articulation may be a single problem to a child or it may be a symptom of a more complex syndrome.

ARTICULATORY DISORDERS AND MATURATION

Because some parents show undue concern about their young children's ability to articulate, teachers must be particularly aware of the need for recognition of the maturing factor in diagnosing articulatory defects. One mother of a five-year-old boy in kindergarten came to a school to demand speech help for him. The only error he made with any consistency was to substitute /t/ and /d/ for the two *th*'s /θ/, /ð/. But at times even these sounds were correct. Occasionally he said a /w/ for /l/. The mother insisted his speech was not "normal," explaining that his sister had spoken better at the same age, that his cousins of the same age spoke very well, and that the neighborhood youngsters who were even younger spoke more clearly. The little boy was a verbal child who expressed himself unusually well with very few articulatory errors.

Prognosis for Improvement Through Maturation

As noted earlier, maturation alone takes care of some of the articulatory difficulties in the primary grades. For some children, the impact of the regular kindergarten curriculum and maturation will bring about satisfactory phonological development. The amount and kind of language stimulation provided in the kindergarten may make a considerable difference in the child's development. Other children, however, even with time do not develop phonologically. Therefore, the clinician needs to be able to predict which of the children will need speech help. Almost all of the studies point to stimulability scores as one index of whether a child will develop a normal phonological system. Therefore, to find out whether children can imitate the clinician's utterance of the target sound in a nonsense syllable and in words seems to be one index of subsequent improvement (Farquhar 1961).

One way of predicting is through the Van Riper and Erickson *Predictive Screening Test of Articulation* (PSTA), 3rd ed. (1973) (Western Michigan University Continuing Education Office, Kalamazoo, Michigan). This test identifies those primary-age school children with functional misarticulations who are not likely to acquire normal, mature articulation by the time they reach third-grade level. As the results of a study of the predictive capability of this test, Barrett and Welsh (1975) conclude that it is a valuable instrument in the speech adequacy screening of the first-grade population. They note that the test can identify first-grade children whose articulation problems are not likely to disappear without therapy by the third grade. Based on this assumption, the clinician can, therefore, efficiently select those children who need clinical help.

Stockman and McDonald (1980) question whether PSTA does consistently and validly predict articulatory improvement. They point out that the accuracy would depend on the type of misarticulated consonants and that this may account for the varying degrees of predictive accuracy revealed in cross-validation studies. They believe, however, that the test may have predictive value for one or more specific misarticulated consonant subgroups. They demonstrated that children with four or more misarticulations obtained noticeably lower PSTA scores than those with fewer misarticulations. Such children then would be among those whom PSTA predicts accurately as needing remediation. They point to the difference in the /r/ subgroup. For example, subjects with 0–3 correct contexts tended to score below 40 (34 is the recommended cut-off score) whereas those with 4–7 correct contexts scored above 40. Whether those at the higher level are more likely to be self-corrected by third grade than those at the lower level is a matter for further research.

The prognosis that maturity alone will take care of articulatory disabilities depends on many factors. Several such factors point to a poor prognosis: (1) poor stimulability, as already mentioned; (2) many articulatory errors—four or more; (3) consistency in making the errors; and (4) possession in the error sounds of more than one feature error.

IDENTIFYING ARTICULATION ERRORS

Various screening devices are used to locate children in a school population who may need articulation therapy. This initial screening is usually planned by the clinician and is often administered by the classroom teacher. The clinician instructs the teacher in the administration of the screening. It includes such items as the following:

1. Giving name and address.
2. Naming of objects in pictures that contain the sibilant sounds /s/, /z/, /ʃ/, /ʒ/, /tʃ/, /dʒ/; the two *th* sounds /θ/ and /ð/; /l/, /r/, and /j/ as in *yellow*.
3. Counting to ten or naming the days of the week.
4. Holding conversations often based on children's books that will hold the interest of young children. These books should contain pictures that will evoke conversation that will include the sounds most likely to be inaccurate. Two such books are:
   Gunella Walde, *Tommy and Sarah Dress Up* (Boston: Houghton Mifflin Company, 1972). Tommy and Sarah find a trunk in Sarah's attic with many old clothes. The two children proceed to "dress up."
   E. Rice, *Oh, Lewis* (New York: Macmillan Publishing Co., Inc., 1974). Lewis and his mother and sister go shopping. Lewis has to

have help buckling his boots, zippering his jacket, finding his mittens, and getting his coat hood on right. He has just as much trouble getting his outer clothes off.

Screening test results, whether the test is administered by the speech/language clinician or by the teacher, are influenced by many factors. As noted earlier in this chapter, the perceptions of even trained assessors differ as to the acceptability of a particular phoneme; the communicative situation involving the attitude of the assessor and his personality make a difference. Also the physical environment, whether it is noisy or quiet, influences both the child's productions and the listener's assessment of the production.

Criteria on which clinicians base their choice of articulation tests include the following:

1. The rationale behind the test (order of development of sounds, distinctive features, frequency of occurrence of sounds, coarticulation of sounds that can indicate the influence of one sound on another, connected speech, single words, or phrases).
2. Administrative facility (time to administer and to score, and ease of administration and scoring).
3. Population to be tested. For example, Drumwright, Van Natta, Camp, Frankenburg, and Drexler (1973) describe the development of an articulation screening test for economically disadvantaged children.
4. Diagnostic purposes.

Winitz (1969, p. 244) sets up clear, more specific criteria for testing:

1. That the test contain a constant set of stimulus words for articulatory subjects.
2. That particular sounds should be elicited by several stimulus words and that they occur in a variety of number of syllables.
3. That the method of elicitation (oral or pictorial) should be consistent for all sounds.
4. That both spontaneous and imitated material be included.
5. That the criteria correctness or inaccuracy be based on more than a single response.

To obtain a sample of the child's language is a profitable exercise in evaluating articulation. The tester should realize, however, that this sample will usually not provide a cross-section of sounds in a variety of contexts but rather those sounds involved in a particular conversation based on particular topics. Connected speech samplings seem to provide a significantly greater number of total errors than single-word testing. Studies by Faircloth and Faircloth (1970), by Dubois and Bernthal (1978) and by Johnson, Winney and Pederson (1980) support this statement. Johnson et al. found that not only did the connected-sampling testing reveal a greater number of total errors than stimulus-word testing, but that it also identified individual defective phonemes not identified through the single-word testing, that it resulted in a greater number of substitution errors than omission errors, and lastly that a significant number of the errors identified by connected-speech sampling were produced accurately in the single-word testing.

Phoneme Production Tests

The following tests are representative of many in the field that test the accuracy of each of the American English phonemes both singly and in clusters, and usually in a variety of contexts.

McDONALD'S SCREENING DEEP TEST OF ARTICULATION WITH LONGITUDINAL NORMS. (Stanwix House, Pittsburgh, Pa.) This test evaluates a child's common misarticulated consonants in various phonetic contexts. It contains norms from a longitudinal study of 521 children based on testing at the beginning and end of kindergarten and first grade and at the beginning of second and third grade. It explains the implications of these norms for case selection.

GOLDMAN AND FRISTOE'S TEST OF ARTICULATION. (American Guidance Service, Circle Pines, Minnesota), in filmstrip format, evaluates all necessary phonemes and obtains an adequate and accurate sample of a child's behavior. Children are asked to respond to pictures by naming familiar objects by answering questions about the pictures. This test is based on the assumption that articulation of speech sounds should be evaluated in words, in sentences, and in imitation of the examiner's correct production in isolation.

THE ARIZONA ARTICULATION PROFICIENCY SCALE. (Western Psychological Services, Los Angeles, California) includes each phoneme of American English and /l/, /r/, and /s/ clusters with the norm age of the acquisition of each sound. It is based on the rationale that the more frequently a misarticulated sound is heard in speech, the greater is the weight of the articulatory problem.

COMPTON-HUTTON PHONOLOGICAL ASSESSMENT. (Carousel House, San Francisco, Ca.). This test provides a structured step by step approach for the linguistic analysis of misarticulations. The clinical application is based on three principles: (1) Misarticulations consist of a system of interrelated deviant patterns, (2) Correction of any deviant production will break down the pattern, and (3) By selecting key patterns and sound for intervention, correct production of consonants will occur more quickly than by using traditional intervention methods.

FISHER-LOGEMANN TEST OF ARTICULATION COMPETENCE. (Houghton Mifflin Company, Boston, Mass.) This test includes eleven cards that can be used to elicit articulatory behavior for screening purposes. It also provides easy distinctive feature analysis and includes an asset: variations of dialect depending on the area of United States and depending on influences of a foreign language.

These tests are used largely to assess the adequacy of the child's articulatory performance—to determine which children need to be in attendance at the school speech clinical facility.

A second type of test, much more detailed, determines the ability of the child to use sounds in various phonetic contexts. In consequence, it provides the clinician with information on the child's ability to produce sounds not only in various positions but also in different phonetic contexts. In addition, it can be used to compare therapy, to evaluate progress, to select case loads, to determine consistency of misarticulations, and to identify factors related to misarticulations such as distinctive features. Brief descriptions of two such tests follow:

THE TEMPLIN-DARLEY TEST OF ARTICULATION, 2ND ED. (Bureau of Educational Research and Service, The University of Iowa, Iowa City, Iowa) is a revision and expansion of the original edition of the Templin-Darley Screening and Diagnostic Test of Articulation. The 141-item Diagnostic Test is subdivided into nine overlapping subtests including a screening test and the Iowa Pressure Articulation Test. A cutoff score is available for each age. This test provides information about a child's general adequacy of articulation, his/her consistency of accurate production of a given type and a detailed description and analysis of articulation. Consonants are tested in initial and final positions and in clusters.

MCDONALD'S DEEP TEST OF ARTICULATION: PICTURE AND SENTENCE FORMS. (Stanwix House, Pittsburgh, Pa.) This test offers a different approach to the assessment and treatment of functional articulatory problems, for it is based on constructs derived from motor and acoustic phonetics, control theory, developmental psychology, and linguistics. It disavows the traditional concept of initial, medial, and final consonants and assesses instead consonants in different syllabic roles (release or arrest), as different consonant types (single, abutting, and compound) and in systematically varied phonetic contexts designed to provide for a diversity of coarticulatory movements.

FACTORS ASSOCIATED WITH ARTICULATORY DIFFICULTIES

Language Deficits

Many authorities believe that most children with deficiencies in articulatory development also have deficiencies in other aspects of language development. Ferrier's (1966) study indicates that children with articulatory difficulties do not do as well in language as measured by all nine tests of the *Illinois Test of Psycholinguistic Abilities* (1st ed.) as do children with normal speech. For the children with articulatory defects, the scores on four tests were substantially lower, indicating that these children do not do as well as normal-speaking children in expressing ideas verbally, using grammatical structures automatically, recalling a series of digits presented to them orally, and recalling a series of geometric forms presented to them visually. Smith (1967) reports a correlated finding on a digit recall test.

Marquardt and Saxman (1972), in a study of language comprehension and auditory discrimination in articulatory-deficient kindergarten children, found that those children with normal articulatory ability performed significantly better than those with poor articulatory ability on *Carrow's Test of Auditory Comprehension of Language*. They noted that the level of linguistic knowledge is less for the poor articulation group than for the high articulation group, and that the children who made the greater number of articulatory errors also tended to make the greater number of auditory comprehension errors.

Other studies point to the ability of normal-speaking children to use more sophisticated syntactical structures than do children with functional articulatory abilities. Menyuk (1964) reports that in comparing children with infantile speech[1] with children with normal

---

[1] This category would seem to be comprised of the more severe articulatory cases. According to Menyuk (1964, p. 119) the most frequent sound errors were omissions and substitutions. Furthermore, 50 per cent of the infantile-speech children omitted initial /s/ and final /t/, and more than 50 per cent of the children used these substitutions: /w/ for /r/ and /l/, /t/ for /k/ and /θ/, /d/ for /g/ and /ð/.

speech (ages 3–5.10), the normal-speaking children used significantly more transformations than the defective-speech group, and the group with infantile speech used more restricted forms and used them much more frequently than the normal-speaking group. The child with normal speech rapidly acquired structures that required increasingly complex rules for their generation over the two- to three-year period, and exceeded in acquisition of structures even the oldest infantile-speech child. There was no significant difference in the mean number of sentences used.

The results seem to indicate that the most meaningful factor is the difference in the two groups' ability to determine the complete set of rules used to generate and differentiate structures at any level of grammar. Examples of transformation types are

> Negation—*He isn't a good boy.*
> Question—*Are you nice?*
> Contraction—*He'll be good.*
> Auxiliary *be* placement—*He is not going.*
> Relative clause—*I don't know what he is doing.*
> Iteration—*You have to drink milk to be strong.*

Examples of restricted forms are:

> Verb phrase omission—*This green.*
> Noun phrase redundancy—*I want it the paint.*
> Preposition substitution—*He took me at the circus.*
> Pronoun subject substitution—*Me like that.*

Similarly, Vandemark and Mann (1965) found that the significant difference between a group of 50 normal-speaking children and 50 children with defective articulation was in the syntactical complexity, which involved grammatical completeness and complexity of response. According to this study, children with defective articulation are not inhibited in terms of amount of verbal output but are deficient in the areas of grammatical completeness and complexity of response.

Shriner, Holloway, and Daniloff (1969), in a study of 30 children with normal articulation and 30 with defective articulation, found that the mean number of words per response was significantly lower for the speech-defective group than for the normal-speaking group. They agree with Vandermark and Mann that the children with defective articulation do not use as developed a syntactical structure as the normal-speaking children. This study used a method of evaluating the complexity of sentences that differed from the Vandermark and Mann study in that these researchers counted the number of noun phrases and verb phrases.

Lee (1966) compared the syntactical development of two boys—one normal, the other deviant in articulatory development. She found marked differences between them. Not only was the speech deviant slower in following a normal pattern of behavior but he failed to produce certain types of syntactic structures.

Linguistic expression is organized centrally as systematic arrangements of syntactic, morphological and phonological elements, which organization controls phonetic behavior. The child with a phonological disorder may be limited in his/her ability to manage his/her linguistic system during complex grammatical encoding and, consequently, may lose control of his/her articulatory processes. Although he/she may exhibit articulatory control in encoding single words and simple phrases, he/she may lose this control as the demands of linguistic processing become more complex in such areas as vocabulary and sentence structure. This lack of development could be related to a neurological impairment, maturational delay, or a defective auditory and/or proprioceptive feedback.

Panagos, Quine and Klich (1979) studied the effects of three structural variables—syntactic structure (noun phrase, declarative sentence and passive sentence), word structure (monosyllable and disyllable), and word position of a sound (initial and final)—on articulatory performance. The children involved in the study misarticulated consonants that were late developing, such as /θ/, /dʒ/, /ʃ/, and /tʃ/. Production difficulties of consonants were compounded when the consonants occurred in phonologically complex words and syntactically complex sentences. Grammatical complexity caused these children to simplify their word production. This study points to attributes of an underlying limitation of organizational ability.

Schwartz et al. (1980) provide support for the hypothesis of Panagos et al. (1979) that some global organization deficit underlies phonological disorders. In this study Schwartz et al. compared the phonological behavior of three normal-speaking and three language-disordered children matched on the basis of mean utterance length, sex, and cognitive ability. The comparison was based on an analysis of the spontaneous speech of the children. The results of their study revealed: (1) There was no substantive divergence in the characteristics of the adult form of the words that the two groups of children attempted; (2) There were minimal differences between the two groups in the syllabic structures of the children's productions; (3) There were more substantial similarities than differences in phonological processes; (4) The two groups did not differ as to the variability in production within words.

Obviously some relationship between language and phonological difficulties does exist. But the exact relationship is not clear. Two studies suggest the complexity of the problem. Arndt, Shelton, Johnson and Furr (1977) point out that their data do not support the hypothesis that children who present articulation problems are consistently deficient in other language measures. They note that the subjects' distribution of scores on many of the psycholinguistic and reading-spelling measures correspond rather closely with the distribution of persons on whom the tests were standardized. They also note that their data do not support the view that children who misarticulate /s/ are distinct from children who misarticulate /r/ in terms of language scores. Singh, Hayden and Toombs (1981) emphasize the role of the heirarchy of distinctive features in differentiating the articulation errors of articulation-disordered children and language-disordered children. They note that evidence exists that the feature profile of the articulation disordered group is somewhat more consistent with normal acquisition than the feature profile of the language disordered group. Their research supports this view. They studied the profiles of over a thousand children enrolled in school remedial speech sessions. The order of features within the heirarchy of this total group were: nasality, sonorancy, voicing, labiality, sibilancy, front/back placement, and continuancy which hierachy implies that nasality and sonorancy are the strongest features and that the front/back placement and continuancy are the weakest. This study showed that in this group strong features were mastered by five years of age and weak features by eight. From this study they make clear that the age differences in processing features in terms of hierarchy are more pronounced in the articulation-disordered group than in the language-disorderd group. They believe these differences suggest that the performance of articulation-disordered children is more age dependent than that of the language-disordered children. They go on to note that this trend supports the idea that articulation problems without language delay represent an inability to manipulate distinctive features correctly and that, perhaps for the language-disordered group, distinctive feature errors are part of a more global linguistic delay.

Low Intelligence

Some studies show a high incidence of articulatory defects among children who are definitely mentally retarded. Undoubtedly, many organic conditions, such as brain injury, contribute to both deficient articulatory and mental abilities.

In a study, representative of others, of the articulatory development of 415 mental retardates, Wilson (1966) found that 53.4 per cent had defective articulation, whereas 46.6 per cent had normal speech. As the mental age increases, the total number of deviant sounds decreases but the articulatory pattern is not orderly. Several sibilant, affricative, and fricative sounds are never produced by 90 per cent of the children through the nine-year mental age level. The articulatory development of the mentally retarded does not parallel the development of normal children even when the mental age of the retardate is matched against the chronological age of the normal child.

When the articulatory defect is typed according to omission, substitution, or distortion, and even to the type of sound substitution, the relationship between intellectual ability and articulatory difficulties is refined. For example, Prins (1962b), in a comparison of speech-handicapped and normal children, found that children with defective articulation errors of the omission type were lower in intelligence as measured by a receptive vocabulary test than were the normal-speaking children. But when the articulatory errors consisted chiefly of interdentalization of /s/ or /z/, or the use of phonemic sound substitutions in which only one articulatory feature is altered, there was no significant difference in intellectual ability as measured by the same test.

Socioeconomic Status

Prins (1962a) also did correlations between a variety of articulatory variables and socioeconomic status. He found that subjects with a high proportion of interdental lisping (where /s/ is produced with the tongue visible between the teeth) tend to come from high socioeconomic levels, whereas subjects with a high proportion of omission-type errors come from low socioeconomic levels.

Adler (1973) in a study involving articulatory deviances and social class membership lists these results: (1) Lower-class children manifested a greater number of omissions and substitutions in all positions than did middle-class children; (2) There was no great distinction between classes for the omission of final consonants; (3) Middle-class children exhibited a higher incidence figure in distortions on all three sound positions in words; (4) Many /θ/ and /ð/ deviances existed regardless of social class; (5) /r/ was incorrectly produced more often by white children than by black children.

Hearing Loss

Obviously a relationship exists between adequate hearing and the ability to learn to speak. Although children's hearing may be sufficient for understanding conversation and what goes on around them, it may be insufficient for learning to make all the sounds. Some sounds children may not hear at all. Their own speech, therefore, reflects their inability to hear. Peripherally deaf children almost always have defective articulation, for they are unable to imitate sounds. They cannot compare the sounds they utter with those produced by others. In fact, they cannot hear the sounds of any model. Their abilities to see and to feel cannot make up for their inability to hear. We discussed the problem of the child with a hearing loss in Chapter 9 and will do so more fully in Chapter 14.

Structural Abnormalities

Anomalies of the tongue, lips, teeth, and palate have long been associated with articulatory difficulties. Recently, however, attitudes have changed on the responsibility of organic deviations of the articulatory mechanism for articulatory defects. For instance, the literature in the field of speech therapy presents opposing viewpoints on the responsibility of dental abnormalities for defective articulation. Undoubtedly, for some children, malocclusion of the teeth or an abnormally large tongue contribute to the child's lack of articulatory development. But some children with similar organic difficulties do not misarticulate the same sounds whereas other children with a normal mechanism do misarticulate them. Poor structures may, however, be a contributing factor in explaining poor articulation.

The Teeth and Gum Ridge

The teeth and/or gum ridge are involved in the sounds /f/, /v/, /θ/, /ð/, /s/, /z/, /ʃ/, /ʒ/, /tʃ/, and /dʒ/. In /f/ and /v/ the upper teeth touch the lower lip. In /θ/ and /ð/ the tongue tip is placed against the biting edge of the upper teeth or between the two rows of teeth. In the sibilant sounds, the air is directed against the teeth in a variety of ways. In some cases the teeth have difficulty reaching the lower lip, the biting edge is badly located, or the teeth are so formed that it is difficult to find a surface of teeth against which to direct the air.

The condition where the upper front teeth protrude abnormally beyond the lower teeth is called an overbite. When the upper lip meets the lower one with difficulty, /p/, /b/, and /m/ may be defective. The tongue lies forward in the mouth, sometimes over the lower teeth. The lower teeth are so far back that they cannot provide the necessary friction to make a good /s/ or /z/. With this condition the lower jaw usually recedes.

In other cases the lower jaw protrudes and the lower front teeth project over the upper front teeth. This is an underbite.

In still other cases, a space occurs between the upper and lower teeth when they are brought together. This condition is called an open bite. Normally the upper incisor overlaps its counterpart on the lower jaw so that about one-third of the surface of the visible lower incisor is covered by the upper incisor. In an open bite /s/ and /z/ are most frequently defective since the narrow stream of air cannot be directed against the cutting edge of the teeth. Sometimes /ʃ/, /ʒ/, /θ/, and /ð/ are distorted. If the lips cannot be brought together /p/, /b/, and /m/ may be defective. When the lower lip cannot touch the teeth easily, /f/ and /v/ may be inaccurate.

Finally, a space may occur between the central incisors or the canine teeth may be irregularly placed. In both these instances /s/ may be defective. When the space occurs, too much air escapes. Where the teeth are irregularly placed, they may interfere with the tongue so that the air is allowed to escape over one or both of its sides. Frequently, however, individuals themselves, finding compensatory movements, speak well in spite of having teeth that are very irregular.

It should be noted that many children with missing or abnormal teeth do make sounds correctly and some children with normal teeth do not make sounds correctly. Teachers and clinicians should also remember that missing teeth usually do not permanently influence the speech production of children.

The Tongue

The term *tongue-tied* is applied when the frenum of the tongue (the little web of tissue underneath the front part of the tongue) is abnormally short so that the tip of the tongue cannot move to points such as the ridge behind the upper teeth. This condition, where it severely disturbs articulation, is comparatively rare in children.

Other conditions may involve the tongue. The sounds that may be disturbed because of the tongue are /k/, /g/, /ŋ/, /θ/, /ð/, /l/, /r/, /s/, /z/, /ʃ/, and /ʒ/. In some few cases the tongue is so large or sluggish that it cannot make the small, precise, and quick movements that are necessary for certain sounds. Sometimes the tongue may be paralyzed or weak. At other times, there may be poor muscular coordination. Occasionally a thyroid deficiency causes sluggishness and poor control of the tongue, the result of generally poor motor coordination.

In /l/ and /r/, the tongue tip points to the teeth ridge. In /s/ and /z/, the tongue is grooved to direct a small stream of air against the teeth. In /n/, /t/, and /d/, the tongue touches the teeth ridge. In /ʃ/ and /ʒ/, the tongue directs a broader channel of air against the teeth. In the sibilant sounds, the tip of the tongue may reach toward the upper gum. In teaching the sibilants, however, clinicians sometimes find it better not to have the child try to reach toward the upper gum but to have him or her reach toward the gum behind the lower teeth. The tongue is obviously an important articulatory agent.

The relationship of the attributes of the tongue to articulatory proficiency are difficult to evaluate. The tongue grows rapidly in the early years and reaches an adult size at about eight years of age. The mandibles to which the tongue is attached mature later.

Tongue Thrust

The relationships between anterior thrusting of the tongue and open-bite malocclusion to lisping are not at all clear. Dworkin and Culatta (1980) measured maximum tongue strength for children with normal speech who exhibited anterior thrusting of the tongue during swallowing and open-bite malocclusions, for children with lisps who exhibited these same characteristics, and for a control group of normal-speaking children with normal occlusion and who did not thrust their tongues during swallowing. Among the three groups, there was no significant difference in protrusive tongue force. The researchers note that other explanations are needed to account for the presence of lisping in children who do thrust their tongues and have open bites than just the presence of these two attributes. The study fails to clarify why some children who exhibit anterior thrusting of the tongue and anterior open-bite do lisp whereas others with the same conditions do not lisp. These findings suggest that tongue-strengthening exercises may be superfluous to the correction of tongue thrust as associated with frontal lisping.

Christenson and Hanson (1981) investigated the assumption that myofunctional services facilitate remediation of articulatory disorders. Some children received articulatory remediation and myofunctional therapy; the others only articulatory remediation. Children in both programs made essentially the same progress in correcting placement of tongue-tip sounds, remediating /s/ and /z/ misarticulation and also remediating general articulation errors. However, only children who received oral myofunctional services remediated tongue-thrust behaviors.

Because of the uncertain status of myofunctional therapy (teaching of proper tongue posturing ad movements), the American Speech and Hearing Association in cooperation with a committee from the American Association of Dental Schools (1975) drafted the following position paper:

> A growing concern with the creation of clinical programs of myofunctional therapy and the involvement of some speech pathologists in these

programs led the American Speech and Hearing Association to seek an assessment of the current status of these clinical management procedures from the Joint Committee on Dentistry and Speech Pathology-Audiology. The Committee is composed of representatives of the ASHA and the American Association of Dental Schools (AADS). Based on a comprehensive study of relevant literature and a thorough evaluation of current clinical methodologies used to manage patients with an allegedly deviant pattern of deglutition frequently called tongue thrust swallow, the Committee developed the following statement:

STATEMENT

Review of data from studies published to date has convinced the Committee that neither the validity of the diagnostic label tongue thrust nor the contention that myofunctional therapy produces significant consistent changes in oral form or function has been documented adequately. There is insufficient scientific evidence to permit differentiation between normal and abnormal or deviant patterns of deglutition, particularly as such patterns might relate to occlusion and speech. There is unsatisfactory evidence to support the belief that any patterns of movements defined as tongue thrust by any criteria suggested to date should be considered abnormal, detrimental, or representative of a syndrome. The few suitably controlled studies that have incorporated valid and reliable diagnostic criteria and appropriate quantitative assessments of therapy have demonstrated no effects on patterns of deglutition or oral structure. Thus, research is needed to establish the validity of tongue thrust as a clinical entity.

In view of the above considerations and despite our recognition that some dentists call upon speech pathologists to provide myofunctional therapy, at this time, there is no acceptable evidence to support claims of significant, stable, long-term changes in the functional patterns of deglutition and significant, consistent alterations in oral form. Consequently, the Committee urges increased research efforts, but cannot recommend that speech pathologists engage in clinical management procedures with the intent of altering functional patterns of deglutition (*ASHA*, 1975, p. 331).

The Palate

In sounds such as /ʃ/ and /ʒ/, the palate plays a part. When the palate is abnormally high and narrow, the child's tongue may have difficulty in making the necessary contacts. When an opening occurs along the middle line of the palate, the condition is serious. Where the velum is inadequate so that the velo-pharyngeal port is not closed, all sounds except /m/, /n/, and /ŋ/ will be distorted—nasalized. This condition is discussed in a later chapter.

Motor Ability

Some children are poorly coordinated. Some youngsters run, go up- and downstairs, and jump much more easily than others. One youngster will put a jigsaw puzzle together and fit the pieces with little or no effort; another will struggle with it. This motor ability develops with maturation. But children of the same age vary widely in this ability. Sometimes poor coordination is evident around the mouth; the tongue, jaw, and palate are awkward. Some studies have shown that children with articulatory defects tend to score significantly lower on tests of motor ability than do children with normal speech. Such a study is one undertaken by Jenkins and Lohr (1964) who compared motor proficiency as measured by the *Oseretsky Test of Motor Proficiency* given to 38 first-grade children with "severe articulatory defects" and 38 normal-speaking controls matched for age, sex, and I.Q. The results of the study showed that the speech-defective group was significantly lower on the total test score and on each of the subtests administered. The tests involve maintaining bodily balance for a given period without gross movements of limbs or torso, performing coordinated hand activities (cutting paper) within a time limit and with accuracy, maintaining balance while performing a given movement of the whole body, as in running or hopping, simultaneously voluntary movements, as in tapping the left and right feet alternately, or performing a given muscular activity without extraneous movements, such as clenching the teeth without wrinkling the forehead.

One study measured one aspect of the motor ability of the tongue of articulatory deficient and normal speaking children. McNutt (1977) measured alternate-motion rate of the tongue for fifteen children with normal articulation, fifteen with misarticulated /s/, and another fifteen with misarticulated /r/. Both groups of children with misarticulations differed from the normal children in motor ability as measured by alternate-motion rate (involving the number of repetitions of syllables in the first two seconds of the first breath group, the first two seconds of the second breath group and the last two seconds of the fifth breath group).

Auditory Discrimination and Auditory Memory

As noted earlier in the discussion of articulatory testing, the examiners, the situation in which the child is being examined, the mood of the child, and the test itself all have impact on the assessment. The assessment is only as effective as are these components. The same attributes apply to the examination of a child's ability to discriminate or to remember sounds. In this testing situation you may find a child who is either consistently negativistic or consistently attempting to please the adult. Or the child may have an off day when nothing is of interest. Lastly, the test may actually test other variables than discrimination.

Many discrimination tests present a series of paired comparisons. About the only place the child encounters paired words is in tests or in clinical situations (see Schwarz and Goldman 1974). Elenbogen and Thompson (1972) pose the question as to whether the *Wepman Test of Discrimination* does not measure a vocabulary factor in addition to auditory discrimination. Their study showed that social class differences in error scores disappeared when a distorted form of the Wepman Test with nonsense words was used. Locke (1980a) explains that both the Templin and Wepman tests contain syllable pairs that do not contrast the phonemes that children often confuse in production; and that they make use of many contrasts in phonemes that children never confuse in speaking. Chapter 7 contains a discussion of tests for perception.

Whether articulatory production depends on correct identification or whether correct identification depends upon production is not completely clear. Perception may well be somewhat more closely related to articulation than to the acoustic stimuli, and consequently phonemic perception may be a function of motor mediation (Monnin and Huntington, 1974). For example, Williams and McReynolds (1975) found that articulatory production training was effective in changing both articulation and discrimination, whereas discrimination training was effective only in changing discrimination. Gottesman (1972) notes that the implication of her investigation is that differences in auditory discrimination between children speaking Black English and those speaking Standard English may be explained by differences in pronunciation; she found no differences between the two groups in auditory discrimination performance on words that could be commonly differentiated in the speech of all the children. Marquardt and Saxman (1972) report that in their study the articulatory proficient group made fewer errors in discrimination than did the poor articulatory group.

Shelton and Johnson (1977) also believe that current clinical description does not satisfactorily specify how various speech sound discrimination measures can be expected to contribute to the understanding of disordered articulation, to the prognosis for improvement of individual clients, or to the process of correcting disordered speech. They report a study where a delayed judgment test of speech-sound discrimination was correlated with measures of articulation status and articulatory improvements in two groups of subjects: one with an /r/ misarticulation and the other with an /s/ misarticulation. While the discrimination measures were reliable and internally consistent, discrimination-articulation correlations were low. This study again points to the need for further investigation of speech-sound discrimination, regardless of measurement procedures used, before it can be used as a base for drawing precise clinical inferences regarding individual children.

Phatate and Umano (1981) studied auditory discrimination of the voiceless fricatives /θ/, /f/, /ʃ/, and /s/ in children between four and six and a half years of age. The subjects were asked to remember the sound and to indicate each time the sound was used. They analyzed two types of errors. They found that the failure to discriminate between the remembered sound and the voiceless fricative decreased with age. The failure to identify the remembered sound and the type of errors did not change with age. They indicate that this study agrees with previous studies, which show that the discrimination between /f/ and /θ/ is difficult for children through the sixth year. It supports evidence that in auditory perception there is a developmental component.

And so, the persistent questions that arise are: Does the perception of speech result in the production of speech? Does the production of speech result in the perception of speech? Or do they go hand in hand? Clinically a child with an articulation production disorder is given production training; simultaneously, however, he is often given perceptual training. Locke (1980a) hypothesizes that the rationale for this perceptual training is:

1. The child is not producing the right phonological segments because he does not know how the right segments sound. (This implies that the child has an efficient articulatory system that is faithfully replicating the wrong sounds.)
2. Perception training can teach the child what the right segments sound like.
3. When the child has learned how the right segments sound, he will begin to produce those segments correctly. (This happens "automatically.") (Locke, 1980, p. 432)

Criticizing this rationale from the past, Locke points out that if it were possible to determine whether the child misperceives speech in much the same way that he misproduces it, one still would not know if perceptual failures were motivating or maintaining the child's production errors. He also points out that there is reason to believe that causality might logically work in the opposite direction. He further points out that in many cases there appears to be little justification for not assessing the child's perception of speech but that questions arise such as "Does the child know that his phonetic forms are not those of the adult community?" Perceptual evidence permits a more complete understanding of the child's phonological system; it also clarifies the broad distinction between articulatory and systemic disorders and, consequently, the extent to which the problem is one of linguistic rules as opposed to production or perception deficiencies.

Consequently, Locke (*ibid.*) has drawn up eight criteria for a clinically useful assessment of speech perception. These criteria are:

1. Examine the child's perception of replaced sounds in relation to replacing sounds.
2. Observe the same phonemes in identical phonetic environments in production and perception.
3. Permit a comparison of the child's performance on target sounds and replacing sounds with his discrimination of target and perceptually similar sounds.
4. Base the test on a comparison of an adult's surface form and the child's internal representation.
5. Present repeated opportunities for the child to reveal his perceptual decisions.
6. Not permit nonperceptual errors to masquerade as perceptual errors.
7. Require a response easily within a young child's conceptual capacities and repertoire of responses.
8. Allow a determination of the direction of misperception. (Locke, 1980b, p. 445)

Locke (1980b) constructs such a test but points to many individual differences. The research indicates that normal-hearing children perceive differentially the sound they produce distinctively and may or may not evidence discrimination of the sounds they collapse in production. He then asks: How do we account for one substituting child failing to discriminate his error contrast, whereas a different but outwardly similar child discriminates the same contrast even though he produces the same substitution? Are there two sources of error—one child erring for perceptual reasons; the other for any one of a variety of nonperceptual reasons? Are there children in different stages of the acquisition process? Do correct and incorrect discriminators differ in the area of their phoneme boundaries, the cognitive processes by which they decide perceptual questions, or the sensitivity of their substitution to syllabic position and phonetic environment?

Locke (*ibid.*) explores the dilemma further. He notes that when one encounters a child who consistently substitutes one sound for another but uniformly discriminates them correctly, one is inclined to think that the production problem is not perceptual in nature. But he indicates this conclusion may well be incorrect. First, children do produce "regressive phonological idiom," isolated forms that do not come up to the child's overall level of phonological progress. And so, if a child's production "disagrees with itself," why should one insist that it coincide perfectly with perception? Second, if we assume that articulatory strategy cannot commence until differential perceptual targets have been established, there would be a built-in lag between the acquisition of correct perception and the emergence of correct production. Further, however, once production capability developed, it still might require time to diffuse through the lexicon to the words used in the assessment procedure. A demonstration that the child had perfect perception, then, would not prove that the child's production disorder was originally nonperceptual. The most one could safely conclude is that whatever the origins of the child's error, it is not presently being maintained by phonetic imperception (Locke, *ibid.*) Obviously the exact relationship between perception and production has not been established.

Similar questions arise as to auditory memory. Locke and Kutz (1975), emphasizing what may be the effect of motor feedback, make the point that whereas speech learning requires memory, memory also depends on speech. Spontaneous speech and subvocal rehearsal both facilitate memory performance. Locke and Kutz found that children who could distinguish between /w/ and /r/, but who consistently spoke /w/ for /r/, made more /w/-/r/ confusions in recall than did children who produced /w/ and /r/ accurately. They suggest that the differences in the production but not in the perception of /w/ and /r/ by the two groups may be the result of the motor experience, which directly or indirectly provides the salient memory clues.

More research needs to be undertaken to determine the roles of auditory discrimination and memory in articulatory production.

Problems

1. List a series of phrases or sentences you use often such as "Have a good day." Transcribe them phonetically as you say them.
   a. Indicate the beginning and end of syllables.
   b. Indicate the assimilation that occurs in such a phrase or sentence.
2. Listen for articulatory errors in a particular child in a classroom. What effect, if any, does it appear to have on the particular child's communication?
3. Listen to a three- or four-year-old's conversation (preferably recording it). Note the omissions and substitutions. Then listen to a six- or seven-year-old child's conversation.
   a. Note the omissions and substitutions.
   b. Compare the omissions and substitutions of the two children.
4. Compare the acquisition of sounds schedule in Arlt and Goodban (1976)

with one set of norms in articulatory acquisition given in Chapter 7, on p. 166.

5. Give an articulatory test to two first graders.
    a. List the substitutions.
       (1) By checking with the norms and by using a stimulability test, indicate your conclusions as to whether the substitution will be taken care of with maturation.
       (2) By using a feature analysis, compare the substitutions with the target sounds. Find out whether you can detect a pattern.
    b. If a distortion exists, indicate the type of distortion phonetically.
    c. By observation or by use of a language test, note what you think the relationship is between articulatory development and syntactical development.
6. Give a sound discrimination test to two children—one in the primary grades and one in the middle grades. Note any differences that may exist.
7. If a case history of a child with an articulatory defect is available, note the information as to the child's:
    a. intellectual and language maturity.
    b. organs involved.
    c. diagnosis.
8. Give a screening test to two kindergarten children, following the procedures suggested in this chapter.
9. Find three children with missing front teeth. Is there a relationship of this condition to their production of /s/ and /z/)

References and Suggested Readings

Adler, S., "Articulatory Deviance and Social-Class Membership." *Journal of Learning Disabilities,* **6** (December 1973), 650–654.

American Speech and Hearing Association Joint Committee with Dentistry, "Position Statement of Tongue-Thrust." *ASHA,* **17** (May 1975), 331–337.

American Speech and Hearing Association, "Task Force Report on School Hearing and Language Screening." *Language, Speech, and Hearing Services in Schools,* **4** (July 1973), 109–119. (Gives basic principles in screening and suggests methods and materials for screening.)

Arlt, P. B. and M. T. Goodban, "A Comparative Study of Articulation Acquisition as Based on a Study of 240 Normals, Aged Three to Six." *Language, Speech, and Hearing Services in Schools,* **7** (1976), 173–180. (Shows that children acquire articulatory proficiency at an earlier age than previously reported.)

Arndt, W. B., R. L. Shelton, A. F. Johnson and M. L. Furr, "Identification and Description of Homogeneous Subgroups within a Sample of Misarticulating Children." *Journal of Speech and Hearing Research,* **20** (1977), 263–292. (Sorts a group of misarticulating children into homogeneous clusters that would be useful in research.)

Barrett, C. M., and H. R. Hoops, "The Relationship Between Self-Concept and the Remission of Articulatory Errors." *Language, Speech, and Hearing Services in Schools,* **5** (April 1974), 67–70. (Studies children who do not spontaneously remit articulation errors in terms of self-concept and discrepancies between self-concept and ideal self-concept.)

Barrett, M. D., and J. W. Welsh, "Predictive Articulation Screening." *Language, Speech, and Hearing Services in Schools,* **6** (1975), 91–95. (Gives results of predictive capability of Van Riper Predictive Screening Test.)

Block, E. L., and L. D. Goodstein, "Functional Speech Disorders and Personality: A Decade of Research." *Journal of Speech and Hearing Disorders,* **35** (August 1971), 295–314. (Includes a section on relationship of articulatory defects to (a) personality and adjustment of parents, and (b) personality and adjustment of children themselves.)

Bond, Z. S. and H. F. Wilson, "Acquisition of the Voicing Contrast by Language-Delayed and Normal-Speaking Children." *Journal of Speech and Hearing Research,* **23** (March 1980), 152–161. (Determines whether the control of the acoustic-phonetic cues for voicing is correlated with language proficiency and compares the pattern of acquisition of these cues in the speech of language-delayed children and normal speaking children.)

Bradley, R. C. and R. J. Stoudt, Jr., "A Five-Year Longitudinal Study of Development of Articulation Proficiency in Elementary School Children." *Language, Speech, and Hearing Services in Schools,* **8** (1977), 176–180. (Reports the results of a five-year longitudinal study of the spontaneous development of articulation proficiency in 60 elementary-school children.)

Bryans, B., J. McNutt and A. R. Lecours, "A Binary Articulatory Production Classification of English Consonants with Derived Difference Measures." *Journal Speech and Hearing Disorders,* **45** (August 1980), 346–357.

Cairns, H. S., and F. Williams, "An Analysis of the Substitution Errors of a Group of Standard English-Speaking Children," *Journal of Speech and Hearing Research,* **15** (December 1972), 811–820.

Christenson, M. and M. Hanson, "An Investigation of the Efficacy of Oral Mysfunctional Therapy as a Precursor to Articulation Therapy for Pre-First Grade Children." *Journal of Speech and Hearing Disorders,* **46** (May 1981), 160–167.

Drumwright, A., P. Van Natta, B. Camp, W. Frankenburg, and H. Drexler, "The Denver Articulation Screening Examination," *Journal of Speech and Hearing Disorders,* **38** (February 1973), 3–14. (Described the development of an articulation screening test for economically disadvantaged children.)

Dubois, E. M. and J. E. Bernthal, "A Comparison of Three Methods for Obtaining Articulatory Responses." *Journal of Speech and Hearing Disorders,* **43** (August 1978), 295–305.

Dworkin, J. P. and R. A. Culatta, "Tongue Strength; Its Relationship to Tongue Thrusting, Open-Bite, and Articulatory Proficiency." *Journal of Speech and Hearing Disorders,* **45** (May 1980), 277–282.

Elbert, M. and L. V. McReynolds, "Aspects of Phonological Acquisition during Artiulation Training." *Journal of Speech and Hearing Disorders,* **44** (November 1979), 459–471.

Elenbogen, E. M., and G. R. Thompson, "A Comparison of Social Class Effect in Two Tests of Auditory Discrimination." *Journal of Learning Disabilities*, **5** (April 1972), 209–212.

Faircloth, M. A., and S. R. Faircloth, "An Analysis of the Articulatory Behavior of a Speech-Defective Child in Connected Speech and in Isolated Word Responses," *Journal of Speech and Hearing Disorders*, **35** (February 1970), 51–61. (Supports the need for testing in connected speech.)

Farquhar, M., "Prognostic Value of Imitative and Auditory Discrimination Tests." *Journal of Speech and Hearing Disorders*, **26** (November 1961), 342–347.

Ferrier, E. E., "Investigation of ITPA Performance of Children with Functional Defects of Articulation." *Exceptional Child*, **32** (May 1966), 625–629.

Gallagher, T., "Revision Behaviors in the Speech of Normal Children Developing Language." *Journal of Speech and Hearing Research*, **20** (1977), 303–318.

Gallagher, T. M., and T. H. Shriner, "Articulatory Inconsistencies in the Speech of Normal Children." *Journal of Speech and Hearing Research*, **15** (March 1975), 168–175. (Shows that inconsistent production of /s/ and /z/ is related to motor sequencing constraints independent of word boundaries.)

——, "Contextual Variables Related to Consistent /s/ and /z/ Production in the Spontaneous Speech of Children." *Journal of Speech and Hearing Research*, **18** (December 1975), 623–633.

Gottesman, R. L., "Auditory Discrimination Ability in Negro Dialect Speaking Children." *Journal of Learning Disabilities*, **5** (February 1972), 94–101.

Hanson, M. L., "Tongue-Thrust: A Point of View." *Journal of Speech and Hearing Disorders*, **41** (1976), 172–184.

Hodson, B. S. and E. P Paden, "Phonological Processes which Characterize Unintelligible and Intelligible Speech in Early Childhood," *Journal of Speech and Hearing Disorders*, **46** (November 1981), 369–373.

Hoffman, P. R., G. H. Schuckers, and R. G. Daniloff, "Developmental Trends in Correct [r] Articulation as a Function of Allophone Type." *Journal of Speech and Hearing Research*, **23** (December 1980), 746–756.

Hoffman, P. R., G. Schuckers and D. Ratusnik, "Contextual-Coarticulation of [r] Misarticulation." *Journal of Speech and Hearing Research*, **20** (1977), 631–643.

House, A. S. "Reflections on a Double Negative: Misarticulation and Inconsistency." *Journal of Speech and Hearing Research*, **46** (1981), 98–103. (Reviews literature in the area. Emphasizes that the seeming variability of speech sounds is not merely a function of the constraints of the articulatory mechanism but must be sought in the social patterns of language.)

Ingram, D. *Procedures for the Phonological Analysis of Children's Language.* Baltimore: University Park Press, 1981.

——, *Phonological Disability in Children.* New York: American Elsevier Publishing Company, 1976.

Jenkins, E., and F. E. Lohr, "Severe Articulation Disorders and Motor Ability," *Journal of Speech and Hearing Disorders*, **29** (August 1964), 286–292.

(Compares motor proficiency as measured by the Oseretsky Tests of Motor Proficiency of 38 first-grade children with severe articulation defects with 38 normal-speaking children.)

Johnson, A. F., R. L. Shelton, W. A. Arndt, and M. L. Furr, "Factor Analysis of Measures of Articulation, Language, Auditory Processing, Reading-Spelling and Maxillofacial Structure." *Journal of Speech and Hearing Research*, **20** (1977), 319–324.

Johnson, J. P., *Nature and Treatment of Articulation Disorders*. Springfield, Illinois: Charles C. Thomas, 1980. Table p. 122, reprinted by permission.

———, B. L. Winney and O. T. Pederson, "Single Word Versus Connected Speech Articulation Testing." *Language, Speech, and Hearing Services in Schools*, **11** (July 1980), 175–179.

Jordan, L. S., J. C. Hardy and H. L. Morris, "Performance of Children with Good and Poor Articulation on Tasks of Tongue Placement." *Journal of Speech and Hearing Research*, **21** (September 1978), 429–439. (Investigates whether a child can learn a nonspeech task of tongue placement when relying on kinesthetic feedback.)

Kresheck, J. D., and G. Socolofsky, "Imitative and Spontaneous Articulation Assessment of Four-Year-Old Children," *Journal of Speech and Hearing Research*, **15** (December 1972), 729–733.

Kupperman, P., S. Bligh, and M. Goodban, "Activating Articulation Skills Through Theraplay." *Journal of Speech and Hearing Disorders*, **45** (November 1980), 542–545.

Lawrence, J. R., and R. E. Potter, "Visual Motor Disabilities in Children with Functional Articulation Defects." *Journal of Learning Disabilities*, 3 (July 1970), 355–363. (Reveals that children with functional articulatory defects show a higher degree of visual-motor integration disability than do normal-speaking children.)

Lee, L. L., "Developmental Sentence Types: A Method for Comparing Normal and Deviant Syntactical Development." *Journal of Speech and Hearing Disorders*, **31** (November 1966), 211–330. (Investigates the development of syntactic structure in two children, one with normal speech development and one with delayed speech development.)

Lencione, R. M., and N. C. Trent, "Evaluation of Articulation Testing Using Spontaneous and Imitative Procedures." *ASHA*, **7** (October 1965), 380.

Leonard, L. B., "The Nature of Deviant Articulation." *Journal of Speech and Hearing Disorders*, **38** (May 1973), 156–161.

———, J. A. Miller and H. Brown, "Consonant and Syllable Harmony in the Speech of Language-Disordered Children. *Journal of Speech and Hearing Disorders*, **45** (August 1980), 336–345.

Locke, J. L., "The Influence of Speech Perception in the Phonologically Disordered Child. Part I. A Rationale, Some Criteria. The Conventional Tests." *Journal of Speech and Hearing Disorders*, **45** (November 1980), 431–444. Reprinted by permission. (a).

———, "The Influence of Speech Perception in the Phonologically Disordered Child. Part II. Some Clinically Novel Procedures, Their Use. Some

Findings." *Journal of Speech and Hearing Disorders*, **45** (November 1980), 445–468. Reprinted by permission. (b).

—— and K. J. Kutz, "Memory for Speech and Speech for Memory." *Journal of Speech and Hearing Research*, **15** (March 1975), 176–189. (Investigates the concept that learning of speech requires the ability to remember phonetic information long enough to use it in reproducing speech.)

Longhurst, T. and G. Siegel, "Effect of Communication Failure on Speaker and Listener Behavior." *Journal of Speech and Hearing Research*, **16** (1973), 128–140.

McDonald, E. T., "Disorders of Articulation." In R. J. Van Hattum, *Communication Disorders*. New York: Macmillan Publishing Co., Inc. 1980.

McNutt, J. C. "Oral Sensory and Motor Behavior of Children with [s] and [r] Misarticulations." *Journal of Speech and Hearing Research*, **20** (1977), 694–703.

McReynolds, L. V. and M. Elbert, "Criteria for Phonological Process Analysis." *Journal of Speech and Hearing Disorders*, **46** (May 1981), 197–203. (Suggests the need for the establishment of reasonable quantitative and qualitative criteria for phonological process identification.)

——, D. Engmann, and K. Dimmitt, "Markedness Theory and Articulation Errors." *Journal of Speech and Hearing Disorders*, **39** (February 1974), 93–101. (Studies whether children's substitutions consist of phonemes that are less complex than target phonemes and whether children's feature errors in substitutions show a consistent pattern wherein features are changed from a marked to an unmarked value.)

——, J. Kohn, and G. C. Williams, "Articulatory Defective Children's Discrimination of Their Production Errors." *Journal of Speech and Hearing Disorders*, **40** (August 1975), 327–338. (Studies seven articulatory defective children wherein a discrepancy in their production and discrimination of error phonemes was found. They discriminated features and phonemes they did not produce.)

Marquardt, T. P., and J. H. Saxman, "Language Comprehension and Auditory Discrimination in Articulatory Deficient Kindergarten Children." *Journal of Speech and Hearing Research*, **15** (June 1972), 382–389.

Mason, R. M. and C. Simon, "An Orofacial Examination Checklist." *Language, Speech, and Hearing Services in Schools*, **8** (1977), 155–163. (Presents a regular and short form of an orofacial examination checklist, supplemented by explanatory comments and bibliographic citations.).

Menyuk, P., "The Role of Distinctive Features in Children's Acquisition of Phonology," *Journal of Speech and Hearing Research*, **11** (March 1968), 138–146.

——, "Comparing Grammar of Children with Functionally Deviant and Normal Speech." *Journal of Speech and Hearing Research*, **7** (June 1964), 109–122.

Monnin, L. M., and D. Huntington, "Relationship of Articulatory Defects to Speech-Sound Identification." *Journal of Speech and Hearing Research*, **17** (September 1974), 352–366. (Compares normal speaking and speech-defective children on a speech-sound identification task that included sounds the speech defective children misarticulated and sounds they articulated correctly.)

Mowrer, D. and A. Scoville, "Response Bias in Children's Phonological Systems." *Journal of Speech and Hearing Disorders,* **43** (November 1978), 473–481. (Determines the extent to which auditory and visual stimuli influence certain sound productions of children. Suggests the use of nonmeaningful instruction material as stimuli when teaching new sounds to young children.)

——, P. Wahl and S. J. Doolan, "Effect of Lisping on Audience Evaluation of Male Speakers." *Journal of Speech and Hearing Disorders,* **43** (May 1978), 140–148.

Norris, M., J. R. Harden and D. M. Bell, "Listener Agreement on Articulation Errors of Four- and Five-Year-Old Children." *Journal of Speech and Hearing Disorders,* **45** (August 1980), 378–389.

Ohde, R. N. and D. J. Sharf, "Order Effect of Acoustic Segments of VC and CV Syllables on Stop and Vowel Identification." *Journal of Speech and Hearing Research,* **20** (1977), 543–554. (Determines the importance of the vocalic transition relative to other acoustic cues in the perception of both CV and VC syllables.)

Oller, D. K., "Regularities in Abnormal Child Phonology." *Journal of Speech and Hearing Disorders,* **38** (February 1973), 36–47. (Examines carefully abnormal articulatory development.)

Panagos, J. M., M. E. Quine and R. J. Klich, "Syntactic and Phonological Influences on Children's Articulation." *Journal of Speech and Hearing Research,* **22** (December 1979), 841–848. (Determines the extent to which sources of grammatical complexity at different levels of linguistic encoding separately and in combination influence articulatory performance.)

Perozzi, J. A., and L. H. Kunze, "Relationship Between Speech Sound Discrimination Skills and Language Abilities of Kindergarten Children." *Journal of Speech and Hearing Research,* **14** (June 1971), 382–390. (Investigates the relationship between two measures of speech sound discrimination skills and specific as well as general language abilities.)

Pflaster, G., "Mirror, Mirror on the Wall —?" *Journal of Speech and Hearing Disorders,* **44** (August 1979), 379–387. (Discusses the use of the mirror in therapy.)

Phatate, D. D. and H. Umano, "Auditory Discrimination of Voiceless Fricatives in Children." *Journal of Speech and Hearing Research,* **24** (1981), 162–168.

Pollack, E. and N. S. Rees, "Disorders of Articulation: Some Clinical Applications of Distinctive-Feature Theory." *Journal of Speech and Hearing Disorders,* **37** (1972), 451–470.

Powell, J. and L. V. McReynolds, "A Procedure for Testing Position Generalization from Articulation Training." *Journal of Speech and Hearing Research,* **12** (1969), 630–645.

Prather, E. M., D. L. Hedrick, and C. A. Kern, "Articulation Development in

Children Aged Two–Four Years." *Journal of Speech and Hearing Disorders*, **40** (May 1975), 179–191.

Prins, D. T. "Relation Among Specific Articulatory Deviations and Responses to a Clinical Measure of Sound Discrimination Ability." *Journal of Speech and Hearing Disorders*, **28** (November 1963), 382–387. (Evaluates sound discrimination in relation to sound production.)

———, "Abilities of Children with Misarticulations." *Journal of Speech and Hearing Research*, **5** (June 1962), 161–168(a). (Compares subgroups of children with different types of functional articulatory difficulties with normal-speaking children on variables such as intelligence as measured by receptive vocabulary and motor skills.)

———, "Analysis of Correlations Among Various Articulatory Deviations." *Journal of Speech and Hearing Research*, **5** (June 1962), 152–160(b). (Correlates aspects of subjects with a high proportion of interdental lisping errors, those with a high proportion of omissions, and those with a variety of other errors with aspects of normal-speaking children.)

Putnam, A. H. B., and R. Ringel, "Some Observations of Articulation During Labial Sensory Deprivation." *Journal of Speech and Hearing Research* **15** (September 1972), 529–542. (Suggests that the relative importance of oral sensory feedback to speech provides information about the motor control of articulation.)

Rampp, D. L. and M. Pannbacker, "Indications and Contraindications for Tongue Thrust Therapy." *Language, Speech, and Hearing Services in Schools*, **9** (October 1978), 259–264.

Sander, E. K., "When Are Speech Sounds Learned?" *Journal of Speech and Hearing Disorders*, **37** (February 1972), 55–63.

Sax, M. R., "A Longitudinal Study of Articulation Change." *Language, Speech, and Hearing Services in Schools*, **3** (January 1972), 41–56.

Saxman, J. H., and J. F. Miller, "Short-Term Memory and Language Skills in Articulation-Deficient Children." *Journal of Speech and Hearing Research*, **16** (December 1973), 721–730.

Schissel, R. J. and L. B. James, "An Investigation of the Assumptions Underlying the Scoring System of the Arizona Articulation Proficiency Scale: Revised." *Language, Speech and Hearing Services in Schools*, **10** (October 1979), 241–245.

———, "A Comparison of Children's Performance on Two Tests of Articulation." *Journal of Speech and Hearing Disorders*, **44** (August 1979), 363–372.

Schwartz, A. H., and R. Goldman, "Variables Influencing Performance on Speech-Sound Discrimination Tests." *Journal of Speech and Hearing Reserch*, **17** (March 1974), 25–32. (Shows that factors in the construction and administration of speech-sound discrimination tests can influence performance.)

———, L. B. Leonard, M. K. Folger, and M. J. Wilcox, "Early Phonological Behavior in Normal-Speaking and Language-Linguistic Disorders." *Journal of Speech and Hearing Disorders*, **45** (August 1980), 357–377.

Shadden, B. B., C. W. Asp, J. D. Tonkovich, and D. Mason, "Imitation of Suprasegmental Patterns by Five-year-old Children with Adequate and Inadequate Articulation." *Journal of Speech and Hearing Disorders*, **45** (August 1980), 390–400.

Shelton, R. L. and A. F. Johnson, "Delayed Judgment Speech Sound Discrimination and [r] or [s] Articulation Status and Improvement." *Journal of Speech and Hearing Research*, **20** (1977), 704–717.

Shriner, T. H., and R. G. Daniloff, "Reassembly of Segmental CVC Syllables by Children." *Journal of Speech and Hearing Research*, **13** (September 1970), 537–547. (Tests the perceptive-resynthesis performance of normal speaking first- and third-grade children.)

Shriner, T. H., M. S. Holloway, and R. G. Daniloff, "The Relationship Between Articulation Deficits and Syntax in Speech-Defective Children." *Journal of Speech and Hearing Research*, **12** (June 1969), 319–325.

Silverman, E., "Listeners' Impressions of Speakers with Lateral Lisps." *Journal of Speech and Hearing Disorders*, **41** (1976), 547–552.

Singh, S., "Perceptual Similarities and Minimal Phonemic Differences." *Journal of Speech and Hearing Research*, **14** (March 1971), 113–124. (Compares the strength of features in noise and quiet conditions.)

––––––, M. E. Hayden and M. S. Toombs, "The Role of Distinctive Features in Articulation Errors." *Journal of Speech and Hearing Disorders*, **46** (May 1981), 174–183 (Analizes articulatory errors of 1,077 children of various ages and etiologies. Gives reasons for acquisition of categories of sounds at a particular time and for the substitution of one sound for another.)

Smith, C. R., "Articulation Problems and Ability to Store Articulation and Process Stimuli." *Journal of Speech and Hearing Research*, **9** (June 1967), 348–353. (Compares the performance of children with nonorganic articulatory problems with children with normal speech as to the short-term storage of auditory and visual stimuli.)

Smith, M. W., and S. Ainsworth, "The Effects of Three Types of Stimulation on Articulatory Responses of Speech-Defective Children." *Journal of Speech and Hearing Research*, **9** (June 1967), 333–338. (Studies whether children with defective articulation produce the same number of articulatory errors when their speech is stimulated by three different methods: picture stimulus, auditory stimulus, and auditory-visual stimulus.)

Snow, K. A., "A Detailed Analysis of Articulation Responses of 'Normal' First-Grade Children." *Journal of Speech and Hearing Research*, **6** (September 1963), 277–290. (Reports on the frequency of substitutions for various sounds.)

Sommers, R. K., S. Cox, and C. West, "Articulatory Effectiveness, Stimulability and Children's Performance on Perceptual and Memory Tasks." *Journal of Speech and Hearing Research*, **15** (September 1972), 579–589. (Contrasts the articulatory deviant, the articulatory defective, and the articulatory superior child on discrimination, auditory closure, memory of sentences, and auditory sequencing.)

Stewart, S. R., and G. Weybright, "Articulation Norms Used by Practicing Speech-Language Pathologists in Oregon: Results of a Survey." *Journal of*

Speech and Hearing Disorders, **45** (February 1980), 103–111. (Ascertains the developmental norms used by speech-language pathologists in Oregon to determine whether a child is functioning at age level in articulation skills and asked the sources for their interpretations of norms.)

Stockman, I. J., and E. T. McDonald, "Heterogeneity as a Confounding Factor when Predicting Spontaneous Improvement of Misarticulated Consonants." *Language, Speech, and Hearing Services in Schools,* **11** (January 1980), 15–29. (Evaluates predictive tests on articulation.)

Telage, K. M., "A Computerized Place-Manner Feature Program for Articulation Analyses." *Journal of Speech and Hearing Disorders,* **45** (November 1980), 481–494.

Toombs, M. S., S. Singh and M. E. Hayden, "Markedness of Features in Articulatory Substitutions of Children." *Journal of Speech and Hearing Disorders,* **46** (May 1981), 184–190. (Defines differences in articulatory complexity. Found that more features moved from marked to unmarked values than from unmarked to marked values.)

Vandermark, A. A., and M. B. Mann, "Oral Language Skills of Children with Defective Articulation." *Journal of Speech and Hearing Research,* **8** (December 1965), 409–414. (Investigates the oral language achievement of children with defective articulation to determine if such children differ from children with normal articulation, as indicated by quantitative language measures.)

Van Riper, C., *Speech Correction: Principles and Methods,* 6th ed. Englewood Cliffs, N.J.: Prentice-Hall, Inc., 1978, chap. 6.

Walsh, H., "On Certain Practical Inadequacies of Distinctive Feature Systems." *Journal of Speech and Hearing Disorders,* **39** (February 1974), 32–43.

Weinberger, C. B., "Successful Tongue Thrust Modification in the Schools." *Language, Speech, and Hearing Services in Schools,* **4** (April 1973), 89–91. (Describes a program of public school tongue-thrust therapy.)

Weiner, F. F., "Systematic Sound Preferences as a Characteristic of Phonological Disability." *Journal of Speech and Hearing Disorders,* **46** (August 1981), 281–285.

———, and A. A. Ostrowski, "Effects of Listener Uncertainty on Articulatory Inconsistency." *Journal of Speech and Hearing Disorders,* **44** (November 1979), 487–493.

Willbrand, M. L., and M. J. Kleinschmidt, "Substitution Patterns and Word Constraints." *Language, Speech, and Hearing Services in Schools,* **9** (July 1978), 155–161. (Presents a case study of a child whose substitution patterns were affected by the constraints of individual words.)

Williams, G. C., and L. V. McReynolds, "The Relationship Between Discrimination and Articulation Training in Children with Misarticulations." *Journal of Speech and Hearing Research,* **18** (September 1975), 401–412.

Wilson, F. B., "Efficacy of Speech Therapy with Educable Mentally Retarded Children." *Journal of Speech and Hearing Research,* **9** (September 1966), 423–433. (Evaluates the articulatory abilities of 777 educable mentally retarded children. Indicates the types of errors that exist in this group.)

Winitz, H., *From Syllable to Conversation.* Baltimore: University Park Press, 1975.

———, *Articulatory Acquisition and Behavior.* New York: Appleton-Century-Crofts, 1969. (Includes material on prelanguage articulatory development, phonetic and phonemic development, variables related to articulatory development and performance, articulatory testing and predicting, and articulatory programming.)

Wimitz, H., and B. Bellerose, "Effect of Similarity of Sound Substitutions on Retention." *Journal of Speech and Hearing Research,* **15** (December 1972), 677–689. (Makes clear the distinct operations in the recall of sounds.)

———, "Interference and the Persistence of Articulatory Responses." *Journal of Speech and Hearing Research,* **21** (December 1978), 715–721. (Tested the effect of phonological interference on short-term recall using non-English phonological sequences that were pronounced easily.)

———, "Phonetic Interference and Motor Recall." *Journal of Speech and Hearing Research,* **15** (September 1972), 518–528. (Suggests that since imitation is highly stable over the intervals listed that "motor memory" does not contribute to articulatory decay.)

11

Articulation Disorders (II) Remediation

We have already discussed the possible causes for articulatory difficulties. Some of these causes point to the need for the assistance of other specialists in solving the problems of the youngster with an articulatory difficulty. The teacher, the supervisor, principal, and the speech/language clinician must be aware of this need, for the child's defective articulation may be but the symptom of another difficulty.

FINDING THE CAUSE

Both the teacher and the clinician take into account the stage of phonological development of the child. The child of six who substitutes a [w] for an [l] is probably in no need of immediate speech help, for in all likelihood maturity alone will take care of this difficulty. But a child of the same age who confuses /p/ and /b/ is in need of help, because by six years of age, a child should distinguish accurately between these two sounds. As children learn to speak, they frequently omit sounds, distort them, or substitute one sound for another. These conditions in young children are usually part of a particular facet of their development. The teacher and the clinician must decide whether a particular child needs speech and language therapy. In the preceding chapter we discussed the part that maturation plays in articulation and how to consider maturation in making a prognosis on a child's articulatory difficulty.

Because the child's speaking mechanism may be inadequate in

311

some instances, the clinician should determine whether the child has an underbite, an overbite, or a malocclusion that may be an obstacle to the child's making certain sounds easily. As a result of this examination, the clinician may recommend that the child sees a dentist or orthodontist. The importance of organic factors should not be overemphasized. As noted earlier, many children with oral anomalies such as marked overbites nevertheless do articulate proficiently. In many instances, oral structural deviations constitute a contributing rather than a sole cause for speech difficulties. The clinician should also examine the child's health record to see whether another medical problem exists or has existed. The incidence of such problems as polio, cleft palate, cerebral palsy, or a thyroid deficiency may appear on the child's record. Furthermore, when obvious difficulty with muscular coordination or symptoms such as constant colds or listlessness suggest a poor physical condition, the clinician refers the child to a doctor through the health officials of the school.

When emotional difficulties seem to exist along with the articulatory problems of children, children may or may not respond to treatment for the articulatory disorders alone. If they do respond to treatment for the articulatory disorders, the symptom but not the cause may be removed. In such instances, the help that will be provided by the school psychologist may come before the child's speech therapy or be given concurrently with it. The psychologist administers tests to such children to assist the school personnel in understanding them and advises the teacher and clinician on handling both the problems and the children. Frequently the psychologist works with the children and their parents to help them better understand themselves and those around them. With the aid of the psychologist, the adjustment of parent and child to one another and to society will generally improve.

In one case, no obvious reason for the many articulatory errors of an eight-year-old girl of average intelligence was evident. But as the school psychologist talked with the family, he found the mother to be over-solicitous, and a sister four years older than the girl was overprotective. The mother, confind to a wheelchair, wanted both girls to do well and set very high standards for them. She was a kind, likeable person, anxious to do all she could for her children. The psychologist conferred with the mother and helped the teacher and the clinician to understand the child and the parents. He suggested to all three ways of assisting the child to develop self-confidence. The child began to take and accept responsibility. The older sister learned to let the younger child work out her own problems and to allow her to play and live with other youngsters more normally. Concurrently with the psychological help, the speech/language clinician worked with the child's speech and the teacher reinforced the work. The psychologist's help made the work of both the clinician and the teacher more effective. Few children with articulatory problems are so badly adjusted that they need help from a psychologist. Most of these children use incorrect sounds simply because of faulty learning. When needed, however, psychological help is important and uniquely effective.

As noted earlier, children with phonemic articulatory disorders are likely to be deficient in language functions. When evaluations indicate deficiencies in language as well as phonology, the clinician plans therapy to help build both the phonological system and the other language systems.

INTERPRETING THE ARTICULATION TEST

Examiners gain considerable information about a child's articulatory difficulty through articulation testing. They find out which sounds are omitted or distorted and what sounds are substituted for what other sounds. They discover whether the deviant sound occurs before stressed or unstressed vowels, between vowels, in initial or final position of a syllable, or in a cluster as /r/ in *street* or /s/ in *lips;* they find out whether the sound is ever correctly uttered and if so, where.

Clinicians also compare the phonetic features of the deviant sound with the phonetic features of the correct sound. This informaton is helpful in determining the kind of involvement of the articulatory difficulty and in determining whether categories of features are occurring in the defects. For example, they learn whether unvoiced sounds are used for voiced sounds, whether stops are used for fricatives, and whether the place of articulation of several sounds is moved forward. They learn whether the child can say the sound accurately in nonsense syllables. For instance, clinicians may say to a child who does not make /k/ correctly, "Repeat after me":

kay may	[ke me]
meekeem	[mi kim]
fawk	[fɔk]

When a child makes a sound correctly in certain positions or when he makes it accurately in nonsense syllables, retraining usually is not too difficult. Stimulability is a very important factor not only in the assignment of children with articulatory disorders for remediation but also in the remediation process itself.

Speech/language clinicians consider various other factors. They

ether the sounds the child is missing are those usually ac-
or late in the phonological development. This informa-
inicians determine the part maturity may be playing (see
They check to see whether or not the sounds the child
says incorrectly are those readily visible. They learn whether they are
high- or low-frequency sounds, for a hearing loss may cause the lack of
perception of these sounds in a particular individual. When the sound
is uttered correctly in some contexts, clinicians analyze in what contexts it is inaccurate: the position of the sound in a syllable, the co-
articulating agents, the length of the utterance, the sound's relationship in position to vowels.

The examiner finds out which incorrect or omitted sounds influence either the child's perception of his/her pattern of speech or the
pattern of speech itself. Bud, a ten-year-old boy who made a /θ/ sound
for /s/, said,"The kith thay I talk like a baby. My eth'th, you know." He
realized that his speech sounded out of place. This boy liked to box,
ride a bike fast, play baseball, and climb the tallest trees. He believed
he was quite grown up. Although he said /t/ and /d/ for /θ/ and /ð/, /t/
and /d/ for /tʃ/ and /dʒ/, /w/ for /l/ and /r/, he himself was most concerned about his /s/. To his listeners the /w/ for /l/ and /r/ was also a
part of the "baby speech." Bud went on to tell the speech clinician
that almost every word has an *s* in it; he pointed out that he lived on
Sycamore Street. In this instance, the clinician attacked the /s/ first.
Bud was so strongly motivated that his improvement was rapid.

Lastly, the clinician records the errors in some systematic way—
perhaps using one of the systems mentioned earlier—and perhaps
even being assisted by a computer analysis (Telage 1980). The analysis and the factors just mentioned are important in the choice of the
plan for remediation.

PROGRAMS FOR REMEDIATION OF DEVIANT ARTICULATION

Many strategies for articulatory training exist. Whatever the clinician has in mind should be planned carefully and should be geared to
the individual children involved and their needs. Some clinicians believe that a one-to-one relationship has the advantage of being truly
individualized therapy. Others work in groups, believing that listening to and watching others achieve are important in the rehabilitative
process. Ritterman's (1970) study concerning the effects of learning by
participation and learning by observation in discrimination training
suggests that children's observation of the speech sound discrimina-

tion practice of other children is generally effective in teaching sound discrimination. Thus, being in a group for sound discrimination practice may well be more efficient for teaching sound discrimination than being taught it individually. Some of these clinicians believe in group communication-centered therapy where successful communicative endeavours reinforce improved articulatory ability. They believe that the reinforcement is real and that the new articulation patterns are carried over into home and school situations readily. Almost no drill as such is present. Other therapists believe in a sensorimotor approach where the accuracy of a sound is related to the type of sound produced and to the kind of overlapping movements that are characteristic of ordinary utterances. These clinicians rarely use the isolated sound but rather the syllable that consists of coarticulated sounds. Still other therapists correct not one sound at a time but a number of sounds with the same deviant feature pattern. Weber (1970) explains this method wherein a child who used stops for the fricatives /s/, /ʃ/, /f/, and /θ/, worked on all four sounds at the same time. Both in discrimination and production, Weber used the strategy of contrasting the features of the voiceless stops with voiceless fricatives; at every stage the child discriminated between and/or produced the error and the target sound.

And still other clinicians use the paired stimuli technique, which begins by finding the contexts in which the children articulate the target sounds correctly and then goes on to modify the sound production in other contexts. Children pair words in which they use the sound correctly with words in which they use the error sound. The clinician then creates a situation wherein the correct existing response will generalize to other words with different contexts.

The clinician frequently emphasizes learning theory involving behavioral objectives. Articulatory therapy lends itself to this process partly because the behavioral objectives are almost always easily delineated and their achievement readily evaluated. One result is that programs involving operant conditioning have emerged and are being utilized in many schools. The steps form a kind of ladder with each step focusing on the acquisition of a particular kind of behavior and reinforcement for its acquisition.

Regardless of the strategies to be followed or the rationale to be employed, certain generalities are valid. Every child's articulatory remedial program should be carefully planned. The objectives for each lesson and for the program as a whole should be carefully stated and their attainment just as carefully evaluated. For example, a child may be expected at the end of the term to use the target sounds /s/ and /z/ and not the substituted sounds /θ/ and /ð/ in both formal and informal situations at home and at school. The clinician by visiting the classroom and observing the child at play can ascertain whether this behavior (learned in clinic) is consistent.

To summarize, the teacher should have a long-range goal, objectives for each lesson, plans for attaining these objectives, and means and standards for evaluating the results of the therapy. There should also be a way of renforcing the acceptable behavior and of providing feedback to the child. Clinicians may base their therapy on a particular rationale and use a single set of strategies to accomplish their goals in therapy. Or they may use an eclectic approach—making use of a variety of strategies and perhaps even changing their rationale.

Because many theories of speech intervention for articulatory disorders do exist, we are summarizing them. We believe that clinicians may well use strategies applicable in many or all of the theories. The clinician makes use of strategies most likely to be effective for a particular child.

The Traditional Approach Based on Feedback

The traditional approach, to be described, has been used for many years and is still being widely followed. In this approach, children establish an auditory image of the phonemes. They refine the image and change some of the characteristics of the image. In other words, they are monitoring their own productions. They match their auditory outputs with their auditory images. They then store these matches and automatic control takes over.

And so, the first step is that children must learn to recognize both their error sound and their target sound. The role of discrimination in this process is not clear, as noted earlier. In general, research indicates that discrimination errors do occur in phonetic contexts that contain the child's error or errors. Articulatory errors may then be related to specific discrimination abilities, or the learning that took place in mastering the deviant sound may be reflected in the discrimination tests. Winitz and Bellerose (1962) seem to support this latter premise.

Before training particular sounds, the clinician often assesses the child's discriminatory ability—perhaps using Locke's (1980b) method. The clinician, then, stresses the discrimination between the target sound and the deviant one, first helping the child to identify the sound.

The clinician or teacher does well to remember that ability to produce an unfamiliar sound may develop as a function of the ability to contrast that sound with other sounds; hence discrimination ability is more a function of the number of available cues (distinctive features) than of the type of cues available. In discrimination teaching the teacher can point to these clues: manner of production, articulatory position, and the vocal component. As the child works on distinguishing [θʌm] from [sʌm], the teacher points to the features that are alike: For a second grader, the teacher might say: (1) "In both sounds the engine is not working. Feel?" (2) "Both sounds can go on and on: /θ/ and /s/" (prolonging both somewhat). (3) "Both sounds have a light, noisy sound. Listen: /θ/ /s/." (4) "But in [sʌm] the tongue is here, whereas in [θʌm] it is here."

At this point you may program discrimination teaching so that all of one category of a child's errors are presented. For example, you may work on discrimination with all of a child's unvoicing errors, all errors where a stop is substituted for a fricative, or all errors where the tongue is moved forward in position.

In your discrimination training, you wish to reinforce the language learnings of the classroom. For example, the teaching of all kinds of morphological structure can take place: adjectivization, adverbial, affirmative, agentive, agreement, comparative, emphatic, genitive, imperative, interrogative, negative, nominalization, passive, past participle, past tense, plural, predeterminer, present participle, superlative. For instance, you might show three sizes of trucks and say, "This is a big truck; This truck is even _____; This truck is the _____ of all." Then, pointing to the smallest truck, you might say, "Of the three trucks, this is the _____." Or you might say, "This man drives the truck. What is he called?"

The second step in this theory is the teaching of the target sound. In some instances, the child may not need to be taught how to make the sound, for he already makes it accurately in most phonetic contexts. When this is the case, usually the only remaining problem is to incorporate the target sound in all phonetic contexts. In such cases, the classroom teacher, who has had speech training, helps the child to be consistent in using the target sound. Where necessary, the clinician advises the teacher and sometimes may even need to include the child in clinical sessions.

In other instances, however, children, even though they hear the unacceptable sound and can identify it, cannot make it accurately in many phonetic contexts. In such cases, the speech clinician teaches the child to make the sound. Because parents, teachers, and classmates have already stimulated children with words, phrases, and the sound itself, and the children have failed to respond, the clinician tries other modes of attack. To this child, *wope* [wop] for *rope* [rop] sounds right. The child, having always made a /w/ for /r/ and having established the habit firmly, must learn the target sound thoroughly, first in simple syllabic combinations, then in words and phrases. Throughout the sound must be a vivid stimulus, sometimes repeated and prolonged.

Normally in articulatory therapy in teaching the target sound, the clinician uses syllables and words (real or nonsense) in phonetic contexts that facilitate the correct production of the target sound. The facilitating feature for a phoneme is often related to place of articulation. The sound before the deviant sound can be chosen so as to provide the same feature of placement and consequently a minimum of movement. The result is a minimal demand on the neuromuscular system. The phrase *one red bag* may be used as an illustration. The tongue in /n/ is near where it is for /r/, provided the /r/ is made near the alveolar ridge. Because feedback is important, the more often children hear themselves say the target sound and feel the parts of their mechanisms producing the sound, the more sensitive they become to the error sound. Whatever facilitates the detection of error, even before it is made, helps. Undoubtedly, the phonetic contexts where the child receives feedback indicating successful performance are important.

Other factors are also important in selecting the syllables, words, and sentences to be used in articulatory therapy. Using the target phoneme in a stressed syllable rather than in an unstressed syllable facilitates accurate production. In addition, except for contrast, to avoid the error sound in practice syllables or words—or even sounds closely resembling the error sound—is wise. For instance, if a child substitutes /θ/ for /s/, to use the phrase *this top* is unwise even though /s/ and /t/ are often made in approximately the same place, for the /ð/ of *this* is produced in exactly the same position as is the error sound /θ/ (see McNutt and Keenan 1970). Furthermore, in choosing words for practice, to select them from a list that indicates their high frequency of utterance is expedient, for the child is likely to hear the target sounds in these words more often than in words that are less frequently uttered. The child will also use these words more frequently than many other words.

Teachers can reinforce the training in a variety of ways. For example, the teacher might ask the child who has been working on /l/ to tell her what he was *glad* about. The child might respond with, "I'm glad for the Good Humor Man," or "I'm glad my Daddy's home." Together the teacher and child might go on to think of all the things they are glad about. Other children in the class might well become involved in the discussion. It is important for the child to have opportunities to use his/her new target sound in meaningful conversation. Adults know that drill and critical listening are needed and recognize that they must carry over their correction of a sound into words and into conversation. But children need renforcement by the classroom teacher.

The last step in any of the remedial programs is carrying over the target sounds into everyday speech. When children incorporate the sounds into words easily, they are ready to begin the transfer of the sounds to their everyday speech. Their clinician, teachers, and parents need to provide as many speaking situations for them as possible. At this stage, teachers are important to the work of the clinician, for they can set up situations wherein the child has many speaking opportunities to incorporate the newly acquired sound. Teachers tell the child to think before making the sound; if the sound comes out inaccurately, the members of the group will wait until it comes out right. After the activity has occurred, the teacher commends the child on the acceptable pronunciations and provides a list of phrases where the substituted sound was retained.

Sometimes the teacher will ask the clinician to work on some words and phrases that occur frequently in the classroom work. For instance, one child, who was working on *s* and at the same time preparing a report comparing a small town in the suburbs to New York City, needed to pronounce these words: *subway, station, supermarket, stores, suburbs, schools, snow, small, success, house, miss, bus, stop,* and *smooth.* Consequently, the clinician helped the child to say these particular words acceptably. Because the child was excited about her research, it also proved a good topic of conversation in the session. The classroom work/remediation helped to motivate the improvement.

Creative activities, including both puppetry and creative drama, encourage children to talk. To give practice in certain sounds, the clinician may use these activities in a therapy session and the teacher may use them in reinforcing work taught by the clinician. For the puppet play or the creative drama, the teacher or clinician can create a situation or use a story that will involve particular sounds. For example, in guiding a dramatic activity the teacher may suggest articles to build a story that contains many *s*'s: a silver scepter, red dress, and a sled.

Other situations for just plain talk arise spontaneously. The teacher takes advantage of these opportunities to promote oral communication. Chapter 8 suggests many speaking experiences for all children.

This traditional approach with its emphasis on training the child to hear the sound and on feedback theory culminating in accurate production may well seem more applicable to the remediation of phonetic errors than to phonemic errors. The techniques, however, of contrasting the input of sensory impressions and the output of speech would seem to make it acceptable in remediation of phonemic errors. This is but one of a number of possible approaches to articulatory therapy.

Van Riper (1978) explains this approach clearly. Obviously, the carry-over procedures are applicable in all approaches.

The Sensorimotor Approach

Whereas the approach just described emphasizes auditory feedback and the acoustic nature of the phoneme to be remediated, the primary emphasis in sensorimotor therapy is to establish the needed sensory-motor reactions. In this theory, the syllable is the basic unit of speech production and articulation is a dynamic, ongoing process consisting of a series of overlapping movements. The proponent of this theory, McDonald (1980) does not believe that work with the isolated sound and one static place of articulation carries much value. Rather he believes in working on sounds in syllables and phonetic contexts that emphasize the patterns of movement that lead to correct production. The complexity is increased until the clients finally work on sentences.

Johnson (1980, pp. 190–193) explains the three phases of McDonald's treatment: The first phase is designed to heighten a child's perceived awareness of the overlapping movements of articulation. Designed to be a preliminary step to work on the error sounds, this step helps the child to get a "feel" of articulatory movement patterns. Questions that "pinpoint" the feel include: What did you feel when you said that? Where did the tongue go? Did the lips touch? Did the tongue move forward or backward? In terms of movement, this training goes from the simple to the complex—beginning with such simple syllables as [bibi]. The second step in this phase involves differentially stressing the first and second bisyllables. This step progresses, using different vowels as [bibu], different consonants as [daga], different consonants and different vowels as [diga] and finally trisyllables as [patiku]. Once again the progression is from the simple to the complex.

The second phase centers on the child's error sound; its purpose is to establish and strengthen the sensorimotor patterns associated with correct production. It begins with selecting a phonetic context in which the child correctly articulates the sound. The child repeats after the clinician the syllable or word, exaggerating the particular correct sound. This emphasizes the correct sensorimotor feedback. The clinician works on firmly establishing the tactile-kinesthetic images associated with the accepted production of the sound.

The third phase systematically increases the number of phonetic contexts in which the child acceptably articulates the target sound or sounds. Hopefully as the sensorimotor apparatus becomes strengthened, additional facilitative contexts appear. The testing for identification of new contexts goes on. This approach is particularly applicable to phonetic disorders.

Using Minimal Pair Contrast Theory

Sometimes children, perhaps because of environmental reasons—including persons involved, experiences that were important and influential, reinforcement by adults and others—seem to resist correct production at the word level and to retain their misarticulations. One six-year-old, very bright—able often to make deductions and use abstractions—substituted /w/ for /r/ although he was perfectly capable of making /r/. With little or no effort, he imitated the clinician's /r/ in a variety of words. For this child, the clinician chose to use the minimal pair contrast theory. She found two pictures, one representing a child who had *won* an award and another showing a boy *run*ning between bases. She did the same with *wail* and *rail*, with *wok* and *rock* (the mother was into Chinese cooking), and *wake* and *rake*. In each instance, the child was to produce the target sound correctly and then to explain the meaning of the picture.

Blache and Parsons (1980) illustrate this theory well, explaining the four steps used to teach the linguistic importance of a distinctive feature.

1. First the child must understand that the two contrasting words differ in meaning. For example, if the clinician is using *tea* and *key*, the child must understand that *tea* is something you drink and that *key* is used to open a door.
2. The second step is that the child be able to hear the difference between the two words. For example, the child may be asked to touch the picture of the word uttered by the clinician.
3. Third, the child must produce the words in response to the objects of pictures. The child says the words and, at the same time, the clinician touches the pictures or objects. Usually the child will first say the word he/she produces easily, as [ti], and then attempt to say the alternate word [ki]. Where needed, the clinician provides traditional techniques such as placement, demonstration and imitation but still stimulates at the word level.
4. Lastly, after the word pairs have been learned, the clinician uses traditional procedures to help the child generalize from treated words to untreated words, from words to connected speech, and from treatment settings to nontreatment settings.

Weiner (1981) provides another example of the child's being confronted with honomymous word pairs and changing the pronunciation of the target word to eliminate the confusion:

PROCESS: Deletion of final consonants.
STIMULI: Five pictures of a *boat* and four pictures of a *bow*.
INSTRUCTION: We are going to play a game. The object of the game is to get me to pick up all five pictures of the boat. Every time you say *boat*, I will pick one up. When I have all five, you may paste a star on your paper. (Weiner, 1981, page 98).

As the child deleted the /t/ in *boat*, the clinician picked up the *bow* picture. The clinician then gave the child instructions on how to complete the *boat* task successfully. The child was reinforced for each correct production.

Using the Paired Stimuli Technique

The paired stimuli technique described above is applicable where children do articulate some sounds correctly, even if only in one word. The correct production is brought to the child's attention by having him/her frequently repeat the word. Then words, limited in number at first, using the same sound in the same position are presented. Each time the child uses the sound correctly, he is rewarded. The repeated pairing of the words and the reinforced correct production in key words results in generalization after a number of trials. The objective is for the child to produce the sound correctly in spontaneous conversation. Sometimes the clinician does well to start with phrases and then to expand the training to sentences.

Applying Distinctive Feature Theory

Distinctive feature analysis (see Chapter 6, p. 126 ff) assesses the child's phonemic system, not his phonetic production capability. Such an analysis ideally reveals what the child knows about the sound system —what features have been acquired and under what rules those features are being used for the perception and production of speech. Articulation disorders do not always reflect simple phonetic production problems but frequently represent inappropriately developed phonemic rules. In such instances, an analysis of the substitutions on the basis of distinctive features and remediation based on the analysis is useful. Children tend to be consistent in their feature errors. Let us suppose that the child substitutes nonfricative sounds for fricatives. The clinician then works on developing the concept of frication. Or let us suppose that the child tends to substitute unvoiced sounds for voiced sounds. The clinician then works on developing the voicing feature.

Training on the feature concept in a single phoneme tends to generalize across phonemes. McReynolds and Bennett (1972) support this statement but note that the degree of generalization in their study varied across phonemes and the position of the phonemes in words. Costello and Onstine (1976) describe a distinctive feature program used in remediation of multiple phonemic errors of two schoolchildren. They reported on the acquisition of two directly treated target phonemes and the improvement of five other nontreated error phonemes. They had predicted this generalization from an analysis of the feature errors of the children.

Even when phonetic errors are involved, distinctive feature training often works. Ruder and Bunce (1981) planned articulation remediation for two children diagnosed as having severe articulation disorders, both of whom could be characterized as having phonetic disorders and one manifesting problems with neuromuscular control of tongue movements. As a result of training with distinctive features, generalizations reoccurred on some untrained target sounds that were predicted to emerge because of the distinctive feature analysis and the sequence of training. Ruder and Bunce conclude that when the clinician structures articulation therapy to enhance generalization, he/she will likely not have to train all deviant or absent phonemes in the child's repertoire. Distinctive feature analysis provides a theory-based methodology for achieving such structuring in articulation theory.

Approach Based on Developmental Phonological Processes

Ingram (1976, page 120) notes that training should not deal with isolated sounds but with phonological processes that affect entire classes of sound. For example, he cites that /k/ may be substituted for /t/ and /g/ for /d/ where in both instances velar sounds are substituted for two alveolar sounds. This type of substitution reflects the use of the fronting process. But the voicing attribute and the manner of production are, however, correct. In this instance, Ingram would deal with the substitution of the velar sound for the alveolar sound. In other instances, more than one articulatory feature are involved. He believes that to attack all segments of a process rather than a single one is wise because this is the way phonology develops.

Having selected the processes for remediation, after a phonological analysis, Ingram (1976) would then hope that an elimination of errors dependent on specific processes, rather than the elimination of the substitution of a particular sound for another would occur. He would determine which processes to attack first from a developmental standpoint. For instance a child may say *poon*, then with help, *soon*, and finally the adult pronunciation *spoon*. Similarly for some children with deviant phonology stages occur in the presence or absence of final consonants. For example, the clinician would be glad to see /p/, /b/, and /d/ used in a final position even though these phonemes replace /t/, /k/ and /g/. At least the child is using a final plosive phoneme with the right voicing characteristic. Then all final consonants except /k/ and /g/ may be added. Lastly, all final consonants are included.

This part of the remediation process is based on the assumption that the clinician has carefully assessed the level of the child's phonological development; in other words, the clinician determines how the child is operating in terms of phonological processes. For example, the reduction of syllable structure such as the deletion or elimination of an element in a consonant cluster is acceptable at an earlier age than other reductions.

Ingram (1976, page 149) also emphasizes that the establishment of contrasts and the acquisition of individual words makes the selection of processes more explicit. The clinician looks at the child's use of actual words and his/her particular system of contrasts, for the child must learn to contrast sounds and to use this contrast in marking one word from another. Using this as a base, the clinician stabilizes the more highly unstable words in the child's speech, determines the forms of the child's speech resulting in the greatest homonymy, and ascertains the sounds that are used contrastively in the child's speech and compares these to those used by normal children at a comparable level of development. Finally, the clinician establishes new contrasts gradually on the basis of this comparison.

This approach is systematic, adapted to the sounds the child already possesses, and is based on normal phonological development. In other words, Ingram (1976) advocates a "gradualness" rather than a "fell-swoop" approach, for the normal child does not learn the production of a sound in a single step but goes through several stages.

PRINCIPLES IN ARTICULATORY TRAINING

We believe that certain principles are important in articulatory remediation:

1. The child's inconsistencies and patterns of articulation should be analyzed and this analysis of processes used as a basis for remedia-

tion. This then involves remediation based on phonological processes, on classes of sounds and sounds in context.

2. Strategies should take place in situations where meaningful communication is occurring. These situations can be so planned that many aspects of language training can be attacked.

3. Different strategies should be planned and adopted for different children. What works well for one child may not work well for another because of a variety of reasons.

4. Provisions for the planning and carrying out of generalization processes should be made. This process may well involve help from other school personnel and from the home.

Using Context Variables and Patterns of Sounds in Remediation

Articulation training studies have shown that as children learn to produce a sound accurately in one context, they are often able to produce it accurately in other contexts (usually in cross-positions) without training. Sometimes, however, they produce the sound in one context but not in another. (See Powell and McReynolds, 1969, and Elbert and McReynolds, 1975)

Hoffman et al. (1977) studied ten children who misarticulated /r/ to survey their inconsistent misarticulatory behavior. They found that /r/ was produced correctly more often in some contexts than others. For example, correct production of an initial /r/ occurred more frequently when preceded by /k/ and when followed by the vowels /i/, /æ/, and /u/ as in these sentences: Dick *r*eads the book. The sick *r*at died. Jack *r*uined his pants. /r/ in clusters was produced more often within /k/ and /t/ contexts (as in *cream* and *true*) than in /p/ contexts (as in *prance*).

A study, however, in which the role of context, (the influence of surrounding sounds on a particular sound in an utterance) in facilitating generalized responses was the primary focus did not support the theory that facilitative contexts are strong. Although there was a slight trend that could be interpreted as supporting possible facilitative contexts caused by coarticulation effects, this trend was not consistent within and across subjects. The data, dependent on various vowel and consonant combinations, did not support the selection of any particular context on the basis of what the children produced correctly most often. Elbert and McReynolds suggest that for evidence for clinicians to use contexts in which one sound facilitates another, more consistent data is necessary. This study, undertaken by Elbert and McReynolds

(1978), emphasized that factors other than context played important roles in the children's ability to generalize: (1) As soon as the children learned to imitate, generalizations occurred in a variety of contexts. (2) Whereas all subjects developed a generalized response, the amount of training required to develop this generalization varied across the group of children. (3) Minimal syllable training resulted in generalizations across positions as well as to different vowel-syllable combinations, to clusters, and to both imitated and spontaneous items. (4) Children with different error patterns revealed different generalization patterns.

As noted earlier, however, clinicians teach the target sound in syllables and words where the phonetic context facilitates the correct production of the sound. Even using the target sound in a stressed rather than an unstressed syllable facilitates production of the target sound.

We further believe that where the articulatory analysis shows that classes of sounds are inaccurate, these classes, rather than single sounds, should be remediated. A distinctive feature or feature production assessment of children's articulatory errors then seems advisable. Weiner and Bankson (1978) describe the remediation of a child who substituted plosive sounds for these fricatives: /ð/, /s/, /v/, /θ/, and /ʃ/. They taught the child the difference between flowing (running water) sounds and popping (dripping water) sounds. They explain in detail the steps in reaching generalization.

Teaching distinctive features can simultaneously teach semantic features. The rationale is similar to that of the minimal word pair theory. Blache and Parsons (1980) use words to teach distinctive features rather than using distinctive features to teach the composition of words. Thus, the communicative function of features becomes important. Blache and Parsons assume that a thorough assessment and analysis of the child's articulation has taken place. They then proceed to a specific feature and a sound pair is selected to create minimal word pairs. They cite the example of a child who may have difficulty with voicing and hypothesize that these minimal pairs could be used: *pea/bee, pack/back, peach/beach, pear/bear, pin/bin, cap/cab, tap/tab,* and/or cop/top. They include four steps:

1. The child must understand that the two contrasting words differ in meaning.
2. The child must be able to hear that the two words sound different.
3. The child must produce the words in response to the pictures or objects.
4. Finally, he/she must incorporate the words into communicative situations outside of remediation.

This study shows: (1) how one program based on a particular theory may borrow strategies from another theory, and (2) how important the communicative situation can be in articulatory intervention. The latter point leads us to our next principle.

Articulation Intervention in Meaningful Communicative Situations

Since in the public schools attention has turned increasingly to language problems, and since evidence exists that at least in some cases of articulatory deficiencies, language difficulties are also present, it seems important to provide some aspects of language training. When clinicians are aware that these problems coexist, it seems advisable to work on the syntactic, morphemic, semantic, and pragmatic language problems at the same time. Matheny and Panagos (1978) studied the influence of intervention programs for syntax and articulation on the articulatory and syntactic skills of public-school children with multiple linguistic problems. One group received a program of syntax only, a second received a program of articulation only, and a third group received no speech/language intervention. The two experimental groups made significant gains in both syntax and articulatory skills. These results indicate that clinical manipulations of a child's linguistic system at any level such as sounds, syllables, phrases, or sentences are likely to produce broader linguistic development than anticipated.

In the chapter on communication we emphasize that language is used for a variety of functions. The speech act may serve many purposes. We believe that the clinician must keep the range of functions in mind. To illustrate, a child may be receiving and giving information about a variety of *trucks* and their functions and at the same time be learning the distinction between /tw/ and /tr/. The clinician can provide through pictures or replicas an oil truck, moving truck, milk truck, power company truck, mail truck, milk truck, dump truck, or parcel delivery truck. The child responds to the variety of trucks, naming a particular truck, such as *oil truck*. Thus, the child has produced a noun phrase. The clinician may go one step further and with encouragement the child may add, "brings heat," or "comes every month," or "parks in the driveway." The clinician, pointing to the power company truck, may ask, "What does this truck do?" The child may answer, "The power company truck fixes lights." No matter that it carries men who do hundreds of other things. You are satisfied that the child has added an idea, and incidentally a verb phrase, and has formed a sentence.

One clinician was working with two children who misarticulated

/r/. He first showed them Dorothy Baruch's book about rabbits, reading part of the story and telling the rest of it. He went on to talk about rabbits as he manipulated the two rabbit puppets. The following conversation ensued:

TEACHER (*developing the automatic habit of pluralization*): Here is one rabbit. Here is another rabbit. Now there are two _____.
CHILD ONE and CHILD TWO: Rabbits.
TEACHER (*developing concepts about rabbits*): What does he look like?
CHILD ONE: He's round, fat.
CHILD TWO: He has long white ears.
TEACHER (*wriggling the puppet's nose and cocking its ears*): Why does he do that?
CHILD ONE: He hears something.
CHILD TWO: He's going that way.
TEACHER: To me he looks like a big marshmallow. What do you think he looks like?
CHILD ONE: Cotton candy.
CHILD TWO: A white muff. A ball of snow. White ice cream.
TEACHER: What does the rabbit eat?
CHILD ONE: Lettuce.
TEACHER: And other things like apples and potatoes. What does he feel like?
CHILD ONE: He feels smooth.
CHILD TWO: Soft like silk.
CHILD ONE: No, more like Mommy's fur coat.
TEACHER (*relating concepts*): Does he feel like sandpaper?
CHILD ONE: (*giggling*) No, that's rough.

Teachers reinforce the articulatory remediation through using various language experiences. Fortunately for one child who had been working on /l/, the teacher was developing the concept of analogies. She asked Jackie, "What is a lemon like?" Using /l/ correctly, he said, "Like an orange but smaller and sourer." Another child responded with, "But it's a different color." That other children in the room became involved in the evaluation of his analogy helped to make his generalization of his new sound meaningful. Too, the reinforcement by the teacher helped; the reinforcement in this instance was only a smile but it was effective. Further, the reinforcement is occurring in meaningful communicative situations.

Older children who are working with the sound of /l/ might learn the meanings of these words: joyful/joyless; meaningful/meaningless; helpful/helpless; graceful/graceless. A variety of language experiences could be used: pantomime, discussion, creative drama. Or working with /r/, they could combine one of the following adjectives with one of the following nouns:

- *Adjectives:* gray, drafty, frisky, bright, proud, pretty, rich, rough, weary, purple, red, bright.
- *Nouns:* ribbon, room, rabbit, Scrooge, brother, eyebrows, picture, car.

They could then go on to build a story around their noun phrase and perhaps to enact the story.

Around Christmastime there might well be a discussion of Christmas trees. In one New York City class, the children talked about the tree at Rockefeller Center, what colored lights it was decorated with and how big it was. In this particular classroom three of the students were working with /r/, so that this the reinforcement was particularly helpful.

Planning a Program to Meet the Individual Needs of the Children Involved

The particular strategy to be used in articulation intervention depends on (1) the type of articulatory disorder, (2) the degree of seriousness of the disorder, (3) what seems to best fit the individual child's articulatory and linguistic behavior.

Hodson (1978) describes an eclectic approach for phonological remediation with severely articulatory-disabled children that is adaptable to individual needs. She notes that this hierachical model for phonological remediation has been developed and implemented at the University of Illinois Speech and Hearing Clinic. We are including Hodson's description of this program, for we believe that it could well apply to a wide variety of articulatory disorders. It has three stages:

Stage 1. This step involves helping children to develop appropriate word-final consonant productions in CVC syllables. These children learn through auditory, visual and tactile stimulation that many words do have consonantal endings. Since /p/ and /t/ are most easily identified and produced, stimulus words with these sounds are used. A child does not necessarily have to produce the final consonant accurately as long as he attempts some consonant.

As the final consonants emerge in the children's speech but where the consonants exhibit velar fronting, the clinician moves on to develop kinesthetic awareness of the back/front contrast. The children usually begin with /k/, since this is the sound they most readily produce. As would be expected, regressive voicing assimilation contributes to sounding an easier prevocalic /g/ over the prevocalic /k/. Neither voicing nor devoicing are criteria for success at this stage. The prime objectives are awareness of contrasts and of kinesthetic differences.

Stage 2. The major goal of the second stage involves teaching the children awareness of stridency and providing limited practice in producing stridency in phonemes by using carefully selected target words. Since the children typically substitute /t/ for /s/, to use /s/ clusters first rather than an /s/ + vowel is more effective. For instance, children who say *tand* for *sand* often say s-tand more readily than *sand*, since they typically deal with the intrusion of /t/ when saying a word such as *sand*. Thus, consonant clusters are taught simultaneously with stridency. The second step of Stage 2 involves word-final /s/ clusters in plurals and in third-person singular verbs. As children become aware of and incorporate stridency in /s/ clusters, most of them are ready for postvocalic /s/ and for copular forms in short phrases such as *it's* and *that's*. Prevocalic /s/ is usually last in this sequence. They then typically proceed to attacking stridency as a whole, targeting such sounds as /f/ and /ʃ/ depending on the individual being remediated.

Since six of the strident phonemes are also continuant—/v/, /f/, /s/, /z/, /ʃ/, and /ʒ/—the continuancy feature is stimulated simultaneously with stridency. This strategy is intended to promote generalization to other continuant phonemes, resulting in overall reduction of the substitution of stops for other sounds. Stage 2 remediation also seems to facilitate reduction of sound omissions even in clusters (for example, movement from [peɪ] to [pweɪ] for *play*).

Stage 3. Assuming that word-final consonants, back consonants, stridency, continuancy, and consonant clusters are beginning to emerge in spontaneous utterances, the children are ready for Stage 3, which involves more traditional remediation of their remaining phonemic deviations, typically *l*, *r*, *th* and the sibilants. By this time, however, marked gains in speech intelligibility are usually noted (Hodson, 1978, p. 237–238).

This model provides for a progression of skills: establishment of word-final consonants, development of front-back contrasts, facilitation of stridency, use of consonant clusters, and reduction of stopping as basic strategies in remediation for unintelligible children. Intervention can begin at any particular level of development.

The Importance of Providing Opportunities for Generalization

The aim of the speech/language clinician is to have the child use the correct articulation in spontaneous speech in a variety of communicative situations. The child will first use the correction in a clinical setting and then use the corrected sound in various positions in the word and in a variety of phonetic contexts. He/she may well change his/her pronunciation of several phonemes as the result of training on one phoneme. In the clinical situation he/she may then be able to use the corrected sound in spontaneous speech. The term generalization is applied to this behavior. The clinician needs to be aware, however, of facets of this behavior. If the child is using the corrected sounds only in a clinic setting, he/she needs to generalize this to other situations. That he/she is receiving praise or some other kind of reward in clinic may be the major motivating force. This motivation needs to expand to other situations. Teachers, paraprofessionals and parents help in this process.

Training by teachers and parents often results from conferences set up by the speech/language clinician. Through discussion, teachers and parents develop an understanding of the child and his handicap. As a result of their talk, teachers and parents find ways to reinforce the training that has taken place in the clinical setting. Often the teacher's and parents' intimacy with the child helps provide the clinician with a better understanding of the child's behavior and gives the clinician important clues to the interests and needs of the child that will increase the success of the remediation program. The program then must be based on a cooperative endeavor, with the teacher, parents and clinician working for the good of the child.

PROBLEMS

1. Visit a school or speech and hearing clinic where you can observe a specialist working with a child with an articulatory disorder. Indicate how a teacher could reinforce in the classroom some of the learning that took place in the clinic.
2. Indicate ways in which one theory of remediation could complement another theory of remediation.
3. How can you, as a classroom teacher, make use of some of the strategies described in this chapter?
4. Find children's books that emphasize a particular sound. How can each book be used in the classroom? in the clinical setting? (Try to find those books that have particular sounds as well as material that will further some aspects of language development.)
5. Devise a strategy that will contrast an error sound with a target sound.
6. Indicate ways you, as a classroom teacher, could help a particular child with a specific articulatory difficulty.
7. Indicate ways you, as a speech clinician, could seek reinforcement from a classroom teacher of a child with a particular articulatory difficulty.
8. Read and report on one of the following: Dworkin (1980), Elbert and McReynolds (1978), Madison (1979).

References and Suggested Readings

Arndt, W. B., M. E. Shelton, and R. L. Shelton, "Prediction of Articulation Improvement with Therapy from Early Lesson Sound Production Task Scores." *Journal of Speech and Hearing Research,* **14** (March 1971), 149–153.

Blache, S. E. and C. L. Parsons, "A Linguistic Approach to Distinctive Feature Training." *Language, Speech, and Hearing Services in Schools,* **9** (October 1980), 203–207.

Bankson, N. W., and M. C. Byrne, "The Effect of a Timed Correct Sound Production Task on Carryover." *Journal of Speech and Hearing Research,* **15** (March 1972), 160–168. (Investigates the feasibility of a program that would encourage the development of the motor skills necessary to produce sounds with ease and speed and the extent of generalization to spontaneous speech from a particular training task.)

Brown, J. C., "Techniques for Correcting /r/ Misarticulations." *Language, Speech, and Hearing Services in Schools,* **6** (April 1975), 86–90.

Carrier, J. K., "A Program of Articulation Therapy Administered by Mothers." *Journal of Speech and Hearing Disorders,* **35** (November 1970), 344–353.

Carroll, J. B., P. Davies, and B. Richman, *The American Heritage Word Frequency Book.* Boston: Houghton Mifflin Company, 1971. (Based on materials to which children are exposed in grades 3–9. Provides a frequency analysis of five million words sampled from textbooks and other materials currently in use in American schools.)

Costello, J. and S. Bosler, "Generalization and Articulation Instruction." *Journal of Speech and Hearing Disorders,* **41** (1976), 359–373. (Studies the treatment of articulatory disorders by mothers in the home under the direction of the speech/language clinician.)

—————— and J. M. Onstine, "Modification of Multiple Articulation Errors Based on Distinctive Feature Theory." *Journal of Speech and Hearing Disorders,* **41** (1976), 199–215.

Dworkin, J. P., "Characteristics of Frontal Lispers Clustered According to Severity." *Journal of Speech and Hearing Disorders,* **45** (February 1980), 37–44. (Determines the relationship among frontal lisping, protrusive lingual force and lingual diadochokinetic rates when subjects are grouped according to severity of lisping.)

Elbert, M. and L. V. McReynolds, "An Experimental Analysis of Misarticulating Children's Generalizations." *Journal of Speech and Hearing Research,* **21** (March 1978), 136–150. (Studies the role of context in remediation.)

——————, "Transfer of [r] Across Contexts." *Journal of Speech and Hearing Disorders,* **40** (August 1975), 380–387. (Points out that training on one specific [r] allophone may result in transfer to other [r] allophones without specific training.)

Engel, D. C. and L. R. Groth, "Case Studies of the Effect on Carry-over of Reinforcing Postarticulation Responses Based on Feedback." *Language, Speech and Hearing Services in Schools,* **7** (1976), 93–101.

Fleming, K. J., "Guidelines for Choosing Appropriate Phonetic Contexts for Speech-Sound Recognition and Production Practice." *Journal of Speech and Hearing Disorders,* **36** (August 1971), 356–367. (Presents guidelines for formulation of context lists that will enhance or challenge a child's discrimination and production abilities.)

Gould, D. G., "Remediation for Articulation Disorders." *Language, Speech and Hearing Services in Schools,* **11** (April 1980), 127–128. (Lists 14 suggestions for successful articulation modification.)

Hodson, B. W., "A Preliminary Hierarchical Model for Phonological Remediation." *Language, Speech, and Hearing Services in Schools,* **9** (October 1978), 236–240. (Describes a model of phonological intervention that facilitates a progression of articulatory skill development adaptable to individual needs.)

Hoffman, P. R., and G. H. Schuckers and D. L. Ratusnik, "Contextual Coarticulatory Inconsistency of [r] Misarticulation." *Journal of Speech and Hearing Research,* **20** (1977), 631–643. (Studies the coarticulatory effects of selected phonetic contexts upon misarticulated allophones of [r].)

Ingram, D., *Phonological Disability in Children.* New York: American Elsevier Publishing Company, 1976.

Johnson, J. P., *Nature and Treatment of Articulation Disorders.* Springfield, Illinois: Charles C. Thomas, 1980. (Explains a variety of intervention procedures for articulatory disorders.)

Kaliski, L., R. Tankersley, and R. Logha, *Structured Dramatics for Children with Learning Disabilities.* San Rafael, Calif.: Academic Therapy Publications, 1971.

Leonard, L. B., and S. I. Ritterman, "Articulation of [s] as a Function of Cluster and Word Frequency of Occurrence." *Journal of Speech and Hearing Research,* **14** (September 1971), 476–485. (Suggests that inconsistencies of [s] in consonantal clusters need not be attributed solely to the transitional motor differences in producing one cluster (such as [sk] as compared to another (such as [st]). These inconsistencies also appear related to the frequency with which these clusters occur, making the more common concatenations more available for the child to discriminate and practice in his language usage.)

Locke, J. L., "The Influence of Speech Perception in the Phonologically Disordered Child. Part 1. A Rationale, Some Criteria. The Conventional Tests." *Journal of Speech and Hearing Disorders,* **45** (November 1980), 431–444. (a)

———, "The Influence of Speech Perception in the Phonologically Disordered Child. Part II. Some Clinically Novel Procedures, Their Use. Some Findings," *Journal of Speech and Hearing Disorders,* **45** (November 1980), 445–468. (b)

———, "Ease of Articulation." *Journal of Speech and Hearing Research,* **15** (March 1972), 194–200. (Asks whether ease of production can account for age of acquisition of sounds.)

Longhust, T. M., and J. E. Reichle, "The Applied Communication Game: A

Comment on Muma's Communication Game: Dump and Play." *Journal of Speech and Hearing Disorders*, **40** (August 1975), 315–319. (Shows how theory of interpersonal communication can be used in a clinical setting.)

McCabe, R. B., and D. P. Bradley, "Pre-and Post Articulation Therapy Assessment." *Language, Speech, and Hearing Services in Schools*, **4** (January 1973), 13–24. (Suggests a way to evaluate articulation therapy.)

McDonald, E. T., "Disorders of Articulation." In R. J. Van Hattum, Ed., *Communication Disorders*. New York: Macmillan Publishing Co., Inc., 1980.

McGlone, R. E., and W. R. Proffit, "Patterns of Tongue Contact in Normal and Lisping Speakers." *Journal of Speech and Hearing Research*, **16** (September 1973), 456–473. (Notes that lispers possess an inability to use tongue muscles accurately. Suggests that causes could be physiological, neurological, or maturational.)

McNutt, L. D. and R. A. Keenan, "Comment on the Relationship Between Articulatory Defects and Syntax in Speech Defective Children." *Journal of Speech and Hearing Research*, **13** (September 1970), 669–679. (Suggests that therapy take account of the use of facilitating phonemes related to place—or other facilitating features—and avoid the phonemes that are frequently found to be substitutions.)

McReynolds, L. and S. Bennett, "Distinctive Feature Generalization in Articulation Training." *Journal of Speech and Hearing Disorders*, **37** (1972), 462–470.

Madison, C. L. "Articulatory Stimulability Reviewed." *Language, Speech, and Hearing Services in Schools*, **10** (July 1979), 185–190. (Examines the clinical value of articulatory stimulability through an analysis of past research and a review of clinical implementation.

Matheny, N. and J. M. Panagos, "Comparing the Effects of Articulation and Syntax Programs on Syntax and Articulation Improvement." *Language, Speech, and Hearing Services in Schools*, **9** (January 1978), 57–61. (Investigates the influence of interventive programs for syntax and articulation on the articulatory and syntactic skills of public school children with multiple-linguistic problems.)

Merton, K., "A Self-Directing Approach to Articulation Therapy and Practical Considerations." *Language, Speech, and Hearing Services in Schools*, **3** (July 1972), 24–31. (Discusses therapy based on sounds in successful contexts, practice, feedback, and expansion in systematically successful contexts.)

Miller, J. L., "Nonindependence of Feature Processing in Initial Consonants." *Journal of Speech and Hearing Research*, **20** (1977), 519–528. (Assesses the location of the voiced-voiceless boundary as a function of place of articulation and investigates the location of the labial-alveolar boundary of a function of manner class. Points to the existence of a mutual interaction in the processing of feature information.)

Mowrer, D. E., "Transfer of Training in Articulation Therapy." *Journal of Speech and Hearing Disorders*, **36** (November 1971), 427–446. (Reviews research having to do with these stages of therapy: (1) discrimination training, (2) sounds in isolation, (3) transfer among words, (4) transfer among sentences, and (5) transfer to spontaneous conversation.)

Mysak, E. D., *Speech Pathology and Feedback Theory.* Springfield, Ill.: Charles C Thomas, Publisher, 1971.

Parker, F., "Distinctive Features in Speech Pathology: Phonology or Phonemics." *Journal of Speech and Hearing Disorders,* **41** (1976), 23–29. (Discusses phonemic theory and generative theory and their role in distinctive feature intervention. Points out that a one-to-one relationship does not necessarily exist between distinctive features and production features.)

Pollack, E., and N. S. Rees, "Disorders of Articulation: Some Clinical Applications of Distinctive Feature Theory." *Journal of Speech and Hearing Disorders,* **37** (November 1972), 451–461. (Suggests the application of distinctive feature therapy as an approach to articulatory training.)

Powell, J., and L. V. McReynolds, "A Procedure for Testing Position Generalization from Articulatory Training." *Journal of Speech and Hearing Research,* **12** (September 1969), 629–645.

Rampp, D. L. and M. Pannbacker, "Indications and Contraindications for Tongue Thrust Therapy." *Language, Speech, and Hearing Services in Schools,* **9** (October 1978), 259–264.

Ritterman, S. I., "The Role of Practice and the Observation of Practice in Speech-Sound Discrimination Learning." *Journal of Speech and Hearing Research,* **13** (March 1970), 178–183. (Reports on the effect of learning by participation and learning by observation on the acquisition of a repertoire of phonetic distinctions.)

Ruder, K. F. and B. H. Bunce, "Articulation Therapy Using Distinctive Feature Analysis to Structure the Training Program: Two Case Studies." *Journal of Speech and Hearing Disorders,* **46** (February 1981), 59–65. (Suggests that phonological processes rather than unrelated sounds need to be the therapy target.)

Ruscello, D. M., "The Importance of Word Position in Articulation Therapy." *Language, Speech, and Hearing Services in Schools,* **6** (October 1975), 190–194. (Evaluates the importance of the position of sounds in words in a typical therapy program.)

Shelton, R. L., A. F. Johnson, D. M. Ruscello, and W. B. Arndt, "Assessment of Parent Administered Listening Training for Preschool Children with Articulation Deficits." *Journal of Speech and Hearing Disorders,* **43** (May 1978), 242–254.

Sommers, R. K., and A. R. Kane, "Nature and Remediation of Functional Articulation Disorders." In S. Dickson, Ed., *Communication Disorders: Remedial Principles and Practices.* Chicago: Scott, Foresman and Company, 1975, pp. 106–193.

Telage, K. M., "A Computerized Place-Manner Feature Program for Articulation Analyses," *Journal of Speech and Hearing Disorders,* **45** (November 1980), 481–494.

Van Hattum, R. J., J. Page, R. D. Baskervill, M. Duguay, L. Schreiber Conway, and T. R. Davis, "The Speech Improvement System Taped Program for Remediation of Articulation Problems in Schools." *Language, Speech, and Hearing Services in Schools,* **5** (April 1974), 91–97. (Describes the use of a particular program.)

Van Riper, C., *Speech Correction: Principles and Methods,* 5th ed. Englewood Cliffs, N.J.: Prentice-Hall, Inc., 1978, chap. 6.

Walsh, H., "On Certain Inadequacies of Distinctive Feature Systems." *Journal of Speech and Hearing Disorders,* **39** (February 1974), 32–43. (Describes the inadequacies of distinctive feature systems in diagnosing and treating speech disorders.)

Weber, J. L., "Patterning of Deviant Articulation Behavior." *Journal of Speech and Hearing Disorders,* **24** (May 1970), 135–41. (Indicates how an entire pattern of articulation can be taught at once.)

Webster, E. J., "Procedures for Group Parent Counseling in Speech Pathology and Audiology." *Journal of Speech and Hearing Disorders,* **33** (May 1968), 127–131. (Discusses use of group discussion and role playing in parent counseling.)

Weiner, F. F., "Treatment of Phonological Disability Using the Method of Meaningful Minimal Contrast: Two Case Studies." *Journal of Speech and Hearing Disorders,* **46** (February 1981), 97–103.

—— and N. Bankson, "Teaching Features." *Language Speech, and Hearing Services in Schools,* **9** (1978) 24–28.

—— and A. A. Ostrowski, "Effect of Listener Uncertainty on Articulatory Inconsistency." *Journal of Speech and Hearing Disorders,* **44** (November 1979), 487–493.

Winitz, H., *Articulatory Acquisition and Behavior,* New York: Appleton-Century-Crofts, 1969, chap. 5. (Discusses articulatory programing.)

——, *From Syllable to Conversation,* Baltimore: University Park Press, 1975.

—— and B. Bellerose, "Self-Retrieval and Articulatory Retention," *Journal of Speech and Hearing Research,* **18** (September 1975), 466–477. (Gives the results of testing the effect of self-retrieval on articulation recall. Self-retrieval indicates saying the name of the object rather than imitating the examiner's production of the word.)

——, "Sound Discrimination as a Function of Pretraining Conditions," *Journal of Speech and Hearing Research,* **5** (December 1962), 340–348.

12

Voice Disturbances

Before considering voice disturbances, the student should review the material on the vocal mechanism in Chapter 5. As supplemental reading, especially for the student who is concerned about his/her voice, we recommend the chapters on voice in Eisenson (1979, Chaps. 3–9).

The incidence of vocal disturbances in the school-age population varies considerably with the age of the group studied, the criteria used to determine abnormal or defective voice, and, we suggest, with the time of the year or season when an investigation may have been undertaken. Primary-grade children would be likely to show a considerably greater amount of denasality and hoarseness associated with common colds than middle-grade children, who may be hoarse instead as a result of vigorous physical activity associated with shouting on school and park playgrounds. Adolescents, males more than females, may have vocal problems as well as problems adjusting to their changing voices, which are associated with physiological factors inherent in adolescence. Curtis and Morris (1978, p. 144) based on data from several surveys, arrive at an estimate of 1 to 2 per cent for voice problems among children in the 6-to-14-year age range "depending on the criteria used." Hull and Timmons (1971) in their report of "The National Speech and Hearing Survey" (NSHS) arrived at 3 per cent of the school age population (grades 1 to 12). The percentage for males was 3.7 per cent compared with 2.1 per cent for females. These percentages are higher than those of earlier reports and are greater than for the incidence of defects of articulation (1.9 per cent) or for stuttering (0.8 per cent). The NSHS survey also noted an age-related prevalence for voice defects, varying from as high as 5.6 per cent among first-grade children to a low of 1 per cent in the twelfth grade. Hoarseness is noted as a particular problem among the younger schoolchildren.

Before considering vocal disturbances, we ought first to appreciate the characteristics and potentialities of a normal voice.

CHARACTERISTICS OF A NORMAL VOICE

A normal voice should be able to communicate reliably the feelings and thoughts the speaker wishes to convey to the listener. When well controlled, the voice should reveal rather than betray the types and shades of feeling that color the speaker's thinking. Through appropriate changes in pitch, force, duration, and quality, a speaker's voice should be able to command attention, maintain interest, and convey changes and emphasis in meaning.

The ability of a speaker to communicate intellectual and affective content will be enhanced if the speaker's voice attracts no attention to itself because of the manner in which it is produced or because of any undesirable characteristics. Vocalization should take place without apparent effort or strain. The acoustic results should be appropriate to the speaking situation. The voice should, in addition, be appropriate to the age and sex of the speaker. Little children may sound like little children, but older ones should not be mistaken for them. Neither should first graders sound like their parents or their teachers.

From the point of view of the listener, a normal and effective voice is one that is *pleasant, clear,* and *readily audible.* It should be heard without listener effort, provided, of course, that the listening conditions are not unfavorable for the purpose.

TYPES OF VOICE DISTURBANCES

The defects of voice most frequently heard are

1. Inadequate loudness.
2. Faulty volume (loudness) control.
3. Loudness inappropriate to the speaking situation or speech content.
4. Defects of quality, especially nasality and denasality, breathiness, huskiness, or hoarseness.
5. Faulty pitch range or too narrow a range of pitch.

6. Voice "breaks."
7. Inappropriate rate.

Each of these defects is considered in our discussion of therapy for vocal disturbances.

CAUSES OF VOCAL DISTURBANCES

Vocal disturbances may be present for a variety of causes. Among the most common are:

1. Poor physical health.
2. Anomalies (abnormalities) in the structure or condition of the voice mechanism.
3. Pathologies in the neurological control of the mechanism.
4. Glandular conditions or other physical conditions that may affect the growth or the tonicity and the responses of the muscles involved in voice production.
5. Defects of hearing that impair the individual's ability to respond to and monitor his/her own voice as it is being produced.
6. Disturbances of personality that reflect themselves in voice.
7. The presence of poor models that the child is imitating, so that he/she acquires a vocal defect through normal process of learning.
8. Poor habits of vocalization.

When a vocal disturbance either recurs or becomes chronic, evaluation *is a must*. The evaluation should be performed by a medical specialist whose training and experience qualify him or her for making medical judgments as to cause and treatment. Fortunately, in many instances, even when the cause is found to be of organic origin or is a result of poor vocal habits that produce organic (physical) changes, appropriate treatment often improves the condition as well as the voice.

The speech language clinician and classroom teacher are most likely to be directly concerned with the last two of the causes. To a lesser degree, defects of hearing may also directly concern them. Vocal disturbances that have a physical basis, as already suggested, are the therapeutic concern of the laryngologist, the specialist in voice problems. The teacher, however, is frequently the first to have an opportunity to recognize that something may be wrong that is causing the child to have a vocal difficulty, and so has a responsibility for bringing the condition to the attention of the parent and speech/language clinician.

Poor Physical Health

Most of us are able to recognize that "something is wrong" with a friend or relative by the way the friend sounds. Sometimes "what is wrong" may be temporary and a matter of momentary mood; occasionally, it may be physical and a matter of health. The interested and sensitive listener, who may be parent, friend, or teacher, is often the first to suspect that a speaker may not be well. Voice, because it is a product of the physiological as well as the emotional and intellectual state of the speaker, is the mirror that reflects the speaker's state of health. The expert speaker may, with awareness, control his/her voice and so succeed in disguising this condition. School-age children, less practiced in concealment and control, frequently reveal both their affective state and the state of their general physical health through their vocalizations.

Physical Anomalies

Perhaps the most frequent cause of vocal disturbances is the common cold. When we suffer from a cold, any or all of the following modifications of the voice mechanism may be present. The nasal cavities may be filled with mucous and so prevent adequate reinforcement of voice. The mucous membranes of the nose, throat, and larynx may be inflamed, and so modify the normal resonating activity of the voice mechanism. The vocal bands may themselves be inflamed and swollen, and so prevent normal vocal activity. The general "run-down" condition of the individual may impair normal functioning and control of the voice mechanism. If the cold is accompanied by a persistent cough, the general condition may be aggravated by the vocal abuse that is caused by coughing.

Persistent coughing may produce laryngitis. The condition of laryngitis may, however, be caused by vocal abuse not associated with either a cough or a cold. Continued overloud talking, or yelling under conditions of competing noise, may also produce laryngitis.

Sometimes vocal difficulties are associated with abnormalities of the structure of the larynx. The laryngeal cartilages may, for congenital reasons or through injury, be so constructed that the vocal bands may not be able to approximate (come together) normally, or the reinforcement of vocal tones may be impaired because of the change in the size and shape of the larynx. More frequently, the vocal bands may have developed nodules on the inner edges as a result of vocal abuse. Sometimes the vocal bands become thickened because of chronic incorrect vocalization. The effect is usually a voice characterized by low pitch, breathiness, and effort in production. Fortunately, these conditions usually improve through a combination of voice rest and a program of training to modify the incorrect vocal behavior of the speaker. Occasionally, the edges of the vocal bands may have slight irregularities, which impair normal activity. Any of the conditions described can be determined only through an examination of the larynx by a competent physician. The treatment of these conditions will call for the active cooperation of the classroom teacher. Voice therapy, if it is indicated, is a problem for the speech/language clinician working in cooperation with the physician.

Hearing Loss

Because we learn to vocalize as well as to articulate "by ear," hearing loss is likely to be manifest in vocal inadequacies. If the hearing loss is appreciable, and of the type that does not permit the child to check on the voice produced, the child may speak in a voice too loud, or not loud enough, for the specific speaking situation. Sometimes the loss may be temporary, and associated with the effects or aftereffects of a cold. Occasionally, as a result of middle-ear involvement, there may be prolonged hearing loss. With proper medical attention, this situation should clear and the vocal disturbance disappear. (See Chapters 6 and 14 for fuller discussion of hearing loss.)

Glandular Disturbances

Thyroid gland deficiency is associated with a falling of the basal metabolic rate. Frequently, though not invariably, decrease in metabolic rate is causally associated with sluggish physical and mental activity, and with a general reduction of body tone. This condition is likely to reflect itself in a colorless, poorly modulated voice.

In contrast with thyroid deficiency, the presence of an excess of thyroid hormone generally results in making the individual hyperactive and "nervous." The condition is likely to be reflected in a rapid rate of speech and in a tense, high-pitched voice.

The teacher and speech/language clinician who observe what appear to be significant changes in the general activity and mental alertness of a child, in association with vocal changes, should refer the child to the school nurse or physician for a medical examination to determine the possibility of a glandular involvement. Caution, however, should be exercised in order that no hasty conclusion be made. Comparable changes in the voice of a child may result from conditions not related to glandular disturbances. Vocal changes may sometimes merely indicate a temporary indisposition on the part of the child.

Pubertal Changes

With the coming of physical adolescence and its associated physiological and growth changes, many children have marked vocal difficulties. These are more likely to be present among boys than among girls. In males, the size and structure of the larynx undergo considerable change, so that boys have to adjust to longer vocal bands as well as a larger larynx. Girls, with a longer and slower pubescent period, and with a smaller amount of laryngeal growth, have less modification and more time for adjustment. The little girl soprano may, during adolescence, become a woman mezzo-soprano or perhaps an alto. The boy soprano may become a tenor or a baritone.

Often the difficulty during puberty is aggravated by problems of social adjustment. The shy youngster may be so embarrassed by his voice "breaks" that he withdraws from his groups or finds excuses for not talking. Some of the difficulties may be related to self-consciousness resulting from a poor skin condition, or an awareness of physical awkwardness. Occasionally, overly passive adolescents may try to vocalize within a pitch range determined for them by their parents or older siblings, or other influential members of their environment. In some instances, dependent and infantile boys and girls may try to maintain their preadolescent voices as an aspect of their general wish to continue to be young children. In other instances, both boys and girls may try to show how mature they are by attempting to establish low, deep-pitched voices incompatible with their own amount of laryngeal growth and general physical change.

The junior high school years, usually the 12–15 age range, is the period for major vocal changes, especially in males. It is also the period for voice or pitch "breaks," which are frequently associated with initiating voice at too low a pitch. This age period, as teachers, clinicians, and parents can attest, is also one during which many changes take place in attitudes and behavior. Thus, adjustments to vocal change are correlated with other dynamics of adolescence. A great deal more than a "new" voice is being tried!

The influence of the speech/language clinician and the classroom teacher in helping adolescents through their period of voice change can hardly be overestimated. The teacher can ward off taunts and help the adolescent build up defenses. If the adolescent has prolonged difficulty in arriving at his/her "new voice," referral to a speech/language clinician may be of help. If there is reason to believe that psychological problems may be part of the difficulty, referral of the adolescent for proper guidance is in order.

Personality Disturbances

Few of us question the general observation that the voice is a mirror of the personality. Temporary emotional upsets are likely to be reflected in the speaker's voice. Similarly, chronic emotional disturbances and maladjustments of attitude are likely to be manifest in disorders of voice.

Part of the early and continued experience of classroom teachers is the need to urge a child to "speak up" because of a weak and timid voice. Other children, in sharp contrast, need to be reminded to "tone down" because thre is no cause for shouting. Children of both voice types may be revealing attitudes toward their classmates in particular and their environment in general that are suggestive of a significant degree of maladjustment. So does the child whose voice is a constant whine; so also does the child whose breathless voice and breathtaking rate of speaking suggest fear of interruption and apprehension that once interrupted the youngster may not be able to resume talking.

Although the vocal defects described briefly in this chapter are not important in themselves, they may be significant as symptoms of chronic personality maladjustments. Occasionally, the child's voice may be reflecting not only his or her own maladjustment but that of an older member of the environment whom the child, consciously or unconsciously is imitating. Whatever the case may be for the individual boy or girl, appropriate treatment calls for determining and dealing with the underlying cause as well as with the vocal symptoms of the cause. With the young child, the voice symptoms sometimes disappear without direct treatment provided that the basic personality problem is relieved. The older child, who may have established vocal traits that have become habitual, may need direct treatment for voice even if the personality problem is treated. The voice may even improve while the underlying adjustment problem remains.

Imitation of Poor Models

The child learns both his/her language and the manner in which his/her language is produced by ear. The mother who teaches her child the name of something also teaches the child the manner in which the naming is done. If mother shouts, so will the child; if mother speaks as though she were not worthy of the evocation, the child is likely to develop the same tone. As the child grows up, other models become subjects for imitation. Friends, liked or respected adults who frequent the home, and teachers become likely models when the child is of school age. Usually the imitation is unconscious; occasionally a child's urge or need to identify with another person is so strong that the imitation may be conscious. Imitation that begins early may continue into and beyond adolescence.

Often a parent will be aware that there is something wrong with a child's voice but have no awareness that the fault is parent-centered. We have frequently pointed out to complaining parents that they must have children who love them because the children speak so much like them. And frequently we have suggested to parents that they accept treatment for their own voices as the best device for improving the voices of their children.

Teachers, obviously, have a great responsibility for the voices of their classroom children. A well-liked teacher is likely to be an imitated teacher. A disliked teacher may be mimicked in manner as well as in voice. So, before a teacher turns to other sources for an explanation of common pupil vocal traits, self-reflection is in order. Beyond this, an objective appraisal by a professionally competent person may go a long way in explaining the positive or negative reasons for common vocal faults among pupils in a given classroom. Though rare, a sudden "epidemic" of hoarseness may be explained by a teacher's hoarseness. Pupil manifestations of breathiness, denasality, or low pitch may indicate the need for teacher correction if the children are to vocalize without these defects.

Poor Habits of Vocalization

The professional speech clinician often treats persons whose vocal habits are poor and are not apparently associated with any present disturbance of personality or any specific or general physical condition. It is possible, of course, that the faulty vocal habits have outlived the cause of their origin, that in a given instance the speaker is presenting the residual of an adolescent "crush," or a once-serious personality maladjustment, or a vocal manner that began with an illness and has persisted long after all physical evidence of illness disappeared. Not infrequently vocal habits may be interpreted as lingering memories of what used to be. If, however, "what used to be" is no longer in need of treatment, the vocal symptoms, or the vocal habits with which the symptoms are associated, may be directly treated. Chief among faulty vocal habits are unsuitable pitch level, inappropriate nasal reinforcement, and poor breath control for speech.

Pitch and Range

Vocal pitch and vocal range are not to be selected by the individual as one might choose articles of dress. Pitch, as pointed out earlier, is determined by the size, shape, and normal functioning of the vocal bands and the resonating cavities. Each of us is potentially intended for a given range of pitch according to individual vocal equipment. Most of us arrive at this without special instruction by doing "what comes naturally." Some of us make the most of our potential by special motivation or by competent instruction. A few of us succumb to pressures to vocalize in a manner not consistent with nature's intentions for us, and difficulties may arise. One of these pressures is one of admiring women's voices that are low-pitched and somewhat breathy in quality (considered a desirable quality a few years ago). The not infrequent result of employing a voice pitched too low for the physical mechanism is hoarseness. Although there is considerable variability in the consequences of the constant use of a voice pitched too low for the mechanism, there is a growing body of evidence indicating that undesirable physical consequences can frequently be expected. Among these consequences are thickening of the vocal bands and chronic irritation of the larynx.

Boys, as well as men, are not at all exempt from the cultural pressure for the low-pitched voice. Unfortunately, just so many women are born to have soprano voices, and only a few to be altos; so it is that many boys and men are by nature intended to be tenors and high baritones, just as some are to be low baritones and basses. The result of confusing virility with vocal depth is frequently low pitch and poor quality. On occasion, chronic hoarseness can result from attempts to pitch the voice at a level too low for the optimum functioning of the vocal apparatus. Strain and fatigue may also occur.[1]

Our emphasis thus far has been on the abnormally low-pitched voice. This does not mean that some persons do not speak at a pitch

---

[1] M. Cooper, "Spectographic Analysis of Fundamental Frequency and Hoarseness Before and After Vocal Rehabilitation," *Journal of Speech and Hearing Disorders,* **39** (1974), inferred that in a population of 155 patients who required vocal rehabilitation, 150 were vocalizing in too low a pitch range. Cooper concluded that ". . . the use of a pitch which is below the optimal or natural level is a major factor in initiating, contributing to, or continuing most types of dysphonia."

level too high for their vocal mechanism. Among speakers with inappropriate pitch they are, however, likely to constitute a small minority. Cultural preference in the United States places a premium on the low-pitched voice and is inclined to penalize the high-pitched voices. Unless there is a strong psychological drive to maintain an abnormally high-pitched voice, the individual is likely to yield in the direction of cultural preference. Interestingly enough, persons who persist in vocalizing at high pitch levels, unless they are also shouters, are usually not as susceptible to some of the physical changes that frequently accompany abnormally low-pitched vocalization. We may appreciate some of the reasons for this by intentionally, but briefly, talking considerably below and then considerably above our normal pitch range. In talking at the low end of our range, we will find that it takes appreciably more effort to produce a loud voice than within our normal range, or at a relatively high pitch. Fatigue is likely to set in quickly, and a feeling of vocal strain will follow if vocalization is continued. We are not, incidentally, referring to the use of a high-pitched falsetto or of a pitch range associated with laryngeal hypertension.

Habitual use of pitches much below or above our natural pitch range is often accomplished at the expense of the abuse of the vocal mechanism. We have worked with preschool children who developed nodules on their vocal bands as a result of vocal abuse. Typically, these children were high-pitched screamers (Wilson 1961).[2] There are always, of course, some individuals who are able to vocalize either above or below normal pitch range without suffering physical consequences. Perhaps these persons are kin to those who do not develop calluses despite poorly fitted shoes, or who do not become sunburned despite what would be overexposure to the sun for most of us. Our only suggestion is that these hardy persons be considered exceptions rather than models for the more susceptible of us to follow. Most of us do better vocalizing within a pitch range suited to our vocal apparatus. How to determine this range is considered later in the discussion of optimum pitch in the section on voice therapy in the next section.

Caution needs to be exercised when judgments are made about pitch levels and ranges. Schneiderman (1959) found that judgments about pitch, including those by listeners with "trained ears," are not always valid. Other aspects of voice—quality or loudness—may produce an erroneous impression as to the "perceived" pitch. This obser-

---

[2] In a survey, E. M. Silverman and C. H. Zimmer, "Incidence of Chronic Hoarseness among School Age Children," *Journal of Speech and Hearing Disorders,* **40** (1975) found that 38 of 162 children in the elementary school grades suffered from chronic hoarseness. A majority of these children were below the fourth grade. On otolaryngological examination, most of them were found to have vocal nodules.

vation emphasizes the need to determine optimum pitch level and range rather than to make arbitrary judgments as to the appropriateness of the speaker's pitch.

Inappropriate Nasal Resonance

The movements of the soft palate largely determine whether the produced voice is characterized by the presence or absence of nasality. Normally, when vocalization occurs with a relaxed soft palate that permits the stream of breath to enter the nasal cavities, the voice is "resonated" there and becomes characteristically nasal. Of course, some nasal reinforcement occurs whether or not the soft palate is relaxed or elevated, so that a degree of nasality is likely to be present even when nasality is not the characteristic quality of the produced voice.

The American-English sounds *n*, *m*, and *ng* are normally produced with a relaxed soft palate and "open nasal cavities." All other sounds of English are normally produced with the soft palate elevated so that the stream of breath is directed and emitted orally. If an individual has a weakened soft palate, he or she will tend to speak with more than a normal amount of nasal resonance, and so has a voice quality characterized by *positive nasality*. The same quality may result from sluggish palatal control and from related activity of the mouth, throat, and nasopharynx in their functions as resonators. Positive nasality may also arise as a result of imitation. The French-speaking child quite properly nasalizes some of the vowels as well as the nasal consonants. The American- or English-speaking child may do the same in imitating the speech of a member of the environment who nasalizes more than most American or English speakers do.

Denasality, or an absence of appropriate nasal resonance, occurs when there is too little reinforcement by the nasal resonators. This may result from a blocking within the nasal cavities themselves, or a partial blocking within the area of the nasopharynx. The result is a pinched, flat quality that suggests the voice of a person with a head cold or an allergic condition involving the nasal cavities. The quality is more than an absence of nasality when it is anticipated in the production of the nasal consonants. It is an overall effect recognizable on sounds that are normally emitted orally. We can produce what approaches a denasal voice by pinching our nostrils in the articulation of such a sentence as "Who is that tall boy with a black coat?" The result, even though the sentence does not contain nasal consonants, should be different in quality if the sentence is articulated without pinched nostrils.

Techniques for recognizing and improving nasal reinforcement are considered in the discussion of voice therapy in the next section.

Breathing Faults

It is unusual for a physically normal child to breathe incorrectly while speaking unless he or she has somehow been trained to do so. Such training may be the result of a child's efforts to be obedient to the direction, "Take a real deep breath before you begin to speak," or "Raise your chest high and pull your tummy in before you begin to speak." Occasionally, but really rarely, a child may speak with a too shallow breath, or attempt to speak while inhaling rather than, or in addition to, exhaling. In such instances, investigation may reveal that we are dealing with an insecure, apprehensive child who fears that pausing for a normal breath will result in an interruption of thought. Someone will break in, and during the interruption the child will forget and suffer the consequent social penalties. The same factors may operate with the child who attempts to speak on inhalation as well as exhalation, or who tries with effort to speak on residual air after "tidal breath" has been expired. However, we should not overlook the possibility that in some instances we may be dealing with a normal child with normal psychological dynamisms, who is simply imitating a member of the environment whose breathing habits for speech are faulty.

We are inclined to agree with Curtis (1967, pp. 193–194) that it is probably of little importance whether the person's breathing is predominantly abdominal or diaphragmatic, predominantly thoracic, or predominantly medial (characterized by activity about the base of the sternum). What seems to be of most importance for almost all speaking occasions is that the speaker has an adequate supply of breath (exaggerated deep breathing is not required) and is comfortable while speaking. Most persons who have not been specially trained to emphasize the activity of one part of the thoracic mechanism are likely to do relatively well in coordinated participation of all parts of their respiratory mechanism. For the rare individual who does not have adequate breath for normal speech purposes, attention may be directed to an emphasis on either diaphragmatic action and control, thoracic action, or medial action. Our own preference is for diaphragmatic (abdominal) control, because it is easy, effective, and readily discernible. The individual may be directed to breathe while speaking as he or she is likely to breathe when relaxed, unless tightly girdled or belted. On inspiration of breath the abdominal area will be noted to move upward if the person is lying down, or forward if the person is sitting up or standing. On expiration, the abdominal area should pull in. A gradual, controlled pulling in of the abdominal muscles helps to bring about an upward movement of the diaphragm and so to produce a well-sustained, steady vocal tone if the action takes place during vocalization.

It is probably best to minimize or to eliminate entirely breathing characterized by action of the upper chest (clavicular breathing). Such breathing frequently results in a strained humping of the chest and shoulders, and so interferes with easy breath flow. In this awkward and strained position, which is associated with neck and throat tension, proper reinforcement of tone in the resonating cavities becomes difficult so that voice production becomes unnecessarily effortful. It is apparently also more difficult to obtain an adequate supply of breath with clavicular breathing; the speaker finds it necessary to pause for breath more often than with abdominal, thoracic, or medial breathing.

Generally, we do not consider it either advisable or necessary to stress manner of breathing. As a practical matter, we have found that it is usually possible to modify and improve breath use for vocalization without direct attention to the individual's breathing activity. Correction of posture and attention to the initiation and maintenance of proper vocal tones are usually sufficient and effective.

THERAPY FOR VOICE DISTURBANCES

The classroom teacher who suspects that a student has a voice disturbance should first make certain that the student's personal preference alone, even though it may be incompatible with the child's physical mechanism, is not being expressed. Personal preference is not the best determiner of vocal quality, and such a student should be motivated to change to a physically appropriate voice. Probably no other therapy will be needed in such a case. Second, the teacher should be certain that no physical condition requiring medical attention is present before any treatment is undertaken. It follows also that if a psychological problem underlies the voice defect, the problem and the child rather than the defect should be treated. With these precautions in mind, the classroom teacher with an understanding of voice production may be a real help to those children with defects of quality, pitch, or loudness of voice. The classroom teacher, as well as the speech/language clinician, will also do well to bear in mind that despite the best of teachings, not all defects are fully remediable. Sometimes the most apparent defect resists specific improvement, but overall improvement may still be attained if other, not so readily apparent, aspects of voice and speech are trained to the fullest extent. For example, a child with a weakened soft palate may necessarily speak with a characteristic nasal quality. If this child is helped to articulate clearly, but not pedantically, and to have a wide and flexible pitch range reflective of changes in thought and feeling, the overall impression is likely to be favorable despite the persistence of nasality. Similarly, a child with a high-pitched voice, especially if the child is a boy, may not be able to do much about lowering his fundamental pitch if he is one who is intended by nature to have a high pitch. Such a child can still be helped if he learns to make full use of his pitch range, and can produce a voice that is readily audible and is meaningfully emphatic according to speech content. With these points in mind, several specific suggestions for dealing with particular aspects of vocal deficiency may be considered.

Pitch Level and Range

As indicated earlier, appropriate pitch for an individual should be determined by factors other than either the listener's or speaker's liking for a given pitch range. The other factors are anatomic, including the length and mass of the individual's vocal bands, the relationship of vocal bands to the laryngeal structure, and the size and shape of the other resonating cavities. We are aware that pitch varies inversely as the length and directly as the tension of the vibrating body. Changes in length and tension enable the speaker to produce a range of normal or natural pitches that comprise a physically appropriate pitch range. The production of vocal tones consistent with the intellectual and affective content of speech comprises an appropriate pitch range for speaking.

The natural or *optimum* pitch is that pitch level at which an individual is able to vocalize most efficiently. This is the level at which good quality, loudness, and ease of production are found. For most persons, natural or optimum pitch level is about one-fourth to one-third above the lowest level within the range of pitch levels at which vocalization can occur.

You can find your own speaking pitch range and optimal or natural pitch by the following procedure:

1. With the musical scale in mind, intone the vowel /ɑ/ at your lowest possible pitch level.
2. Go up the scale, a level at a time, until you reach falsetto.
3. Repeat, using the sound /m/. The two levels should match. If not, take the wider range. Within your pitch range your optimal pitch is about the third or fourth level from your lowest pitch. Thus, if you can intone 12 levels, optimal pitch is about level three or four.

Perkins (1977) observes that the idea of optimal pitch is a notion that "seems to have clinical validity but persistently escapes scientific verification."

If a child's habitual pitch is found to be more than two levels below or above the natural or optimal level, then it is advisable to help the youngster to initiate voice at the optimal level.[3] The same advice, of course, holds for adults. It is well to remember, however, that young growing children have changes in their natural pitch as laryngeal growth takes place. After physiological adolescence, growth changes are not so great and natural pitch should become pretty well stabilized.

From our point of view, the determination of pitch range and one's natural pitch is an initial step in establishing effective voice. For most persons, the most effective range seems to be between natural or optimal pitch and a level about one-third below the highest within the total range. This, we admit, is our clinical impression, one shared by Boone (1977, p. 92) and by Perkins (1977). When indicated, as when a child has difficulty because his/her pitch range is too narrow, or too high, or too low to be comfortable or effective, or appears to have learned to imitate someone's voice that unhappily was not a good vocal model, we do recommend training for pitch "control." Most children can learn to initiate voice for conversational purposes on their natural pitch level and to use several levels above that and, if possible, a level or at most two below it for variety, emphasis, and appropriate expression of feeling. There is no objection to the initiation of voice at a level or two below natural level if the child has a fairly wide range. If the range is narrow, it is probably best to avoid dropping more than one level below natural pitch. The danger of dropping two levels below natural pitch for a person with a narrow pitch range is that an effortful, breathy voice may be produced that actually may be harmful to the speaker.[4]

Breathiness

Vocal quality characterized by breathiness results from air "leakage" between vocal bands during voice production. The ultimate of breathiness is intentionally whispered speech. Voiceless consonants are, of

---

[3] It is important for us to make it clear tht we are not recommending that the procedures for determining optimal pitch and optimum pitch range need to be instituted for all children. We have in mind children, and adults for that matter, who are having problems in voice production.

[4] Alternate methods for determining habitual and optimal pitch and pitch range may be found in J. Eisenson, *Voice and Diction: A Program for Improvement* 4th Edition. (New York: Macmillan Publishing Co., Inc., 1979), pp. 95–97.

course, breathy, and appropriately so. Vowels, however, and voiced consonants should be produced without any obvious breathiness.

Breathiness may result from overrelaxed vocalization with associated partial approximation of the vocal bands. If a person's voice is pitched too low in terms of his natural pitch range, the tension of the vocal bands will be less than optimum, and the voice is likely to be breathy. If a person is suffering from laryngitis, attempts at vocalization are frequently associated with pain because of contact between the swollen inner edges of the bands. To avoid or reduce pain, the speaker is likely to keep the vocal bands in a partially approximated position, and so will speak with breathiness. Figure 11 shows the position of the vocal bands when they are not sufficiently approximated for good voice production, and yet too closely approximated for purposes of normal breathing.

Sometimes a breathy voice is associated with shyness or timidity. A child who speaks quietly because of fear of speaking aloud may not bring the vocal bands close enough to vocalize without excessive breathiness. Occasionally a "good" but not necessarily timid child will imitate a teacher's low voice used to keep the class quiet. Such a child, in the attempt to speak "low and quiet," may also speak breathily.

There are several reasons for children to avoid a breathy voice quality. First, the breathy voice is frequently too low in pitch, and vocalization may become effortful and unpleasant. Second, breathiness is wasteful in terms of length of phrase in speaking. The child, or the adult for that matter, who speaks with excessive breathiness will need to pause for inhalation more often than would otherwise be necessary. In the attempts to establish normal phrasing, the child may speak on residual breath, and the speech efforts will sound strained and be strained.

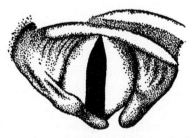

FIGURE 11. Diagram, adapted from a high-speed photograph, showing vocal bands not sufficiently approximated for good voice production, and too closely approximated for normal breathing. Courtesy Bell Telephone Company Laboratories, New York.

To overcome breathiness it is frequently necessary to have the child become aware of the difference between a breathy and a normal voice quality. This may be done by having the child place his/her hand in front of his/her mouth while saying a sentence such as "My bunny's name is Lanny." Normally, such a sentence, which has no voiceless sounds and only one voiced stop, should be produced with a very minimum of breath felt on the hand placed a few inches in front of the mouth. The child should then be directed to "feel" the breath accompanying a sentence such as "Polly likes to eat thin crackers," which has both stop and fricative sounds and is, therefore, necessarily produced with accompanying breath. If there is no distinct difference in the child's vocalization of the two sentences, another child whose voice is not breathy should be asked to speak the two sentences while the breathy-voiced child holds his/her hand about six inches in front of the second child's mouth, and notes the difference.

After the concepts and the feeling of breathiness and nonbreathiness are established, other techniques may be employed to produce normal vocalization. A very simple and often effective approach is to direct the child to speak as if breath were precious and to emit as little breath as possible while talking. Then, for contrast, the child may be instructed to be as breathy as possible, so that the difference can be clearly appreciated.

Another helpful technique is to have the child intone a vowel such as /i/ (ee) and to hold the vowel as long as comfortable on a single breath. The vowel /i/, because it is relatively tense and high-pitched, is likely to be produced with a minimum of breathiness even by the child who is inclined to be breathy. If this is done successfully, the child may then be directed to intone /ɑ/ (ah) and to maintain the sound until the child begins to become breathy, or until he/she needs to inhale. Then the effort should be repeated with reduced loudness but without obvious breathiness. In this way the child can learn how "quietly" it is possible to speak without becoming breathy. The same technique may be used with a change in pitch rather than loudness so that the child and clinician may learn at which level or levels breathiness occurs, and so the child may be helped to vocalize without "waste" of breath.

Other recommended exercises include saying as much of the alphabet as possible or counting as long as is comfortable on a single breath. When quantity of production becomes the objective, the child spontaneously is likely to conserve breath. As soon as possible, of course, the child should be given an opportunity to apply what has been learned in the exercises to other situations, such as reading aloud and conversational speech. Although the child should not be interrupted in normal speaking efforts because of breathiness, the clinician should work out a system of signals to tell the youngster whether the effort to control breathiness has been successful. The teacher, working with the speech clinician, may apply this approach in the classroom situation.

Organic Causes of Breathiness

Figure 11 shows the vocal bands in a position of incomplete approximation for good voice production. This position would in and of itself produce a breathy or semiwhispered voice. Figure 12 shows vocal nodules that because of their mass would prevent normal approximation of the vocal bands. Discomfort on contact of the nodules would increase the likelihood of insufficient approximation and consequent breathiness. Any other growth or a thickening of the bands would produce breathiness. Laryngitis, which is accompanied by vocal band thickening and pain on contact between the bands, is also characterized by breathiness. Figure 13 shows contact ulcers on the vocal folds. This condition also results in breathiness and low pitch. Pain in the laryngeal area is likely to be felt, especially after prolonged talking.

Because of the possibilities of organic causes of breathiness, including malignant growths, it is important that the child be examined by a physician and cleared medically before any corrective measures are undertaken.

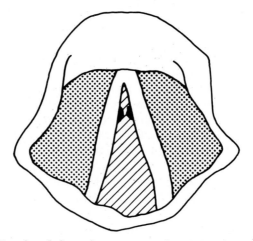

FIGURE 12. Vocal nodules, often associated with high-pitched shouting. Note typical paired formation in upper (middle third) of vocal folds.

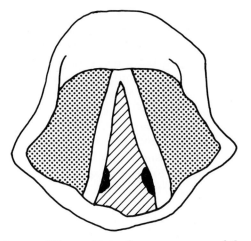

FIGURE 13. Contact Ulcers. Note the appearance of the ulcers at the lower portion of the vocal folds in contrast with the typical position of vocal nodules, as shown in Figure 12.

Nasality

Positive or excessive nasality as a characteristic voice quality, as we pointed out earlier, is associated with a relaxed soft palate during the act of vocalization. In the absence of specific anomaly involving the palate, nasality may occur either because of generally slow or sluggish palatal action or because of specific "retarded" action of the soft palate after the articulation of appropriately nasal sounds. If there is generally sluggish soft palate action, speech as a whole is likely to sound nasal. If there is a limited failure of the soft palate to be elevated quickly immediately following the production of a nasal consonant, the sound or sounds produced after the nasal are likely to be partially nasalized. In the latter case, words such as *me, many, and, among, nine,* and *mine* are likely to be produced as if all the sounds were nasal.

In some cases, the excessive nasality appears to be associated with a general expression of lassitude and an air of indifference to the environment. Such children, except possibly in their playground activities, seem to lack the energy for any physical effort, including the elevation of the soft palate. We should not, however, overlook the possibility that the expresson of lassitude and apparent indifference may have a physical basis. The contrast in the child's playground behavior may be the effect of strong and specific motivation.

Children who have had their adenoids removed frequently change from having markedly denasal voices to having characteristically nasal voices. This change can be appreciated when we realize that when enlarged adenoids are present, a child does not need to elevate the soft palate very much to obstruct the opening to the nasal cavity. After the removal of the adenoidal tissue, the habit of partial elevation of the soft palate may persist, and nasality may then occur during the production of all speech sounds.

Regardless of the cause of nasality, if therapy is in order it should begin with giving the child awareness of how a nasal voice sounds and, if the child is capable of such understanding, how nasality occurs. The child can easily learn to recognize nasality by listening to the teacher intentionally nasalize a sentence such as *The sailor shouted "All aboard!"* or *This is the house that Jack built* and then listening to the same sentences spoken without intentional nasality. Both of these sentences, incidentally, contain no nasal consonants and so provide no temptation to nasalize because of proximity of a sound to a nasal consonant (assimilation).

The child inclined toward nasality may also learn how nasality feels by pinching the nostrils while speaking one of the sentences that follows. If the child becomes aware of pressure, or a feeling of stuffiness in the nose, or of fullness in his ears, it indicates that breath has entered the nasal cavity that should have been emitted through the mouth.

> Bob took Ted to the zoo.
> Please take care of the kitty.
> The dog chased the bird up the tree.
> Polly likes crackers with cheese.
> Joe played baseball.
> The baby played pit-a-pat with his daddy.

The same sentences may be used to help the child *see nasality*. This can be accomplished by placing a cold hand mirror under the child's nostrils while he/she repeats one of the sentences having no nasal consonants. Clouding of the mirror by the warm air that escapes from the nostrils is visual evidence of positive and inappropriate nasality.

Once awareness is present in a child, who is not organically involved and is motivated to overcome nasality, the following techniques may be employed:

Raising the Soft Palate

Have the child stand before a mirror and yawn with the mouth wide open. The child should be directed to note that the soft palate tends to lift up. The youngster should learn how this feels as well as how it looks for the soft palate to elevate. The child may also be directed to blow up a previously stretched balloon and note the feeling and movement of the soft palate.

The child may be directed to say /ɑ/ (ah) with nostrils pinched. All sound should come through the mouth, and no stuffiness should be felt. Then the child should be directed to produce a nasalized /ā/. The procedure should be repeated with other vowels and for such words as *boy, girl, tree, tall, big, go, bread, hot, skip, stop,* and *dog,* and short phrases such as *go away, pretty girl, big boy,* and *a slice of bread.* Older children, who can understand the difference between nasal and nonnasal sounds, should be encouraged to make up their own list of words and phrases for practice.

Ear Training

One of the ways that children can be helped to distinguish between appropriate and inappropriate nasality by listening to appropriate articulation of the following pairs of words are examples that can be used:

moo	two	an	at	him	hit
me	bee	wing	wig	pen	pet
my	by	I'm	I'll	can	cat
no	go	in	it	bean	beat
may	pay	aim	ape	seem	seat
mall	ball	home	hope	boom	boot

It may also help if the clinician informs the child that occasionally words in the second column will be intentionally nasalized and the child is to signal his/her awareness of such nasalization. The clinician with good control, who can turn nasality off and on at will, may go beyond single words to pairs of phrases and sentences.

If a tape or cassette recorder with playback is available, ready use may be made of such an instrument in helping the child to recognize his/her own nasality. A sentence or two may be recorded by the nasal child and the same material by another child without the defect. The child "in training" may then hear the difference in voice quality in comparison with a peer. Later, recordings may be used to help the child recognize improvement in exercises and for parts of readings or conversation. Many children enjoy a chance to do intentionally what they are seeking to improve. Permission "to do the wrong thing" should be given so that the child may practice and so gain voluntary control over nasality. The same approach, of course, is also relevant for other aspects of voice therapy as well as for the improvement of articulation.

General Articulatory Activity

Often the child who speaks nasally will also be one whose overall articulatory activity lacks precision and clearness. For this child, in the interest of improving articulation in general as well as nasality in particular, more precise and energetic articulatory activity is recommended. With increased activity of the lips and tongue, there will also be a reflexive increase in energetic activity of the soft palate. The child should also be instructed to direct all nonnasal sounds through the mouth and to increase the feeling of front-of-the-mouth activity. Certain words and phrases such as the following might be used in drill work and incorporated into practice sentences and conversational speech.

two	do	pet	trip
treat	tweet	pit	peep
pooh	boo	step	bend
chew	food	slip	flip
tuck	buck	tent	tune
see	saw	spot	nail
lick	tick	tack	hide
bing	bang	stuck	clip

come along	sing a song	kick the tin can
take some tea	beat the drum	Pat likes to eat
red rose	don't trip	do come soon
all aboard	pickled peppers	see the birds
leave the boat	hit the deck	step lively now
stay away	broken bones	throw the big ball
let's go	pack of sticks	a stack of papers

Denasality (Hyponasality)

Some children speak as though they have either chronically stuffed noses or enlarged adenoids that block the entrance of sound into the nasal cavities. These children need to be helped to become aware of adequate nasal resonance when it is appropriate.

Humming with lips relatively relaxed so that a sensation of tickling is experienced is a recommended technique for establishing nasal resonance. Another useful device is the intentional lengthening of nasal consonants. The child may be instructed to hum and then follow the hum with a vowel. Specifically, the exercise might proceed as follows:

1. Hum gently on a sustained breath, first with the sound *m*, then *n*, and then [ŋ]. Repeat each hum three or four times.
2. Begin a hum and then blend with a vowel.
3. Prolong an initial nasal sound and blend with a vowel as in *mmm-a*, and *nnn-oo*.
4. Begin with a lengthened nasal, blend with a vowel, and end with a lengthened nasal as in *mmmannn, nnnoonnn*.

Other exercises might include articulating such words as *me, my, moo, may, meal, nail, now, new, never, nice, sing, long,* and *running* with intentional lengthening of the nasal consonants.

Sentences incorporating words with more than a usual number of nasal consonants should be made, and conversation with such words and sentences should be practiced. Whenever possible, the child should be encouraged to make up words and sentences so that he/she may have the pleasure of creative activity as well as practice.

Following are some additional materials for practice:

mine alone	man in the moon
running down	many candies
nine and one	Monday noon
round and round	morning at ten

Amanda ran home.
The moon shines on the barn.
Nine and nine make eighteen.
Only Tom may come.
Molly found a new penny.

There was a monkey who climbed a tree,
When he jumped down, he jumped on me.

Demanded the Pieman of Simple Simon,
"Young man, now show me your penny."
Answered Simon to the old Pieman,
"I'm sorry, I haven't any."

London Bridge came falling down, falling down, falling down;
London Bridge came falling down,
I'm glad it did not strike my crown.

Inappropriate Loudness

Most children whose speech patterns are a result of identification with normal adults speak loudly enough to be heard. Those who

speak with inadequate loudness or with a louder voice than the occasion demands reflect either their own personalities or the personalities of the adults with whom they identify. Only in the rarest instances is there an organic basis for either a weak or an overloud
voice. The comparatively rare organic causes include hearing loss,
weakness of the muscles of the larynx, and weakness of the muscles
involved in respiration. Furthermore, it is extremely unlikely that
the carrying power of the voice is significantly related to the individual's breath capacity or the manner of breathing while speaking.
As Van Riper and Irwin (1958, p. 258) emphasize, "So long as sufficient air pressure is engendered below the vocal folds, it does not
matter how it is created, at least so far as adequate loudness is concerned. But we must have a greater air pressure to have louder
speech." In the absence of organic pathology, the will to be heard
is sufficient to supply the energy to provide for the necessary pressure below the vocal folds so that they are closed firmly, held together firmly for an appropriate length of time, and then blown
apart from their occluded (approximated) position to produce a
vocal tone that is loud enough to be easily heard.

Occasionally we find chilren who, because of poor posture, or
from anxiety, get in the way of their own efforts to breathe effectively for speech. A child with a "caved-in" abdominal area may not
be able to breathe comfortably and deeply enough for purposes of
speech. Obviously, the slump and the associated cave-in need to be
corrected. Similarly, any other postural defect that interferes with
adequate air intake and easy control of breath output needs to be
corrected. Such correction might well be directed to emphasizing
the need for the abdominal area to be relaxed and to "push out" in
inhalation and to contract and "pull in" gradually in controlled exhalation.

Another fault found in some children is the attempt to vocalize
and speak during inhalation. This fault, in the absence of neuropathology, is usually a result of an anxious effort to continue talking
when the child's breath supply has been expended. The creation of
awareness of what the child is doing can be established by directing him/her to do intentionally what he/she is doing unconsciously. Such a child is also likely to gain from breathing exercises
that emphasize abdominal control of outgoing breath.

The Overloud Voice

Aside from the possibility of a hearing loss that prevents proper
monitoring of the voice as it is being produced, the overloud voice
is likely to be a product of imitation or an aspect of the personality

of the speaker. Our experience as clinicians suggests that most children who speak too loudly are either imitating their parents or competing with their siblings for attention from their parents. Some parents, who complained to us about their children's loud voices, presented their complaints in our offices in voices that were loud enough to reach the last row of a 40-row auditorium without electrical amplification.

Children who identify with loud-speaking persons, their parents included, speak more loudly than do children who identify with persons who speak with adequate loudness. The overloud voice, especially if it is accompanied by rapid speech production, suggests excitement, anger, or aggressiveness.

Sensorineural hearing loss is associated with an overloud voice. Such impairment makes it necessary for the speaker to vocalize loudly in order to hear and monitor voice. Occasionally, we find a child with normal hearing who speaks in a way to suggest nerve hearing impairment. Investigation, however, may reveal that the child may have been brought up in a noisy environment, or in competition with siblings who were habitual shouters. The child then may have developed a loud voice in order to be heard and share the attention of the parents. These vocal habits may carry over to relatively quiet noncompetitive situations.

The Weak Voice

In the absence of organic involvement, we may assume that a weak voice is a reflection either of a timid personality or of the reaction of the individual to a given speaking situation. Most children who are unsure of themselves, or of what they have to say, tend to talk with a weak voice. The voice, regardless of the particular speech content, is also saying "Maybe if I don't talk loudly I won't be noticed, or what I have to say won't be heard, and I will be left alone." Occasionally, however, the weak voice may be the result of imitation, and the inadequate loudness has become habitual. The reproduction of such a voice on a playback is a necessary first step in the modification of this manner of voice production.

A possible organic cause of weak voice is the existence of a conductive hearing loss. Persons with conductive loss, in contrast to those with sensory-neural loss, tend to perceive themselves as speaking more loudly than do their listeners. In general, we recommend that any child whose voice is either inappropriately loud or inadequate as to loudness be checked for possible hearing impairment. There may be some value, too, for the parents to have a similar evaluation.

Treatment for Inappropriate Loudness

Except for children whose hearing difficulty impairs their ability to monitor their voices, or who have some other organic basis for their weak or overloud voice, an adequately loud voice should be attainable for all children. Treatment should include the following aspects:

1. An assessment of the voices of the members of the family and other key persons in the child's environment.
2. An evaluation of the personality and adjustment factors that may be associated with the child's manner of vocalization.
3. An evaluation of the specific situations (for example, the child's voice in the classroom compared with the voice in play activity) that may be associated with inadequate voice.
4. An evaluation of the overall characteristics of the child's voice, in addition to the degree of loudness.
5. An objectification of the voice through recording and playback so that the child may hear himself/herself approximately as others hear him/her.

In many instances, children who have been brought to our clinic for their voice problems have been treated through their parents. We have permitted parents to hear their recorded voices and invited them to accept treatment—*in the interest of their child.* Sometimes we accepted the child for treatment only if the parent or parents accepted concurrent voice therapy. Occasionally, we have encouraged parents to subdue a sibling just enough to give the child concerned a fair chance in the vocal competition. Sometimes, we have had to advise counseling for the parents while the child, *after medical clearance,* was undergoing symptom treatment.

In instances where we felt that an adjustment problem was basic to the voice difficulty, we have recommended treatment by a qualified psychotherapist. Whenever possible, we prefer that the choice of a psychotherapist be made with the help of the family physician. Occasionally, we have found that a child's voice problem was limited to the classroom. For reasons that developed out of the relationship between a child and a teacher—and sometimes it is a previous rather than a present teacher—the child had become anxiously concerned about his/her adequacy as a student. Obviously, in such instances, treatment should be directed at the improvement of the child-to-school relationship rather than to the vocal symptoms.

When, after investigation, we are convinced that there is nothing organically or emotionally wrong with the child who is speaking either not loudly enough or too loudly, direct treatment of the symptoms is in order. As suggested earlier, an overall evaluation of the vocal characteristics of the child is then undertaken. Our experience suggests that the weak voice is often also a breathy voice, and one likely to be too low in pitch. Often, but not always, we find that the loud voice is likely to be too high in pitch. The first order of the procedure for correcting the degree of loudness is to determine the child's normal pitch range and the optimum pitch. When these are determined (see pp. 350–351), the speech/language clinician should help the child to become aware of them, to initiate voice habitually at or close to optimum pitch, and to vocalize within the optimum pitch range. Breathiness, if it is found to be present, should be treated by procedures indicated in the section on breathiness.

Ordinarily, after following the procedures outlined and after the child has been made aware of the loudness level of his/her voice through playback, adequate loudness is attained. Occasionally, however, old habits are maintained and the child's voice, though appropriate in pitch and not characterized by breathiness, is still not appropriate in loudness. If it continues to be weak, procedures such as the following should be productive of improvement.

1. Record successively the voice of the weak-voiced child and a peer with adequate voice. Have the child make the comparisons and make new recording of the voices until both clinician and child are satisfied with the results.
2. If available, employ visual feedback apparatus so that the child may see when his/her voice is at the proper level. Most tape recorders and many cassette recorders are equipped with "magic eyes" (volume meters) that may be employed for this purpose. An oscilloscope may serve both to impress the child and to provide a basis for visual monitoring. A simpler and more readily available apparatus, though perhaps not quite so impressive, is the raised hand and approving look of the teacher or clinician when the child's voice at a proper level and the lowered (thumb-down) hand and disappointed (but *not* disapproving) look when the voice level is not loud enough.
3. Emphasis on clarity of articulation with lengthening of the vowels and nasal consonants is often of considerable help. By emphasizing clarity of articulation, the child is likely to use greater energy not only for articulatory activity but also for the accompanying respiratory behavior while speaking. The result is a reflexive increase in air pressure below the vocal folds, and a louder voice.
4. The game of *competitive speaking* or "Who can talk loudest in the group without shouting?" may be employed as motivation and play. It may be of help if some of the competitors are encouraged at

the beginning of the game to give the weak-voiced participant a chance to be heard. Later on, the erstwhile weak-voiced member should be permitted free and open competition.

5. The need for the child to adjust his/her voice level to the listener in terms of distance between listener and speaker may need emphasis. A teacher may bring about such an adjustment by asking a child a question when standing close to the child and then intentionally moving away from the youngster. Another technique is to have the child stand at the front of the room and speak just loud enough to be heard by the classmates in the first third of the room, then in the second third as well, and finally throughout the room. This procedure impresses the child with the need to change voice level according to the number of listeners and the distance between himself/herself and the farthest listener.

6. Pretended situations, such as announcing the arrival of a train or plane, giving orders to a military group, or speaking in a crowded and noisy place (a train station or an airport waiting room), can also be useful to help the child to be heard under difficult situations. Artificially competitive noise situations, such as speaking against a masking noise or buzzing noise, may also be used. If these techniques are employed, *care must be exercised that the optimum pitch range is maintained.* We would not want a child to speak loudly at the risk of acquiring vocal nodules.

The Strident, Harsh Voice

In sharp contrast with the weak voice is the one that is harsh and strident. Van Riper (1978, p. 244) characterizes the strident, harsh vocalizers as "so rasping and piercing that they repel listeners." Boone (1977, p. 185) describes the strident voice as "unpleasant, shrill, metallic-sounding." Stridency appears to be related to excessive tension of the muscles of the pharynx and larynx. Almost always the strident voice is both high in pitch and excessively loud. It is the voice we associate with the carnival "barker" who must be heard over the noise of the crowd.

Initial therapy involves creating awareness and motivation to change. The strident vocalizer needs to be faced with the question "Do you want to be heard, no matter the cost?" The cost includes being considered excessively aggressive, repelling listeners after you first attract them, and the real possibility of developing vocal nodules.

Specific vocal therapy includes:

1. Establishing optimal pitch and optimum pitch range.
2. Appropriate breathing (usually avoiding clavicular breathing).

3. Vocalizing with a relaxed throat and mouth "wide open" but not so wide as to distort articulation.
4. General bodily relaxation if pharyngeal relaxation alone is not possible. (This is recommended in any event as good for anybody, and particularly for the strident vocalizer.)
5. Occasional negative practice with the vocal result played back to be certain that the client does not forget how he/she sounds and feels when voice is produced stridently.

REVIEW OF PRINCIPLES FOR CORRECTING VOICE DEFECTS

1. *Medical clearance is a must* for any child who presents a voice problem and for whom vocal therapy is contemplated. A child who develops a vocal disturbance should be examined by a physician and, if at all possible, by a throat specialist for the detection and treatment of possible physical pathology before consideration is given to voice training.
2. When a child's vocal defects seem to be associated with personality disturbances, referral to a competent counselor or psychotherapist is in order. It should not be overlooked, however, that poor vocal habits may persist after the initial cause is no longer present. This principle holds true for vocal defects of both physical and psychological origin.
3. Often vocal defects are temporary and of short duration and call for patience and understanding rather than active treatment.
4. A voice is a product of the mechanism that produces it. The mechanism belongs to the individual, and the product should be consistent with its features. Neither the professional speech clinician nor the teacher, nor any other person who may influence the child, has a right to decide what kind of voice the child should have. Fundamentally, this decision was made by the way the child was physically endowed. The object of vocal therapy is to help the child to make the best possible use of his/her vocal endowment.
5. The classroom teacher, especially if he/she is respected and liked, has a personal responsibility that his/her own voice be free of undesirable traits that the children may imitate.
6. Vocal habits, both good and bad, tend to persist. Considerable motivation is necessary to help a child to wish to change a defective voice and to maintain vigilance that the improvements are maintained.
7. The child with a vocal defect should be helped to become aware of his/her voice as it is produced. The child needs to be aware of how

his/her voice sounds *and* feels when it is at its best as well as its worst. Objective attitudes and objective listening to one's own voice and comparing one's own voice with others by listening to "on-the-spot" recordings are of help.

8. Often a "negative" approach is helpful. By creating awareness of the nature of the undesirable vocal traits and how they are produced, voluntary control may be established. Thus, a child, by intentionally *doing what is wrong,* learns to know what he/she is doing, and so becomes conscious of what should not be done. By contrast, awareness must be created of the right way to produce voice and to replace the undesirable characteristic with a desirable one. *Negative practice must be replaced by positive practice at the earliest possible time.*

9. Both the classroom and the home situation should be studied for evidence of an atmosphere of undue tension. However, normal enthusiasm and excitement should not be confused with tension. Continued competition for the right to be heard may result in tension and consequent vocal penalties.

Problems

1. Review the section on the vocal mechanism. From the viewpoint of the production and reinforcement of sound, what musical instrument is most directly comparable to the voice mechanism?
2. Good vocalization is the product of *periodic vibration.* What does this term mean? What kind of human sounds are *complex and aperiodic?* You may consult Curtis (1978, pp. 29–31) for your answer.
3. What are the characteristics of a normal, effective voice?
4. What is the most frequent physical cause of defective voice?
5. Why is puberty often a period of frequent voice disturbance? Why are males more likely to be affected than females?
6. What is the role of identification in the formation of vocal habits?
7. What is nasality? How do you distinguish this characteristic from denasality? How would you check for each?
8. Why is it important that every child who may be considered for voice therapy first be given medical clearance?
9. What is optimum pitch? How would you determine this for a child? Are you vocalizing within your optimal pitch range?
10. What is the evidence that breathing faults are a cause of vocal disturbance?
11. What is negative practice? Describe how the technique of negative practice may be applied to changing an undesirable vocal habit.
12. Read Moore (1971) on environmental factors and voice disturbances. Are there any factors in your home environment conducive to vocal problems?
13. What is the danger of high-pitched screaming in young children?

14. What are two indications of personality disturbances discussed by Murphy (1964)?
15. What are cultural pressures that might be conducive to voice disorders in adolescents?
16. Describe the strident voice. Have you ever resorted to "stridency" in order to be heard? What were the effects?
17. Boone (1977, p. 19) says: "In the strictest sense, denasality could be considered as an articulatory substitution disorder." What are Boone's arguments for this position? Do you agree with him?
18. Blonigen (*Language, Speech and Hearing Services in the Schools,* 9 (1978), pp. 142–150) describes a program for the management of vocal hoarseness caused by vocal abuse. What is the nature of the abuse? What are the roles of the clinician and the classroom teacher in the treatment of the child? What are the main features of the program? Compare these features with those recommended in our text.

References and Suggested Readings

Bloodstein, O., *Speech Pathology: An Introduction.* Boston: Houghton Mifflin Company, 1979, Chap. 5. (Includes a discussion of the nature of sound, the respiratory mechanism, and the most prevalent types of voice disorders; well-drawn diagrams clarify the exposition.)

Boone, D., *The Voice and Voice Therapy* 2nd ed., Englewood Cliffs, N.J.: Prentice-Hall, Inc., 1977. (A clinical approach to the treatment of common voice problems. Practical and clearly written.)

Brodnitz, F. S., *Keep Your Voice Healthy.* New York: Harper & Row, Publishers, Inc., 1953. (A physician offers suggestions as to how to have a good and "healthy" voice.)

Cooper, M., "Spectographic Analysis of Fundamental Frequency and Hoarseness Before and After Vocal Rehabilitation." *Journal of Speech and Hearing Disorders,* **39** (1974), 286–297.

Curtis, J. F., in W. Johnson et al., *Speech-Handicapped School Children.* New York: Harper & Row, Publishers, Inc., 1967, chap. 4.

Curtis, J. F. and H. L. Morris. In J. F. Curtis, Ed., *Processes and Disorders of Human Communication.* New York: Harper & Row, Publishers, Inc., 1978, Chap. 6.

Eisenson, J., *Voice and Diction: A Program for Improvement,* 4th ed. New York: Macmillan Publishing Co., Inc., 1979 (Chaps. 3–9 are concerned with voice. Contains a considerable amount of practice materials.)

Greene, M. C. L., *The Voice and Its Disorders,* 2nd ed. Philadelphia: J. B. Lippincott Co., 1964. (An authoritative presentation for the treatment of voice problems by a practicing clinician.)

Hull, F. M. and R. J. Timmons, "The National Speech and Hearing Survey, Preliminary Results." *ASHA,* **13** (1971), 501–509.

Moore, P., *Organic Voice Disorders.* Englewood Cliffs, N.J.: Prentice-Hall,

Inc., 1971. (Includes brief but clear and authoritative information on the vocal mechanism.)

Moses, P. J., *The Voice of Neurosis*. New York: Grune and Stratton, Inc., 1954. (A psychiatrist and otolaryngologist describes his approaches to persons with voice problems. Despite the publishing date, still an up-to-date book.)

Murphy, A. T., *Functional Voice Disorders*. Englewood Cliffs, N.J.: Prentice-Hall, Inc., 1964. (A clear introductory consideration of personality disturbances and voice disorders.)

Perkins, W. H., *Speech Pathology* 2nd ed. St. Louis: The C. V. Mosby Co., 1977.

Philips, B. J., "Disorders of Voice." In R. J. Van Hattum, Ed., *Communication Disorders*. New York; Macmillan Publishing Co., Inc., 1980, Chap. 6.

Schneiderman, N., "An Investigation of Selected Factors Affecting the Judgment of Pitch Placement of Defective Voices," Unpublished doctoral dissertation, New York University, New York, 1959.

Silverman, E. M., and C. H. Zimmer, "Incidence of Chronic Hoarseness among School-Age Children." *Journal of Speech and Hearing Disorders*, **40** (1975), 211–215.

Van Riper, C., *Speech Correction*, 6th ed. Englewood Cliffs, N.J.: Prentice-Hall, Inc., 1978, Chap. 7.

——, and J. V. Irwin, *Voice and Articulation*. Englewood Cliffs, N.J.: Prentice-Hall Inc., 1958.

Wilson, D. K., "Children with Vocal Nodules." *Journal of Speech and Hearing Disorders*, **26** (1961), 19–25.

Zemlin, W. R., *Speech and Hearing Science*, Englewood Cliffs, N.J.: Prentice-Hall, Inc., 1968.

13

Stuttering

GENERAL OBSERVATIONS

Stuttering, a term we shall use as synonymous with *stammering*, occurs in about 1 per cent of school-age children. Leske (1981, pp. 217–225) reports both higher and lower prevalences depending upon the period of the survey, the criteria used to identify stuttering, and the ages of the children involved in the sample. If transitory stuttering, or more likely, abnormally high incidences of disfluency are included, the prevalence may be as high as 2 per cent. If adults are included in the sample, the reported prevalence drops to .5 per cent. The National Speech and Hearing Survey (Hull and Timmons, 1971) found a prevalence of .8 per cent. This percentage was based on a survey of 38,802 pupils in grades 1 to 12. The sex ratio in this report was 3 to 1, male to female (1.2 per cent for boys and .4 per cent for girls). Other reports indicate a ratio of 4 to 1, male to female in children and 8 to 1 in adults (Andrews and Harris, 1964).

If we accept the prevalence to be about 1 per cent among children of school age, it is likely that almost every classroom teacher and certainly every speech/language clinician with more than a year or two of experience has had some dealings with a child who at one time was identified as a stutterer. These and other professional persons concerned with stutterers may have shared their perplexities as well as their attitudes about the children and their aberrant speech. They may have exchanged observations and opinions about a form of behavior that varied considerably in amount and degree of severity. They well

369

may have expressed bewilderment about the comparative ease and fluency some stutterers have for brief or long periods of time, and about their sudden relapses. Those who have made private and comparative observations may have noted that fewer adults stutter than do children, but that almost all adults who stutter began doing so when they were children and almost always before adolescence. They may also have noted that relatively few elderly adults stutter. All of these observations, and some others mentioned later, have been made by professional investigators. They too, continue to be perplexed about stutterers and stuttering, even though they have strong opinions, if not theories, about the problem.

Much about stuttering is still to be learned. If we cease to regard stutterers as a total and "homogeneous" population, we will begin to learn considerably more in the near future than in the hundreds of years that we have spent in speculations, critical observations, and even carefully designed investigations. For the moment, however, we present several observations that have withstood the test of time about persons whose speech is characterized by rhythm and fluency that are different from those of most other speakers, who repeat and hesitate, and who prolong sounds, or block on sounds, more than most of us do in our talking.

Tentatively, we define stuttering as abnormally self-interrupted speech flow or utterance characterized by word "fragmentation," excessive sound repetitions and/or prolongations (blockings maintenance of articulatory positions), and "struggle" reactions. Covertly the speaker usually experiences anxiety or apprehension about speaking. This definition follows closely that of Van Riper (1978, p. 257). However, we are aware that stuttering is otherwise defined by different theorists. For a review of such definitions and theoretical positions, the reader may consult Van Riper (1971, Chaps. 2 and 11–15).

Accepted Observations About Stutterers

1. As already indicated, there are more stutterers among boys than among girls. Research on the prevalence of stuttering show ratios of from two to eight males to one female, depending upon place and age range included in the sample. Probably an average ratio is three to four males to one female.
2. The severity of stuttering tends to be greater among boys than among girls. We are, of course, talking about individuals. We have, in fact, known many severe female stutterers, but not nearly so many—even considering the ratio difference for the incidence of stutterting—as males.

3. Stuttering tends to be more persistent, to endure for more years, for boys than for girls. This explains the ratio difference noted in our first observation.

4. No stutterer, regardless of the severity of difficulty, stutters at all times. Almost all stutterers have times when their speech is relatively, if not completely, free of significant hesitancies, blocks, repetitions, or prolongations. In group-speaking situations, and in singing, stutterers are likely to do about as well as other children. Similarly, situations that require no on-the-spot formulation or hold little or no communicative responsibility are likely to be relatively easy for most stutterers.

5. Stuttering is more likely to begin in the nursery, kindergarten, and primary grades than in the secondary grades. It is comparatively rare for a child to begin stuttering after age 12. Andrews and Harris (1964, p. 186) report that 50 per cent of the children in their survey were stuttering (stammering) by age five, and 95 per cent were doing so by age seven. "Onset after the age of ten is rare." Van Riper (1971, p. 64), based on a review of the literature of several countries, also concludes that "the overwhelming consensus is that most stuttering begins in the preschool years."

6. Many young children in the kindergarten and first grade seem to have been on the verge of stuttering without becoming stutterers. They were hesitant and repetitious, but apparently had no awareness of their manner of speaking. By the time these children reached the age of eight or nine, their speech seemed to be "normal" again.

These observations are among the relatively few generalizations or "facts" accepted by students of stuttering. Beyond these, there is considerable difference in opinion as to the cause of stuttering and the choice of treatment. We do not attempt to resolve these differences. Instead, we present several of the more prevalent points of view, and suggest what the classroom teacher can safely do about children who are considered stutterers. We also suggest therapeutic approaches that are widely used with some success by speech clinicians in and out of school settings.

THE NATURE OF STUTTERING: STUTTERING AND FLUENCY

Communicative, informative speech is the product of a creative, planned utterance that is specific to the situation. The less informative the content, the more the content can be "retrieved" from memory with little or no revision with respect to a given situation, the more fluent or free-flowing the utterance is likely to be. Relatively free-flowing utterances include the reproduction of memorized material, counting, reciting the days of the week or the months of the year, swearing (providing there is no inhibition in this regard), singing, and reading or reciting in chorus. In contrast, whenever linguistic content has to be organized for a truly communicative-informative effort or interchange that is not charged with emotion, the utterance is likely to be less fluent. In other words, when we have to think of what as well as how we are to say whatever it is we are about to say, and whenever we have to say what we think with due awareness of the listener and the over-all speaking situation, we are less fluent and should expect ourselves and others to be.

Some of us are more linguistically facile and fluent than others. Nevertheless, for each of us there is a continuum of fluency that is generally predictable. As we will note later, the linguistic situations that are easiest and most fluent for nonstutterers are also usually easiest for stutterers; those situations likely to be associated with some degree of disfluency for nonstutterers are associated with a greater amount of disfluency *and* stuttering for those of us who are inclined to be stutterers.

Van Riper (1978, p. 257) states with certainty:

> "The essence of stuttering lies in its disruption of fluency. *Stuttering occurs when the forward flow of speech is interrupted by repetitions or prolongations of a sound, syllable, or articulatory posture, or by avoidance and struggle behaviors.*"

To support this assertion Van Riper argues:

> "The research shows rather conclusively that stutterers have more syllable repetitions and sound prolongations than normal speakers. They have more syllable repetitions per hundred words, and they have more of them per word."

We are inclined to accept Van Riper's view of the stutterer in regard to kinds and incidences of disfluency. However, a different point of view is provided by Williams (1978) who believes that differences in fluency do not distinguish stutterers from nonstutterers and so holds that ". . . a definition based on fluency can only be a partial definition, and one that may be extremely ambiguous when applied" (1978, p. 177). We should note, however, that Van Riper emphasizes *kinds of disfluencies* and that we emphasize situational differences that are associated with variations in fluency.

THE DEVELOPMENT OF STUTTERING

Do children demonstrate typical histories, characteristics, or stages in their acquisition of oral language that permit us to predict who is most likely to become a stutterer, or for whom excessive disfluencies and/or early stuttering may be transitory? Retrospective research does suggest some tendencies for populations of children, but also indicates that there is considerable variation for individuals in the population studied. Some children who have a history of excessive disfluency and evidence of struggle behaviors do spontaneously improve and cease to stutter. Others with a similar history resume stuttering for a period of time, sometimes associated with stressful experiences, and then become essentially normal speakers. But a few continue to stutter after an early onset, or after a few transitory episodes, and become "confirmed" stutterers into their adolescent and adult years. Children may go from "hard" symptoms at outset to "soft" symptoms to no symptoms and others appear to reverse the process. Many will have no memory, unless their parents remind them, that they were ever so disfluent as to be regarded as stutterers. Perhaps the only conclusion we can come to now— and it is still a tentative conclusion—is that the longer stuttering-like behavior persists from early childhood into the preadolescent and adolescent years, the more likely the individual is to become a confirmed stutterer. The confirmation will come from members of the stutterers' environments and from the stutterers themselves. What is confirmed is that the individual identified as a stutterer has difficulty in speaking and usually exhibits some or most of the speech behavior included in our definition of stuttering.

If there are no reliable developmental stages, are there any patterns that occur with sufficient frequency to permit prognosticating about stutterers and their stutterings? At least two respected authorities believe the answer to be "yes" though they are not in complete agreement as to the symptoms and patterns, and whether there is a developmental chronology. We review the positions of Bloodstein and Van Riper as to their respective concepts of "Phases of stuttering" and "tracks of stuttering."

Three Descriptions

Bloodstein's Phases of Development
Bloodstein (1975b, pp. 57–84) describes four phases of stuttering, as well as therapeutic approaches for individuals in each of the phases. However, Bloodstein acknowledges that there is considerable overlap in the phases and that some stutterers move back and forth from one

phase to another. A few stutterers seem to fit nowhere, moving from one phase to another, and occasionally defying stable description or characterization.

PHASE 1. Age range: usually from two to six years. The child's difficulty is usually episodic, with repetitions being the chief characteristic. Prolongations, forcings, and hard contacts and various associated symptoms ordinarily found among advanced stutterers may also be present. Many of the repetitions occur at the beginning of sentences or other identifiable syntactic units (phrases or clauses). An unusual feature is the tendency to stutter on function words and pronouns.

In general, Bloodstein (p. 57) observes that Phase 1 stutterers appear to do what children might be expected to do if they were fragmenting whole syntactic structures rather than individual words.

Bloodstein notes that children in Phase 1 do not avoid speaking and usually do not show any special awareness or concern about their speech. Some, however, do on occasion show that they are frustrated when blocked in speech and may even ask "Why can't I talk?" Fortunately, the questions do not deter them in their efforts as speakers. Beyond the questions, "They give little evidence of having formed any distinct self-concepts as stutterers or defective speakers" (p. 57). Bloodstein believes that children in Phase 1 of stuttering are essentially indistinguishable from almost all other children from whom episodes of increased disfluency are transient early childhood phenomena.

The main goal of therapy for the Phase 1 stutterer is the prevention of more advanced forms of stuttering. Basically, this dictates that "We must at all costs prevent the child from developing a self-concept as a defective speaker" (p. 58). Counseling of parents is, therefore, the major therapeutic approach.

PHASE 2. Age range: mostly children in elementary school years, but may include adults.

The speaker's difficulty has become fairly chronic though varying in degree of severity. Fragmenting of words rather than of syntactic structures becomes characteristic of the interrupted utterances. Fragmentation and repetition are distributed throughout the sentence or phrase (unit of meaning) rather than occurring on the first word of the unit.

Interestingly, even though the children who are identified as Phase 2 stutterers regard themselves as defective speakers, they do not appear to avoid speaking situations. Bloodstein observes that these children are easy to treat. Moreover, the evidence indicates that "throughout the age range at which Phase 2 stuttering is most prevalent, children recover from stuttering at a very high rate spontaneously." Bloodstein also observes that therapeutically "almost anything works."

From the point of view of therapy, since "almost anything works" the less done the better. Bloodstein suggests that it is important to avoid directing attention to symptoms that might produce anxiety. On the positive side, Phase 2 stutterers should be helped to develop feelings of self-worth. Along this line, parent counseling and teacher cooperation are important.

PHASE 3. Age range: from about eight years to adulthood; highest incidence during adolescence.

The speaking problems reported by the stutterers begin to be anticipated according to situations identified as difficult. Such situations include talking to strangers and reciting in school, and generally where and when communicative responsibility is involved. Some words and some sounds may be regarded as difficult and approached with anticipation of stuttering. Devices such as word substitutions and circumlocutions may be used to avoid the "bogey" words. Except that stutterers give little or no indication of avoiding involvement in speaking situations, they begin to manifest the speech behavior characteristics of Phase 4 (the confirmed, "chronic" adult stutterer). Bloodstein (p. 67) observes that "In the school environment we soon recognize the Phase 3 stutterer as the familiar boy or girl who seems to have an advanced form of stuttering problem, yet continually volunteers to recite in class and may be communicative and gregarious, even to the point of being 'popular'."

Bloodstein recommends that emphasis in therapy for the Phase 3 stutterers should be on symptom modification and general speech improvement. Because Phase 3 stutterers appear to be free of anxiety about speaking, Bloodstein considers it at best a waste of time to become involved with anxieties and apprehensions that these stutterers, most of whom are adolescents, fortunately do not have. If they were apprehensive and anxious about speaking and about themselves as speakers because of their stuttering manifestations, they would be Phase 4 stutterers.

PHASE 4. Age range: approximately ten years to adulthood; mostly adolescence to adulthood.

Phase 4 stutterers are chronic and confirmed about their difficulties. Their speech shows the characteristics of disfluency, blocking, repetition, self-interruption, and the like incorporated in our definition of stuttering. They are anxious and apprehensive about speaking. They have feared sounds, feared words, and feared situations, and employ strategies, usually not effective, to deal with their speech fears.

Therapy for Phase 4 stutterers is directed to reducing anxiety about their stuttering and to a modification of stuttering behavior.

Van Riper's Observations

Van Riper is aware that there is considerable individual variation as to the course of stuttering. Nevertheless he observes that the majority of persons who become chronic or "confirmed" stutterers follow a sequence that begins between ages two and four. The sequence usually begins with: (1) initial, effortless, syllabic repetitions and sound prolongations. These become (2) associated with tension, forcings, and struggle that are followed by (3) the development of interrupter or avoidance reactions. Paralleling these overt developments, we find (4) a change from unawareness to surprise, to frustration, and finally to fear and shame. (Van Riper, 1978, p. 261).

Van Riper notes that not all beginning stutterers show this developmental pattern or sequence of morbid development. In common with other investigators, he shares the observation that four out of five children who exhibit early signs of stuttering or who actually began to stutter are able to attain normally fluent speech "with or without therapy." However, though many stutterers attain and maintain normal speech, others, all too many, do not. "They get caught in the whirlpool of self-reinforcement, the disorder becomes self-perpetuating." So. Van Riper recommends "Our most important job . . . is to prevent this morbid growth of the disorder, to keep it in its early stages, to prevent the struggle and avoidance that are the result of communicative frustration and social rejection." (Ibid., p. 261).

Despite the frequency of spontaneous recovery in young stutterers, Van Riper recommends early intervention. He reports a high incidence of success if clinical intervention begins early, especially if there is good cooperation with the parents. However, the older, confirmed stutterers present more complex and difficult problems because the emotions of fear, shame, and frustration become prevalent. Van Riper cautions: "It is important that . . . all who work with stutterers understand the role played by these negative emotions."

We cannot argue this position with Van Riper. Neither can we confirm that these negative emotions "come to be ever present." Most studies of the attitudes, adjustments, and personality traits of stutterers lead to a more moderate conclusion summed up by Bloodstein (1979, p. 130) that ". . . there is little evidence of any specific character or personality traits that stutterers tend to have in common. . . .

Most stutterers score within the normal range on tests of personality adjustment."

Perhaps the difference between Van Riper's position and that of Bloodstein is that tests and inventories that purport to measure personality traits and adjustments do not tap the involvements of stutterers. Perhaps in formal testing situations stutterers have become "test wise" and so do not reveal their maladjustments. Some stutterers may develop a "benign indifference" to their stuttering. Whether this attitude represents a problem or a solution may in itself present a problem.

Brutten and Shoemaker's Stages in the Disintegration of Speech

One way of looking at Bloodstein's phases of stuttering and Van Riper's "tracks" of stuttering is to see the problem developing as an aspect of difficulty in speech acquisition in children. This position, which happens to be consistent with our own bias and perception, views the stuttering as an inadequacy in the early organization of speech—especially where syntax and appropriate creative communicative messages need to be formulated and expressed to one or more listeners. Brutten and Shoemaker (1967, pp. 31–35) take what may appear to be an opposite position. They postulate three stages in the development of stuttering based on conditioning. Stage 1 is characterized by predominantly fluent speech with occasional fluency failures that may be the result of adverse (noxious) conditions, but not the result of learning (conditioning). Stage 2 is characterized by an increase in fluency failures and qualitative modification "that are indicative of emotional conditioning." Stage 3 is characterized by "the development of conditioned negative emotional reactions to the act of speaking, the words employed, or the speech produced."

It may well be that speech disintegrates in individuals because initially it has not become well organized and well integrated. Thus, the highest incidence of stuttering is in young children. Adults who are identified as stutterers may never have had well-organized speech. Under stress, or under conditions that stutterers respond to adversely, a weakly organized function (oral language) may "disintegrate" and be expressed in the abnormalities of stuttering.

Common Developmental Factors

As indicated earlier, stages, phases, tracks or developmental sequences in stuttering represent the judgments of the individual who is concerned with stuttering and its development. We are able to observe considerable overlapping between positions. Perhaps what really matters is the answer to the questions: (1) "Does it really matter?" and (2) "If it does matter, what are the prognostic and therapeutic implications for the individual child?"

Our own view is that it does matter. Further, careful and long-term study of the "developmental" data may tell us whether and when therapeutic intervention is needed, and possibly what the emphasis of the therapy should be.

In reviewing the positions of Bloodstein, Van Riper, and Shoemaker and Brutten, several factors appear to us to be common:

1. Early disfluencies are in excess of normal in most children who are identified as stutterers.
2. There is a difference between children who repeat whole words and those who repeat sounds and syllables. (Children who do the latter are more likely to become stutterers.)
3. The presence of anxieties and fears about speaking differentiate children who are identified as stutterers. The nonanxious children may in fact be clutterers. (See the last section of this chapter for a discussion of cluttering.)
4. The individual histories of many stutterers reveal periods of remission ranging from days to years.
5. Many stutterers and most clutterers seem to have difficulty in the early organization of their language. Early disfluencies occur between ages two and four, a period when children normally begin to become aware of and use conventional syntax (grammar).

ASSOCIATED SPEECH AND LANGUAGE DEFICIENCIES

Our review of the overt speech and related behavior of stutterers suggests that though stutterers vary considerably in their individual backgrounds, there are common factors, which we enumerated. There are also several associated speech and language differences between most stutterers and most children who are not stutterers and yet not normal speakers. These differences include delayed onset of speech, persistence in so-called infantilisms in articulation (lisping, lalling, sound distortions, and substitutions). Perhaps most important from our point of view is the delay in syntactic proficiency found by both Bloodstein and Van Riper (cited previously) and by Wyatt (1969, pp. 105–106), who regards stuttering "as a disturbance in the learning of speech and language."

Andrews and Harris (1964, p. 191) are impressed with both the late onset of talking, the "poor" talking, and the familial background of stutterers (stammerers) as distinguishing factors. They say:

Late and poor talking and family history together effectively discriminate stammerers from nonstammerers, and as information about these
items may be available prior to the onset of stammering, one might well
identify the nonfluent preschool children who are 'at risk' of stammering.

LANGUAGE DELAY AND THE ONSET OF STUTTERING

We have made several references to the possible relationship between the onset of stuttering and delay in early language acquisition.
Along this line Bloodstein states: "Perhaps the only thing we have
learned about people who stutter that distinguishes them from nonstutterers is that as a group they are more likely to have an early history of delayed language development and . . . a functional articulation disorder of childhood." (Bloodstein, 1979, p. 106) However,
Bloodstein hastens to add "Even this characteristic is only a group
tendency, reliable as it appears to be. The majority of children seem to
develop speech at a normal rate." (Ibid.) From our point of view,
Bloodstein's observation suggests that there may be many causes of
stuttering, and perhaps many pathways or "tracks" to stuttering, with
improficiencies in early language one of the routes. We will review
briefly some evidence to support this assumption.

In his book *The Nature of Stuttering* (1971, p. 108) Van Riper reports that "What is distinctive is that the disorder appeared when they
began to talk consecutively. . . . The onset of stuttering came with
the onset of connected speech."

Language Organization, Normal Hesitation, and Disfluencies

Van Riper's observation, with which we concur, is compatible with
the results of several studies on language proficiency as well as with
investigations of normal hesitation phenomena in the speech of nonstutterers. In a series of studies Goldman-Eisler (1961) found that
many of the hesitations of normally fluent persons occurred at places
in their utterance that indicated *language planning* (how to continue
to say what needed to be said according to plan). McClay and Osgood
(1959) observed that hesitations often appear at points in the flow of
utterance (in effect, interruptions in the flow) of greatest uncertainty
relative to content and appropriate syntactic construction. These studies and others along a similar line are reviewed by Luper and Ford
(1980 pp. 265–269) in their discussion of "Stuttering as a Breakdown
of Speech-Production Processes."

Language Improficiencies in Young Stutterers

Emrick (1971) studied the language performance of three groups of kindergarten and first-grade children: stutterers, nonstutterers, and highly disfluent children who were not regarded as stutterers. Each group consisted of five kindergarten and five first-grade boys. The subjects were required to describe pictures and to respond to items in the 1966 edition of the Torrance Test of Creative Thinking. Emrick found that the stuttering and highly disfluent children obtained significantly lower vocabulary scores, made significantly more grammatical errors, and had more incorrect responses than did the typical nonstuttering children. Interestingly, Emrick found no significant differences between the children identified as stutterers and those who were regarded as highly disfluent.

Emrick found no differences between groups in the number of communication units used (CU's), the number of words per CU, and the use of auxiliaries, negative and interrogative constructions, and subordinate clauses. Emrick speculates that the pragmatic (situational) variables may account for more disfluencies than the surface structure of language.

In another doctoral study Pratt (1972) investigated 17 stutterers and a matched group of fluent children in the age range of 3.4–5.8 years. Pratt employed an experimental battery of eight linguistic tasks to measure aspects of receptive and expressive phonological, vocabulary, and syntactic skills and the "operation of three perceptual cognitive strategies." Pratt's findings indicated that:

1. The performance of the stutterers was significantly below that of the non-stutterers on almost all linguistic tasks. Exceptions included the mean length of response and the production correlates of the act-action-object perceptual cognitive strategy.
2. Older subjects performed better on expressive and receptive syntax and vocabulary tasks than did the younger subjects.
3. Both the production and perceptual aspects of tests that are concerned with vocabulary size, phonology, and syntax significantly differentiated the stutterers from the nonstutterers.
4. The speech of the nonstutterers contained a significantly greater number of sentences with multiple clauses than did the speech of the stutterers.

Muma (1971) analyzed language samples of thirteen highly disfluent four-year-old children and a matched group of fluent children. Muma found that the fluent group used a significantly greater number of double-based (complex) transformations that did the disfluent children. We should note, however, that the disfluent children were not identified as stutterers.

On the basis of these findings, which suggest trends if not conclusive evidence of differences between young stutterers and normally fluent children, and on the basis of additional evidence on a population of seven stutterers (age range 5.0 to 8.8 years) studied by Stemach as a pilot study employing language sampling, we present the following summary of our inferences:

1. Young stutterers are not significantly different from normally fluent children when the measures are mean length of utterance in "spontaneous" (really elicited) speech or in the number of communicative units per response.
2. Young stutterers do differ from peer age nonstutterers in regard to:
   a. Greater number of single-word responses.
   b. Simpler syntactic structures.
   c. Number of grammatical errors.
   d. Later onset of speech.
   e. Greater number of errors of articulation.

CONDITIONS ASSOCIATED WITH STUTTERING

We are aware that no stutterer, regardless of the severity of stuttering, stutters with each utterance. Even the most severe stutterers are often free of stuttering, and sometimes even free of anxiety that they may stutter. Parents of stutterers, teachers, and even the stutterers themselves may be aware that they can engage in choral activity without stuttering, that they can talk aloud to themselves with normal fluency, and that they can usually talk to pets or other animals without difficulty. Many stutterers can talk fluently while playing, especially if the talk is a nonsense level. Some stutterers can talk normally to younger persons, and a few can talk to a selected peer or even an adult without difficulty or with less than usual difficulty. Stuttering, then, may be regarded as a situational problem. We have suggested some situations conducive to relatively free-from-stuttering speech. Are there any general situations that are conductive to stuttering? A review of research suggests an affirmative answer.

Brown (1945), in several studies, found that stutterers tend to have verbal cues or indicators that are related to increased stuttering. These include initial words in sentences; longer words in sentences; more nouns, verbs, and adverbs than other parts of speech; and accented syllables within words.

Eisenson and Horowitz (1945) found that stutterers had increased difficulty with reading material as the intellectual significance of the material was increased.

Lanyon (1969), however, found that the likelihood of a stutterer having difficulty (stuttering) on any given word depends not on how much information the word conveys but on word length and how much speech (articulatory) production is required to say the word.

These and other studies that are available in the literature strongly suggest that two factors or situations are conducive to increased stuttering. These are (1) awareness that what is to be spoken has intellectual, informative content; and (2) awareness of communicative responsibility for the speech content. Conversely, we find that stutterers report that they are relatively free of what characterizes their stuttering when they feel no need to make a favorable impression on their listeners or when they do not feel individually responsible for their utterances. This is in line with the observations of teachers and clinicians who have observed stutterers in their periods or relative fluency and under conditions associated with virtually normal fluency.

Beyond these linguistic and environmental situations, which tend to be related to the incidence of stuttering, there are other factors that apparently influence speech control. Most stutterers have increased difficulty when they are fatigued. Stutterers tend to stutter more when they expect to stutter than when such expectancy does not exist. On an individual basis, some stutterers expect to stutter in special situations or with specific persons more than they do in other situations or with other persons. By and large, these expectancies tend to be confirmed by actual experience. Even when other speech and associated stuttering manifestations are not present, stutterers experience feelings of apprehension and anxiety because of their anticipation of stuttering. The result is that they respond to themselves as if they had stuttered even though the listener-observer may have seen no external evidence of stuttered speech.

The last point suggests an aspect of stuttering that is deserving of consideration. Although what the listener-observer hears and sees may be important in the evaluation of stuttering, much goes on within the stutterer that cannot be evaluated by anyone but the stutterer. How stutterers feel about themselves when they anticipate the need to speak is important. How much effort and anxiety do stutterers expect when they are successful in controlling their stuttering? Is it less rather than more than when they stutter? Do stutterers feel better when their speech seems to be normally fluent than when their speech is marked by an abnormal amount of hesitations, blocks, repetitions, prolongations, and any other type of behavior that accompanies or characterizes stuttering? How stutterers feel about their speaking is a subjective aspect of stuttering that may be of extreme importance to the individual stutterer. The overt characteristics affect the listener's responses to the stutterer. The covert feelings, unless directly translated into some form of readily observable behavior, are not likely to affect the responses of the listener. If we appreciate this, we can begin to understand why some adolescents and adults who seem to speak without any of the speech and associated mannerisms of stuttering nevertheless regard themselves as stutterers. They do so, we may conclude, because they feel like stutterers, even though they do not overtly behave like stutterers.

THEORETICAL POINTS OF VIEW AS TO THE CAUSES OF STUTTERING[1]

Theories as to why people stutter are numerous and diverse in their points of view. Many theories that were influential, if not dominating, have become reduced in importance, not because they have been disproved or discredited but because their proponents have ceased proposing them or have changed their minds. The attempt in this chapter is to present several current points of view. This is done with responsible awareness that we are not including many other points of view, which, in a larger or more specialized text, might well be mentioned. The points of view considered in this chapter may be broadly classified along the following lines:

1. Stuttering is a constitutional problem. There are physical reasons that predispose a person to stuttering or that make him/her a stutterer.
2. Stuttering is essentially a learned form of behavior that may happen to anyone.
3. Stuttering is a manifestation of an underlying personality disorder.

---

[1] C. Van Riper in *The Nature of Stuttering* (Englewood Cliffs, N.J.: Prentice-Hall, Inc., 1971) reviews several historical and current theories of stuttering. He also presents his own position on stuttering in his chapter "The Nature of Stuttering: An Attempted Synthesis."

J. Eisenson, *Stuttering: A Second Symposium* (New York: Harper & Row, Publishers, Inc., 1975) includes several theoretic positions on stuttering.

G. Jonas, *Stuttering: The Disorder of Many Theories* (New York: Farrar, Straus & Girous, Inc. 1977) presents several positions on the nature of stuttering and approaches to its "cure" and what he found to be effective for his own treatment.

Stuttering as a Constitutional Problem

The proponents of the theoretical position that there is a constitutional predisposition to stuttering point to research studies to support their stand. Some of the findings suggest that, as a group, stutterers' familial histories include the following incidents as occurring more often than in the population as a whole: (1) more stutterers; (2) more left-handedness; (3) more twins; (4) later onset of speech; and (5) higher incidence of illnesses and traumas that might cause damage to the nervous system. Support for this position comes from some of the older investigations of Berry (1939) and Nelson (1939) and later from the findings of the Andrews and Harris survey (1964, p. 101). The last report includes the presence of significant genetic and neurologic predisposing factors and a higher than usual incidence of birth traumas or evidence of subsequent brain injury. In addition, it reports findings of delayed onset of speech and a high incidence of speech and language problems other than stuttering, ". . . but by far the most important predisposing factor is the inheritance from either parent of the genetic predisposition to stammer."

Findings of studies by Curry and Gregory (1969) and Perrin (1969) have implications that suggest that stutterers may be different in their neurophysiological organization from nonstutterers. Both investigations employed a special perceptual-listening task (dichotic listening) to compare the responses of stutterers and nonstutterers. The dichotic listening task requires the listener to attend to two different auditory signals presented simultaneously, one to the left ear and one to the right. In essence, the ears of the subject are engaged in competitive listening. Earlier findings indicate an interesting difference in ear-reporting depending upon the nature of the auditory signal. Speech signals, such as digits or words, when presented dichotically are reported by most subjects as being received in the right ear. Nonspeech signals such as clicks, snatches of melody, and other nonspeech environmental noises are usually reported as being received in the left ear (Kimura, 1967, p. 20). The systematic differences between the ears in dichotic listening are interpreted as reflecting the functional differences between the two cerebral hemispheres, consistent with the fact that each ear has its greatest number of connections with the contralateral hemisphere. Findings have been fairly uniform that when the subject reports differences in perception of auditory signals, speech signals tend to be referred to the right ear (processed by the left and normally dominant hemisphere), whereas nonspeech signals are referred to the left ear (processed by the right or nondominant hemisphere). These findings occur only in binaural competitive (dichotic) listening tasks.

This, of course, is a laboratory technique and not the one that pertains to usual listening situations.

Curry and Gregory (1969) and Perrin (1969) found that stutterers did not make the referrals to the right ear for speech signals along the expected lines. Although there was some variation for individuals, the Curry and Gregory data indicate that taken as a group, "stutterers had smaller difference scores between ears on dichotic verbal scores than did nonstutterers. Seventy-five per cent of the nonstutterers obtained higher right-ear scores on the dichotic verbal task, whereas 55 per cent of the stutterers had higher left-ear scores." Perrin's findings confirmed those of Curry and Gregory.

Specifically, Perrin found that stutterers showed a clear left-ear preference for words and sentences in dichotic reception, whereas nonstutterers showed a right ear preference for such materials. As a group, the stutterers were not different from the nonstutterers in regard to their ear preference for vowels and for noises. As a general observation Perrin (1969) notes, "When a hemisphere exerts some control over speech function in the stutterer, it is the right, which is the reverse of that found in normals." We appreciate, of course, that ear preference is contralateral to cerebral control.

Sommers, Brady, and Moore (1975) compared groups of stuttering children and adults (age range four to 48) with nonstuttering controls on dichotic listening tasks. They found a trend for the stuttering children to show a lack of ear preference for words and digits presented dichotically as compared with nonstuttering children. Further, the study found considerably more left-ear preference by the stuttering children. An additional interesting finding was that the left ear preferences and no-ear preference decreased with the age of the children. In general, the nonstuttering children and adults performed alike on the dichotic tasks. However, right-ear dichotic scores were significantly smaller than those for adult stutterers. The investigators speculate that "the speech perceptual function and/or hemispheric lateralization of speech may continue to develop at a slower rate than in nonstutterers."

A dichotic listening study by Slorach and Noehr (1973) with a group of primary-grade children in Brisbane, Australia, showed varying lateralization among stutterers who were compared with children with defective articulation and another group considered to be normal in speech. The dichotic listening task consisted of pairs of three-digit series. All three groups showed a right-ear preference but some of the stutterers showed special patterns of lateralization at variance with the other children.

The trend of the findings using dichotic listening studies strongly suggests that stutterers as a total population differ from nonstutterers in their differential cerebral dominance for language. Discussions of cerebral dominance, as related to language functioning, that review techniques other than dichotic listening may be found in Eisenson (1975b, pp. 411–416) and Van Riper (1971, pp. 351–359). Our impression is that the findings tend to support the assumption that the cerebral organization of most stutterers for speech (language) control is different from that of nonstutterers.

Van Riper (1971, p. 404), although not certain as to the etiology of stuttering, nevertheless says:

> We should like to suggest that stuttering be considered a disorder of timing . . . when a person stutters on a word, there is a temporal disruption of the simultaneous and successive programming of muscular movements required to produce one of the word's integrated sounds or to emit one of its syllables appropriately . . . or to accomplish the precise linking of sounds and syllables that constitute its motor pattern. . . . When, for any reason, that timing is awry and askew, a temporarily distorted word is produced and when this happens, the speaker has evinced a core stuttering behavior.

In his chapter "The Nature of Stuttering: An Attempted Synthesis" (1971, 404–441), Van Riper reviews the literature that indicates why stutterers have defective timing behavior for speech, and when they can overcome the effects of this defect. Van Riper does not minimize the psychological factors that may maintain stuttering. However, we believe that the majority of the evidence presented by Van Riper supports a constitutional factor on the etiology of stuttering.

Andrews and Harris (1964, p. 191) suggest a psychobiological theory of stuttering along the following lines:

1. In some instances, a predisposition may be sufficient to initiate stammering (stuttering).
2. "Emotional stress at an age when adequate speech function is precarious may result in a disturbance of this balance of speech maturation and so produce a repetition of sounds and syllables characteristic of stammering. In a child with abnormal speech development, this period of vulnerability will be prolonged. If there is sufficient genetic and neurologic predisposition only minor anxieties will be sufficient, whereas if there is minimal predisposition a more severe emotional stress will be required to initiate stammering."
3. Once the involuntary repetitions of sounds and syllables have begun, the child soon learns to anticipate those words and situations that are difficult for him. "It is this anxiety about specific word

and situational cues, and its reduction as they are passed, that results in the development of both the severity and complexity of the stammer syndrome."

This position may explain why all children who may have a predisposing background do not necessarily become stutterers. If a child is fortunate and is free of severe illness and physical or psychological trauma during the developmental stages of speech, he/she may be reasonably "safe" from becoming a stutterer.

If however, conditions are less fortunate, and either illness or emotional disturbance upsets the child during the speech-development stage, stuttering is likely to result. In other words, constitutional factors provide a subsoil for stuttering. Stuttering itself is a product associated with both the subsoil and the specific environmental, physical, or psychological factors that tend to nurture it.

Recent support for a constitutional predisposition for stuttering comes from research on hereditary (genetic) factors associated with the prevalence of stuttering in family constellations. Kidd *et al.* (1973) found an incidence of more than 20 per cent stuttering in the fathers of male stutterers, more than 7 per cent in the mothers and more than 17 per cent among brothers as well as more than 7 per cent among sisters. If we compare these percentages with less than 1 per cent in the population as a whole, the figures are most persuasive. Similar findings are reported in later studies by Howie (1976) and Records *et al.* (1976).

Stuttering as a Form of Learned Behavior

The proponents of the point of view that stuttering is a form of learned behavior are, as we might expect, opposed to believing that stutterers as a group are significantly different constitutionally in any way from nonstutterers. Instead, children who stutter are considered to be essentially normal children in regard to heredity, physical development, health history, psychological traits, intelligence, or any other single factor in which the first group of theorists we discussed found important differences. Johnson (1967), who was a leading proponent of the "normality of the stutterer" school, held that stuttering is a *speech disturbance which can happen to anyone.* How stuttering has its onset and how it becomes established as a reaction to some but not all speaking situations are explained through principles of learning that apply to behavior in general as well as to stuttering in particular.

The early stages of stuttering are explained as resulting from a misevaluation of the disfluencies normal in young children. Young children of preschool age and in the early primary grades are inclined to be repetitious and hesitant when they talk as well as in other forms of behavior. Parents, teachers, or other adults who mistake these disfluencies for stuttering symptoms, and who show concern or anxiety about them, are likely to transmit this attitude to the child. When a child becomes aware of adult anxiety and permits it to affect him, he may approach a speaking situation with an attitude of apprehension. It is not the hesitation or repetition but the speaker's reactions to them and to the reactions of other persons to which he, in turn, reacts that make the child into a stutterer.

In another publication Johnson (1961, p. 138) explained that:

> The problem called stuttering begins, then, when the child's speech is felt, usually by the mother, to be not as smooth or as fluent as it ought to be. There seems as a rule to be a quality of puzzlement mixed with slight apprehension and dread about the mother's feelings. She uses the only name she knows for what she thinks must be the matter with her youngster's speech, and that word is "stuttering"—or, if she has grown up in England or certain other parts of the world, "stammering."
>
> . . . She may not be sure of herself at first in deciding that her child is stuttering, but her use of the word crystallizes her feelings and serves to focus her attention on the hesitations in the speech of her child.

Johnson emphasized that the mother's feelings and apprehensions tend to become apparent to the child and in time the child "takes from the mother the feelings she has about his speech."

Williams (1978, p. 183) continues to argue for Johnson's basic position. Says Williams: "A *problem of stuttering* may develop, depending upon the ways important listeners communicate both verbally and non-verbally their attitudes and feelings about the ways a child speaks specifically and their expectations about the child as a speaker more generally."

Eisenson (1966) "tested" Johnson's assumption that stuttering is a result of maternal reaction to the child's speech by investigating the incidence of the disorder among preschool and primary-grade children brought up in kibbutzim (communal organizations) in Israel. Children in these settings were cared for by nurse-teachers throughout the day. They saw their parents in the late afternoon and on some holidays. They slept, ate, were trained and taught in cottage facilities by the nurse-teachers. There was no conscious differences in the treatment of the children along sex lines. The incidence and sex distribution for the presence of stuttering in children brought up in kibbutzim were essentially the same as those found in the United States and those reported by Andrews and Harris in England. The total incidence was about 1 per cent, with a sex ratio of about four boys to one girl.

To return to Johnson's and Williams' position, stuttering may be considered a learned and specific anxiety reaction associated with speaking situations. But stuttering and its consequences seem to be unpleasant and apparently more penalizing than rewarding. Normally, behavior that persists is behavior somehow rewarded. Are there any rewards or pleasant aftereffects (reinforcers) in stuttering? There are, if we look for them. One of the possible reinforcers is the attention a child may receive that may not otherwise be available. Stutterers may learn to enjoy the intensity of reaction, and the disturbance they cause by their speech. If they need such reactions more than they do normal speech, stuttering is likely to persist. In the classroom stutterers may be excused from recitations or win sympathy that they may learn to enjoy. A stutterer may become a "special child" and be reluctant to give up that status. Until ready to do so, the child who began to stutter through no fault of his/her own is likely to continue to stutter. Unfortunately, when the penalties of stuttering begin to exceed the rewards, the habits and attitudes of the stutterer may persist and many stutterers need help in overcoming them. Many, however, seem able to stop without outside help. These children may have taken an accounting of the assets and liabilities associated with stuttering and reached a conclusion that became translated into self-modified behavior. Certainly, many experienced teachers know youngsters who stuttered in the early grades and who became normal speakers in later grades without any outside help.

For those stutterers who do not or cannot stop, a theoretical explanation for the continuance of stuttering can be made along these lines: Stutterers continue to fear that they will stutter in a given situation or on a given word. They become tense and apprehensive in anticipation of the situation or word. If, with great effort, they finally manage to speak despite the initial tension and anxiety, this brings about a momentary reduction in the anxiety-tension state. This brief period of relief may be sufficiently pleasurable to reinforce and to perpetuate not only the stuttering but also the entire attitude and pattern of behavior associated with it.

In a critical and provocative article Sander (1975) challenges most current theories of stutterering and attempts to set things right. Sander suggests that the problem of stuttering, or the problem related to stuttering, may arise from a subliminal anticipation of speech difficulties "of whatever sort." Sander considers the possibility that stuttering is or brings about a *protruding emotion*. He argues that "stuttering is a speaking disruption prompted by the expectancy of speech difficulty but not in itself a reinforced instrumental behavior." Sander characterizes the "moment" of stuttering as an expression of a breakdown in the speaking plan. "Plans for complete motor acts requiring the skilled patterning of movements may be disrupted or aborted by evaluations of impending difficulty" (p. 260). Sander believes that children who stutter may want to communicate but fear that they will be rejected. We assume that the fear is a consequence of a history of failures in communicating. What still needs to be explained is why the successful communicative efforts, presumably ones that occur more often than the failures if we use fluency periods as a measure, are overbalanced by the failures.

In *Stuttering: A Second Symposium* (Eisenson 1975, Ed.) essays by Brutten, Ingham, Shames, and Sheehan represent related but somewhat different views of how stuttering becomes a learned (conditioned) form of behavior. Therapeutic approaches that are compatible with conditioning theories are also explained. Gray and England (1969) also present several conditioning theories and therapies for stutterers. Gregory (1968) edited a monograph on *Learning Theory and Stuttering Therapy*.

Stuttering as a Personality Disorder[2]

The position that stuttering is primarily a manifestation of an underlying neurotic personality is not as widely held as it was up until the 1960s. Nevertheless, many psychologists and psychiatrists, mostly those who are identified as psychoanalysts, still emphasize the maladjustment and do not appear to be concerned with the possibility that stutterers are constitutionally different from normal speakers. They regard stuttering as a manifestation of personality disorder and are inclined to agree that the stutterer speaks as he does because of some psychological need that is better satisfied through stuttering than through normal speech. Stutterers are likely to be characterized as infantile, compulsive, dependent, ambivalent, regressive, anxious, insecure, withdrawn, or by some other adjective or combination of adjectives consistent with the specific theoretic formulation or bias of the theorizer. For example, the psychoanalyst Coriat (1943) viewed stutterers as ". . . infants who have compulsively retained the original equivalents of nursing and biting." The equivalents, we might note, are the specific oral characteristics of the stutterer, the way in which he repeats, hesitates, blocks, or prolongs on the sounds he utters or stops himself from uttering.

Travis (1971, pp. 1009–1033), in an essay entitled "The Unspeak-

---

[2] Even if we view stuttering as an expression of a personality disorder, we still need to explain the nature of the learning—how does the person learn to become a stutterer?

able Feelings of People with Special Reference to Stuttering," traces the development of neurotic behavior and the responsibility as well as the fear of speaking in stutterers. "Stuttering is the consequence of the young child speaking with his mother and father. In his utterances he asked to be known and he understood. In their reply they told him of his unacceptability in his current verbalized forms" (p. 1009). Travis uses learning theory to explain how stuttering behavior becomes reinforced. Basically, however, "stuttering is a manifestation of a fear to speak the truth to oneself or about oneself to another. It occurs most frequently in those families that place a high premium upon the truth and then punish its verbalization. To the extent that a child can be self-conscious comfortably, he will not stutter."

Therapy for Travis emphasizes the need to help stutterers accept their feelings, however hostile and "unspeakable" they may be. Most of the stutterers were adults by the time they were seen by Travis for psychotherapeutic help, and so were able to express their feelings. There is a note of preventive therapy in the Travis position. It is for parents to learn to listen so that their children's feelings may be expressed and not become repressed and "unspeakable."

Van Riper (1971, pp. 265–284) reviews the literature on "Stuttering as a Neurosis." We agree with Van Riper's conclusion (p. 277) that "The case for stuttering as a neurosis and only a neurosis has not been made."

Theorists who believe that stuttering is a manifestation of a personality disorder are able to point to a large number of studies to support their position. The results of many, but by no means all of these studies, suggest that adolescents and adults who stutter are, on the whole, not as well adjusted as nonstutterers. We might add, however, that seldom do the studies provide evidence to indicate whether the stuttering is the cause of, or is caused by, the maladjustment. The possibility that the stuttering preceded the maladjustment must be considered by those who look objectively on the overall problem of the stutterer and his/her stuttering.

Two Multiple Origin Viewpoints

The points of view just presented each sought to explain stuttering as having a single cause. Obviously, theories that are inconsistent with one another cannot all be correct at all times. There is a possibility, however, that each of the theories, and the theorists, is correct at some times—often enough, we would gather, to satisfy himself or herself, but not often enough to persuade those holding opposing or even supplementary viewpoints. Before leaving the discussion of theories as to the cause of stuttering we consider two points of view of practicing speech clinicians who currently believe that stuttering may have multiple causes. Why any given individual stutters can best be estimated by his/her individual clinical history and the cause that seems most likely to fit his/her case.

Stuttering as a Manifestation of Perseveration

Eisenson (1975) believes that persons tend to persist in a given mode of behavior even when such behavior is not appropriate, when they are confronted with conditions that call for more rapid change from previous or ongoing actions, than they are capable of making. The tendency for an individual to resist change, and for a mental or motor process to dominate behavior after the situation that originally evoked it is no longer present, is termed *perseveration*. The perseverating phenomenon is normal for all of us. Most often we experience it when we are tired or sleepy, or under conditions of pressure or tension. We do the same thing or feel the same way even when we are able to recognize that the cause for the doing or feeling has ceased to exist. So, often many minutes after we have gotten off a bicycle, we may still feel that we are riding on it. When we are tired, and required to talk, we tend to repeat utterances more often than the intellectual aspect of the situation requires. If we do not become anxious or apprehensive about our normal inclination to perseverate, we are not likely to fear recurring or similar situations because we have perseverated. There are, however, physiological and psychological conditions that are conducive to more than a normal amount of perseverative behavior. Among these conditions are brain damage, brain difference, lowered vitality, the aftereffects of physical or mental shock, and emotional tension and anxiety.

According to Eisenson (1975), if an individual is required, or feels required, to speak under a condition conducive to perseverative behavior, the perseveration will be manifest in his/her speech. Unfortunately, the awareness of blocked or repetitive tendencies in speech may increase the individual's apprehension about speaking and so aggravate the condition that was initially responsible for the speech perseveration. The result is a generalized reaction toward speaking that transforms what might otherwise be hesitation, block, repetition, or prolongation (perseverating manifestation) into stuttering.

As indicated earlier, speaking conditions that are associated with a feeling of responsibility are more likely to be associated with perseverative speech than speech that is devoid of responsibility. Communicative language content is also associated with perseveration in speaking. Persons who find themselves pressed by their environment, or by their own inner compulsions, to speak (communicate) on an intellectual (informative) level when they have nothing to say, or are not completely prepared to say what they would like, are likely to perseverate in speech. In general, these speech situations are all productive of some degree of anxiety.

It is also possible that some persons with atypical neurological mechanisms are unable to respond with spoken language as rapidly as some speech situations require. In such situations, and for such persons, perseveration in speaking tends to occur. These may be persons with a constitutional predisposition to stutter. It may also be anybody who lacks the language or lacks confidence in his/her language abilities for a given situation.

As noted, most stutterers have periods of relative fluency, and others in which they are normally quite fluent. Such conditions include speaking to animal pets, responding as a member of a group (where communicative responsibility is shared, reduced, or lacking), speaking nonsense intentionally, singing (singing is not really speaking because it is devoid of responsibility either for the formulation of the word sequences or its "communication"), and often reciting memorized material. All of these conditions share a common feature—the lack of formulating and the responsibility of uttering a thought, or a propositional statement (it may be a question) to which an answer might be expected. Stuttering, unless it is patently of neurotic origin, almost always occurs when a speaker is engaged in propositional talking. It has its parallel with the normal hesitations of nonstutterers who are talking about something of importance, even if only of momentary importance, while they are thinking of how to say it. These are normal hesitation phenomena.

In summary, most stuttering behavior is expressed when the speaker is engaged in propositional or communicative interchange. At such times, either because of an anxiety specific to the situation, or a more generalized anxiety about speaking when there is any degree of communicative responsibility, perseveration in speech tends to occur. Only a neurotic individual who feels that he has a commitment to stutter whenever and to whomever he talks or nontalks is likely to stutter in many other situations. Normal speakers, and stutterers when not under stress, may engage in normal hesitations. However, despite superficial resemblances, normal hesitations, regardless of who produces them, should not be confused with stuttering.

In essence, according to Eisenson, stuttering as a manifestation of perseveration may take place whenever the speaker finds himself inadequate or unequal to the demands of the speaking situation. The perseverating tendency may have a physiological cause, a psychological cause, or a combination of both. Initially, the onset cause for most stutterers is a neurological difference along lines considered in our discussion of cerebral dominance for language. Early stuttering is a manifestation of difficulty some children have in the organization of language for purposes of communicating their thinking.

Van Riper's Eclectic Position

Van Riper reminds us (1978, Chap. 8) that stuttering has been identified for thousands of years and has been studied intensively for many years but we are still without an adequate answer to the question "What causes stuttering?" Van Riper—he believes in common with most speech pathologists—maintains an eclectic point of view. He states that

> stuttering may have different origins in different individuals, and that the original causes are not nearly as important as those that maintain the disorder. The River of Stuttering does not flow out from only one lake. (pp. 260–261)

Earlier in this chapter we reviewed the development of stuttering and indicated Van Riper's observation that those children who continue to stutter after early onset into their adolescent and often adult years tend to follow a sequence along this line: hesitations, repetitions, and prolongations; associated tension and struggle behavior; interrupter and avoidance reactions; ultimate reactions of fear and shame. Stutterers, says Van Riper "Get caught in the whirlpool of self-reinforcement; the disorder becomes self-perpetuating." But Van Riper knows that this pessimistic prediction does not always hold. With or without therapy, many stutterers do improve, at least in the overt manifestations that are expressed in speaking.

Van Riper accepts the possibility that stuttering may have its origin in either a constitutional predisposition, and/or a neurosis (deep-seated emotional conflicts), and/or learned behavior as a result of classical conditioning. He does not reject the possibility of other causes. But, because he is not certain of the possible cause or combination of causes, Van Riper also takes an eclectic position about therapy. Essentially, his is a view that the therapeutic approaches must fit the needs and problems of the individual stutterer. He does distinguish between the treatment needs of the young stutterer, who should be approached both directly, through play therapy, and through the family, and the "confirmed" stutterer.

Treatment of the "confirmed" stutterer will probably include modification of speaking to "stutter as easily and effortlessly as he did when the disorder first began." In regard to psychotherapy, referring to himself, Van Riper admits that psychoanalysis helped him to solve many personal conflicts "but left him stuttering as severely as ever. . . . It was only after he stopped trying to avoid stuttering but instead learned to stutter openly but easily, that he was able to solve his problem." (p. 279).

THERAPY FOR STUTTERERS

Although the burden of therapy for stutterers is one that should be carried by the professional speech-clinician, the classroom teacher is necessarily an important member of the therapeutic team. In the following discussion, we consider the objectives of therapy for both the beginning stutterer and the confirmed stutterer, as well as the specific role of the classroom teacher in regard to each.[3]

Objectives for the Early (Incipient) Stutterer

In characterizing the early (incipient) stutterers, we stressed that their disfluencies, even though they may be excessive, usually occur without evidence of either awareness or special effort in speaking. Emphasis in the treatment of the early stutterers is on preventing them from becoming aware that their speech is in any way importantly different from that of others around them or a cause for concern. Awareness of negative difference, whether it be of speech or any other form of behavior, arises from observed reactions. Young children will have no way of knowing that their speech is atypical unless some person important to them says or does something to direct their attention to the difference. A child who is disfluent is not likely to compare himself/herself with other children until after some older person has made or suggested a comparison. Disfluencies become something for a child to be concerned about only if he/she has responded to another person's concern. To prevent the child's awareness and concern, we must somehow control the reactions of persons who may show and so create such awareness.

---

[3] One of the confounding observations about stutterers is that a great variety of approaches, some without any apparent rationale, have been used on stutterers with varying degrees of success—at least for a time. Another, as we have noted, is the frequency of spontaneous recovery. So, J. G. Sheehan in "Conflict Theory and Avoidance-Reduction Therapy," in *Stuttering: A Second Symposium* (New York: Harper & Row, Publishers, Inc., 1975), p. 187, asserts: "In 80 per cent of the cases in which it begins, stuttering is not perpetuated but disappears without treatment by the time the person reaches college provided he has faced the problem." We assume that "facing the problem" is a form of therapy that does not always require the help of a professional person who is identified as a therapist.

Essentially, therefore, the early stutterer, if not of school age, is to be treated through the parents. If the stutterer is of school age, the child's teachers as well as parents become the recipients of direct treatment. The early stutterer should be given no direct speech therapy or any other form of therapy that can be related to the production of speech. Nothing should be done or said to the child that suggests that his/her speech is in any way in need of change. If the early stutterer is to be involved in therapy, it is only to permit the trained speech clinician to observe what possible pressures exist in the child's environment that disturb his speech production. For this purpose, a permissive play group is recommended, in which a clinician is able to observe conditions that are conducive to increased disfluency. The clinician's observations are, of course, later discussed with the parents with a view toward modification of comparable home conditions so that pressure and excessive disfluencies can be reduced, or, if possible, eliminated.

Some of these specific aspects of treatment, and some of the information to be given to the parents of the early stutterer, or to the child believed by the parents to be a stutterer, are now considered. Many of these aspects, incidentally, are also relevant for the classroom teacher. Later we will have more to say about how a teacher or clinician may "teach" a child how to organize and use correct syntactic constructions without making him/her self-conscious or rejecting his/her verbal offering. Examples of constructions that children normally acquire in the two-to-four-year age range may be found in our chapter on The Development of Language, pp. 155–157. Additional examples may be found in Eisenson, *Aphasia in Children* (Harper & Row, Publishers, Inc., 1973, Chap. 9).

Distinguishing Between Disfluency and Early Stuttering

Often parents are unduly sensitized about stuttering because of their own family history. One or both of the parents may have stuttered or may still be stuttering. Older children or relatives may be stutterers.[4] Perhaps the parents are being pressured by their own parents to "do something" about the child's speech. The parents, understandably concerned, are "doing something" about what they believe to be stuttering.

A first step in the direction of treatment of the parents is to deter-

---

[4] Although we believe that there is a constitutional predisposition for stuttering, even when a family constellation suggests such a predisposition, there is no compulsion for any child to become a stutterer. The approaches that we will suggest should help the family to help the child to get through the most vulnerable period.

mine whether the child's disfluencies are within the limits of normal or, in terms of incidence and the nature of the situation, in excess of normal. Are we, in other words, dealing with normal disfluency, which includes some amount of so-called disfluency, or early (incipient) stuttering? Information is obtained from the parents' description and, if possible, imitation of an actual tape recording of the child's speech. The parents are asked to recall when disfluencies most often occur and when they are least likely to occur. The child's speech should be observed when talking to the parents, with a special note made as to whether there is any difference in ease of speaking when the response is made to the mother or to the father. The child should also be observed in a play situation when away from the parents as well as in their presence. If the total observed speech behavior adds up to normal speech flow—normal ease of speech disfluencies included—this should be stated and explained to the parents. We have found that parents are frequently able to understand and accept hesitancies and repetitions in speech when these are compared with hesitant and repetitious nonspeech behavior. We are usually able to get from parents their observations that not only their child but most children repeat activites when at play, that young children enjoy hearing the same song or the same story repeated many times. We try to make parents realize the normality of repetitions in all aspects of a young child's behavior so that repetition does not seem abnormal when it occurs in speech.

We have found effective the technique of recording and playing back part of the interview held with the parents about the child. In listening to the playback, parents are able to hear their own hesitations and repetitions as well as those of the interviewer. If they do not consider themselves stutterers, the parents are then able to compare their own speech with that of their child in regard to the incidence of "disfluencies." If the parents are disturbed about their own hesitant speech, they should be assured that few if any persons are always fluent, except possibly when they are reproducing memorized material. Even actors, it can be pointed out, have occasional "disfluencies," so that nonprofessional speakers should certainly be permitted some of their own.

Nothing in the interview with the parents should suggest, by words or manner, that the parents were either foolish or overanxious or in any way exercised poor judgment in coming for help about their child's speech. We believe that parents have a right, if not an obligation, to be concerned. We also believe that each child has his/her right not to be disturbed by things that may concern the parents. The child's hesitations, if they are normal in frequency and not excessive for the situation, are among those things about which the child should not be concerned. We think that parents are usually able to appreicate that most disfluencies are normal. Furthermore, it is possible that the difference between normal hesitation and stuttering may be made by the awareness and anxiety that young children who are not indifferent to their parents may get from them. Stuttering, is often enough the sum of disfluency plus awareness plus anxiety, whereas disfluency alone is usually developmentally normal speech behavior.

It is possible that in some instances the child may really be disfluent, more than normally hesitant and repetitive in speech. The advice, nevertheless, still holds. There is much greater likelihood that a child will modify this manner of speaking without direct attention being paid to it, than with intervention. The only positive suggestion we would make for "correction" is to observe whether a child is trying to arrive at a new and syntactically more complex way of saying something than he/she did before the occurrence of the hesitations and repetitions. For example, a child at age three might say "Johnny is my brother. Johnny and I go to school together." The same child when a year or so older might try to indicate the same meanings with a single sentence formulation such as "My brother Johnny and I go to school together," or "I go to school with my brother Johnny." While trying to figure out the new "grown up" way to say things, hesitations and repetitions may well take place. If this seems to be the situation, then the mother or the nursery school teacher should give the child a "model" sentence to imitate. The model sentence should not be too obvious or too directly offered. We would suggest that the parent or teacher might take an opportunity to make a parallel statement for the child. If our little Johnny's brother is bright, he will get the idea. If not, no harm will be done.

What we are suggesting has more general implication. We believe that most adults have hesitations in speaking when they try new formulations. Certainly observers of the language acquisition of children may readily note this phenomenon. Most children readily learn new formulations such as embedded phrases and clauses, for example, "Mary, my very dearest doll, broke her arm today." However, while "reaching" for this new formulation, this new way of saying two sentences (thoughts) in one, the child may indeed become somewhat disfluent. So may the child in trying out a "big" word, or the expression of any new "big" thought. Hesitations, repetitions, and even backing up and starting again, are all quite normal for adults. Certainly they should be considered normal for children. To repeat an earlier observation, normal fluency should include an amount of so-called disfluencies, which are really normal hesitation phenomena. However, in some instances, which we believe include most young children with a constitutional predisposition toward at least incipient or early stage stuttering, children may be delayed in their early proficiency for syntactic development. Their inner linguistic formulations, and so, of course, their expressions may be inconsistent with their age and intellectual level of expectations. So they have difficulty in "mature" expressions of their thoughts.

The child who is found to be delayed in language development, and particularly in syntactic competence, deserves and should be given help in how to say a few words well. The child at the outset needs many models of simple but "complete" language formulations. When these formulations of from three to five words are mastered, then more elaborate constructions should be provided. These constructions may be incorporated and practiced in play situations. At first it may be a role-playing situation in which a child talks to a doll, a stuffed animal, or some other toy object. Ultimately, of course, we want communicative interchanges with a peer or an older person. Give the child ample time to formulate and produce the utterances. Interchange roles with the child so that "grown-up talk" and "grown-up behavior," even though it is play behavior, will go together in a mutually enjoyable situation.

Sharing Information About Language Development and Speech Functions

Many parents become anxious about their children's speech because they are either uninformed or misinformed about how speech and language develop in children. They are likely to have some vague notions that children begin to talk somewhere about the time that they begin to walk. Most parents have heard about children who talked reasonably plainly at one year of age and may show disappointment if their own children seem slower. We believe that properly informed parents are likely to be less anxious parents, and so, either in an interview situation or in a larger parent group situation, we inform the parents about the normal expectancies in regard to language development, speech proficiency, and the function served by speech. Among the points we emphasize for parents are the following:[5]

1. Every child has his/her own rate and pattern of language and speech development just as he/she has an individual rate and pattern of physical growth and motor development. A slower than

[5] The teacher or clinician might at this point review Chapter 7 on the development of language in children.

"normal" developmental pattern does not necessarily mean that the child is retarded.

2. Language and speech development are related to some factors over which the child has no control. These include the position and number of children in the family, the linguistic ability and intelligence of the parents, the child's sex, and the appropriateness of motivation and stimulation for the child to talk. A first child tends to begin to talk earlier than a second, and second earlier than a third. Girls, by and large, talk somewhat earlier and more proficiently than boys. The child who is urged to talk too soon may be more delayed in beginning than the child who begins to talk when he/she is ready and needs to talk.

3. Attentive and available parents are much more helpful for the development of language and speech than are either anxious or non-available parents.

4. Language is not likely to be used unless its use is associated with pleasure.

5. Children should enjoy making sounds before sounds are used as words. Even after children begin to use words, they continue to enjoy making sounds though they have nothing "informative" to communicate.

6. Some children do not establish articulatory (speech sound) proficiency until they are almost eight years of age. A young child is entitled to lisp, hesitate, and repeat without being corrected except by good example.

7. Children must hear good speech if they are to become proficient speakers.

8. Fluency does not become established all at once, if indeed it is ever established. Most preschool children speak with some amount of hesitations and repetitions much of the time. Hesitations and repetitions, even up to 10 per cent of utterance, are not abnormal provided they do not abruptly interrupt or fragment the flow of speech. In very young children who are just beginning to speak and in many three- and four-year-olds who are striving for grown-up sentence formulations, disfluencies may exceed 10 per cent of utterance.

9. Absence of speech fluency becomes important and a matter for concern when it is associated with specific recurring situations or events. Parents should note whether the child becomes increasingly hesitant when frustrated, when fatigued, or when talking to particular persons. If the child's disfluencies increase sharply in these situations, control of the situations, if possible, is recom-

mended. Control may take place either by avoiding the situation or by doing nothing that requires the child to communicate in these situations. By communicating, we mean having to answer questions that call for precise answers. Nothing, however, should be done to give the child a feeling that he/she is not to speak if the wish to speak is present.

Parents should also note whether the child becomes increasingly disfluent when bidding or competing for attention. If this is so, *parents should be alert to give the child prompt attention when the child is normally fluent*. This is important so that increased disfluency by the child does not result in greater satisfaction than normal fluency.

Parents should know that children do not always want to say something specific or to share information when they talk. They may wish to use words as they once used sounds, merely for the sake of the pleasure derived from utterance. Adults also do this when they sing nonsense songs or talk nonsense words to their children.

Parents should be at pains to watch how often they unconsciously or consciously interrupt their children. Interruption may produce frustration, and frustration, in turn, produces disfluency. The child who is brought up to become silent when an adult wishes to talk may interrupt speech attempts and become hesitant in fear of talking out of turn.

Modification of Reactions to the Child's Disfluencies

If the child is in an early phase or stage of stuttering, or is excessively disfluent, or is showing any of the speech characteristics associated with stuttering, it is essential that parents avoid revealing their anxiety. First, of course, we try to assure the parents that despite our acceptance that the child may be in the first stage of stuttering, later phases or stages are by no means inevitable. By relieving parental anxiety, we hope to reduce the occurrence of displays of anxiety. Parents are encouraged to listen patiently and without tension when the child speaks. They are instructed not to do or say anything that may be interpreted by the child as a sign that his/her speech is not acceptable. Among the important *do nots* are the following:

1. Do not permit the child to hear the word *stuttering* used about his/her speech. This holds for any synonym or euphemism for stuttering.
2. Do not tell the child to speed up, slow down, think before speaking, start over again, or do anything that makes it necessary for the

child to inhibit speaking or to conclude that he/she is not speaking well.

3. Do not sigh with relief when the child speaks fluently, or look with wide-eyed fear that the youngster may speak hesitatingly.
4. Do not show impatience if the child blocks, hesitates, or repeats.
5. Do not ask the child to speak in situations where disfluencies are likely to occur.

Among the important *positive suggestions* for the parents of the early-stage stutterer are the following:

1. Establish as calm a home environment as can be achieved. Try to avoid exposing the child to situations that are overexciting, embarrassing, or frustrating.
2. Encourage the child to talk, but do not demand talking even in situations where the child is usually fluent and at ease.
3. Listen to your child with as much attention as you would like shown to you when you are talking.
4. Speak to your child in a calm, unhurried manner, but not in a way that is so exaggerated as to be difficult to imitate.
5. Keep your child in the best possible physical condition and check for possible ailments if he/she suddenly shows excessive hesitations and repetitions.
6. Expect that your child will sometimes begin to say things he/she cannot finish. If the child seems to be groping for a word to complete the thought, offer the word. Do not, however, anticipate what the child may want to say by completing the thought in your own words.
7. Do all you can to make speech behavior pleasurable. Tell amusing anecdotes and read aloud to the child stories that you know he/she enjoys. If you note that at a certain time of day your child has an increase in disfluencies, try to make that the time when you do the reading. This reading has two results. It removes the opportunity for the practice of disfluent speech, and with it the possibility that the child may become aware of disfluencies. It also affords the child an opportunity to be passively engaged in an enjoyable speech activity.
8. Assure your child, if he/she asks you whether there is anything wrong with his/her speech, that you think the speech is just fine. If he/she tells you that sometimes he/she has trouble getting words out, make him/her understand that everybody has such trouble at some time so that there is nothing to worry about. Avoid overexplaining and overtalking your assurance, or your child, as a wise child, may suspect that you do not really mean what you say.

The Role of the Classroom Teacher

Virtually all that has been outlined or suggested as appropriate attitudes and behavior for the parents of the early-stage stutterer may be applied to the classroom teacher. The problem of an early stutterer is one that the teacher is likely to meet in the nursery and kindergarten grades and in the first two grades of school. In these grades, the teacher has an opportunity to observe the pressure situations that are conducive to increased disfluencies and to control them in the child's behalf. The teacher, by being a patient and attentive listener, can help the child considerably. The child who shows signs of early stuttering should not be corrected in his/her articulation or have any other aspect of defective speech called to his/her attention. The teacher should avoid calling upon the child when it is likely that the child will be excessively disfluent and should go out of the way to call upon him/her when relatively fluent speech may be expected.

The attitude of calm recommended for the early stutterer's home should also prevail in the classroom. This applies to all children and, of course, to the teacher. A teacher who shows ready anger, ridicules a child for an error, or permits children to ridicule one another, creates an attitude of apprehension. On the other hand, the teacher who accepts error as a normal way of life and indicates that it is better to try even though a mistake may be made sets a tone that most children will accept with pleasure. If any child responds to a mistake with ridicule, the child should be corrected in a private session.

The teacher should be generous with praise for any special abilities shown by the early stutterer. If no special abilities are apparent, praise those abilities that are the child's chief assets.

If the child has been teased because of his/her speech, or dubbed a stutterer by classmates, the teacher should assure him/her that the classmates are mistaken. The early stutterer should be told that everyone has the same kind of speech trouble at some time just as all children stumble occasionally when they walk or run. It might help considerably if the teacher, in a not too evident way, does some intentional hesitating or repeating. Beyond this, the teacher should explain to the class that teasing and name calling are not permitted and that some privilege will be denied to any offending member of the class.

Perhaps the teacher's role can best be summed up in a single directive. Be accepting, permissive, and kind; do only those things to and for the early stutterer, or any other child in your class, that you would want another teacher to do to and for your own child—or for any child you may love. *Beyond this, special language instruction is in order if it is evident that the child has difficulty with learning how to combine words into acceptable constructions (syntax).*

Objectives for the Confirmed Stutterer

Confirmed stutteres, as noted previously, are aware that their speech is atypical and react to themselves and to their environment in terms of their awareness and evaluation of their speech. Therapeutic objectives, therefore, include a modification of the speech pattern as well as a modification of the attitudes that the stutterers have developed toward themselves, their speech, and their environment. How much can be done depends upon the professional resources that are available to the stutterers and their readiness for making use of the resources. In some instances, little more than superficial treatment of speech symptoms can be attempted. Unfortunately, this is not enough for many confirmed stutterers, especially for those who have evident personality maladjustments associated with their stuttering. In some settings, psychotherapy as well as speech therapy is available, and more than speech modification can be attempted in a treatment program. When the family of a confirmed stutterer has no financial problem, private help can be sought outside of the school.

Where the confirmed stutterer shows no evidence of significant maladaptive behavior of attitudes requiring modifications, treatment may be limited to the speech symptoms. The assessment of what is needed should be made by a psychologist, speech/language clinician, or other professional worker *trained in personality evaluation.* The clinician should undertake the assessment of the patient with an objective attitude without assuming either (1) that every stutterer, by virtue of his/her stuttering, necessarily has a personality disorder; or (2) that stutterers need treatment only for their speech symptoms to become wholly normal persons.

One basic understanding must be established with the confirmed stutterer if treatment, either for stuttering symptoms or for behavioral maladjustments, is to be successful. The stutterer, at the outset, must accept himself/herself as a person who stutters and is in need of treatment. The stutterer must not try to conceal stuttering or fight against the notion that he/she is a stutterer. When control over stuttering symptoms is established, and attitudes and behavior are modified, the once confirmed stutterer can then discard this label along with the speech characteristics, attitude, and associated traits.

Another area of understanding that stutterer and clinician must establish is one of possible gains or values that may have grown out of stuttering. The stutterer must be helped to ask, and to answer honestly and objectively, the question, "Am I getting anything out of my stuttering that I don't want to give up?" If the stutterer realizes that his/her speech may serve as an excuse from social situations that may not be enjoyable, from running errands when there are other things to do more to his/her liking, or from preparing for daily recitations because he/she is not called on in school, then he/she will be in a position to weigh the advantages as well as the disadvantages of the speech defect and be prepared for further therapy. When the stutterer ceases to entertain fantasies and never uses stuttering as a ready-made alibi for what he or she might do, or might have been, except for the speech difficulty, then he/she has traveled a long way toward achieving the objectives of therapy.

Treatment for the Family

Often the parents of the stutterer are in need of counseling if the stutterer is to obtain maximum help from therapy. In some instances, the attitudes of the stutterer's parents are characterized by high aspiration, rigidity, and unconscious rejection of the child. If the study of the familial picture shows this to be the case for the individual stutterer, appropriate treatment should be undertaken. Our experience indicates that parental resistance to treatment must be anticipated. Many parents want and expect their children to improve without their active participation in a therapy program. Parents must be made to realize that their participation is essential. The aims of therapy for parents are to give them an understanding about the problem of stuttering in general, their child's stuttering in particular, and the relationship of their evaluations and attitudes toward their child's speech, and to reduce their own anxieties and possible guilt feelings about their child's speech difficulty. Parents must be helped to appreciate that stuttering is not likely to disappear all at once. Frequently, in fact, speech becomes apparently worse rather than better in the early stages of treatment.

Speech Goals

Stutterers as well as their parents must accept the virtual certainty that stuttering will not stop with the beginning of therapy. The immediate objective for stutterers is to encourage them to speak more rather than less despite their stuttering. While speaking more, stutterers need to be helped to take an objective view of their difficulty so that the following intermediate objectives may be attained:

1. A weakening of the forces and pressures with which the individual stuttering is associated.

2. Elimination of the secondary, accessory symptoms of stuttering.
3. Modification of the form of stuttering so that relatively easy, effort-less disfluencies replace the specific blocks, marked hesitations, strained prolongations, or repetitions.
4. Modification of the faulty habits directly associated with speaking such as improper breathing, rapid speaking, or excessive tensions of the speech mechanism.
5. Modification of the attitudes of fear, anxiety, or avoidance asso-ciated with the need for speaking or that occur after speech is ini-tiated.

Therapeutic Approaches for Symptom Modification and Control: The Role of the Speech Language Clinician

Some of the objectives of an overall therapeutic program for stutterers, regardless of the possible etiology for the individual stutterer's diffi-culty, should include modification with the ultimate hope of eliminat-ing the major speech symptoms manifested by the stutterer. Although the rationale for the use of the specific approach may vary consider-ably with the theorist or the clinician, a number of approaches are widely used with a considerable degree of success. We review those we have used and that have wide application.[6]

NEGATIVE PRACTICE. We have previously referred to the princi-ple of negative practice, an approach in which an individual learns to control a habit he or she would like to discard by practicing intention-ally and purposefully that very habit. For a stutterer this would mean that the clinician will direct him/her to become aware of the particular manner of stuttering and to practice one or more of the features of the manner. Thus, a stutterer will practice blocks by imitating his or her own particular way of blocking. When he/she learns this technique of self-imitation, modification of the blocks may be achieved through one or the other approaches we discuss. Through the technique of negative practice the stutterer is helped to undo by consciously doing what he/she presumably prefers not to do. This approach may be em-ployed to overcome facial or bodily tics, faulty breathing, or any other mannerism that characterizes the speech behavior of the individual stutterer.

[6] In their monograph (1980) Guitar and Peters indicate that in recent years most therapeutic approaches for stutterers involve either teaching the stutterer an "easier," more fluent manner of speaking, or teaching initial pattern that is not normal and gradu-ally shaping the flow to normal sounding speech. The techniques to be described fall into these two major categories. Guitar and Peters believe that the two approaches can be combined for effective treatment (see Table on p. 412).

VOLUNTARY STUTTERING. This approach in effect helps stutterers to learn a new, easier way of stuttering so that they can get on with the business of saying what they have to say with a minimum of blocking or spasm. One technique is to direct the stutterer *voluntarily to repeat* the first sound or the first syllable of each word. At first the stutterer may repeat the sound or syllable two or three times, or as many times as necessary to complete the rest of the word. The repetitions should be easy and "nonsticky." Stutterers usually find it easier to engage in voluntary repetition when reading material aloud while observing themselves in a mirror. With practice, the number of repetitions is reduced to the minimum needed to enable him/her to feel prepared to move along and to finish the utterance. Finally, the stutterer reduces the repetitions to the sounds of the words on which a block is anticipated. We usually proceed with the stutterer from reading to paraphrasing and then to a conversation that incorporates the words that carried the key ideas in material previously read. Ultimately, the technique of voluntary repetition is applied in free conversation. This technique is particularly useful in group sessions in which stutterers observe how successful the members of their group are in their efforts at voluntary, easy repetition. A good repetition (easy and "nonsticky") is given a positive value; involuntary repetition earns a minus score.

PROLONGATION. Prolongation or the intentional *lengthening* of initial sounds that are capable of being lengthened (vowels, dipthongs and continuant consonants) is another approach to voluntary stuttering. The lengthened sound must be produced in an easy, relaxed manner. The stutterer must use the lengthened sound production as a preparatory set to move into the next sound and so to complete the utterance. The modifications from reading to free speaking may follow the sequence suggested for volunatry repetition.

EASY ARTICULATION. Though clarity of diction may suffer somewhat, many stutterers find it helpful to learn a relatively lax, "nonsticky" manner of articulation. This is especially helpful in the production of stop sounds. With reduced articulatory tension, it may become possible for some stutterers to move from sound to sound and word to word without abrupt pauses that suggest mild spasms.

ARTICULATORY PANTOMIMING. Some stutterers need to be convinced that there are no real difficult sounds but only "bogey sounds" that the individual has somehow come to believe are difficult for him. For such stutterers, initial pantomiming of words or phrases—going through the articulatory activity without uttering the words aloud—

may be of considerable help. After pantomiming, the stutterer is directed to add voice and to speak (read or engage in free conversation) what had previously been pantomimed. In the second phase, ease of articulation and moving through the utterance are stressed.

FAKE STUTTERING. A useful group technique is to have a stutterer imitate a speech feature of another stutterer. Many can do this with considerable success. For those who can, a feeling of control is achieved. Such control may then be used to imitate speech free or relatively free of stuttering behaviors.

IMPOSED RHYTHM AND TIMING. Speaking to an imposed rhythm has long been known to facilitate speech flow in stutterers. However, there is no encouraging evidence that normal fluency is maintained with the benefit of rhythmic pattern that is not consonant or relevant to the contents of the utterance.[7] A modification of imposed rhythm is syllable timed speech.

SYLLABLE TIMED (ST) SPEECH. In syllable-timed (ST) speech, the subject (stutterer) is taught first to speak each syllable of an utterance to the accompaniment of a metronome. When the subject is able to speak (syllabicate) without stuttering, he/she is encouraged to speak *as if* to a metronome in comunicative situations. At this stage speech is slow, monotonous, and far from normal. In a later stage of ST therapy, the stutterer is encouraged to speed up the rate, add syllable stress, and phrase pauses more in the manner of normal speech flow.

Ingham (1975, pp. 354–379) describes a program of syllable-timed speech employing operant procedures in a population of 16 adults. Ingham reports improvement with nine of the 16 nine months after the end of the treatment program. However, Ingham has considerable reservation about the long-term implications of ST therapy, and just what aspect of the program brought about the demonstrated improvement.

DELAYED AUDITORY FEEDBACK (DAF). Nonstutterers can be made to stutter by having them listen to themselves after an imposed delay in auditory feedback. Interestingly, a delay in auditory feedback improves the fluency of stuttering when the delay is about one quarter of a second and speech rate is slowed to about 30 words per minute.

---

[7] Evidence and arguments for and against imposed rhythm are reviewed by R. J. Ingham in *Stuttering: A Second Symposium*, J. Eisenson, Ed. (New York: Harper & Row, Publishers, Inc., 1975), pp. 346–347.

At the present time, we consider Delayed Auditory Feedback an experimental laboratory approach and not one we recommend for use with school-age children. Reviews of DAF experiments may be found in Van Riper (1971, pp. 382–403), Sheehan (1970, pp. 216–217), and Bloodstein (1979, pp. 127 and 154).

AIRFLOW CONTROL. Recently an "airflow control" technique to teach the stutterer a relaxed form of breathing in anticipation of and during speaking was revived and revised by Schwartz (1977). As it is stated in possibly oversimplified terms, the stutterer is taught to initiate vocalization with a "sigh" in order to avoid or reduce the occurrence of laryngeal spasm. Diligent daily practice is required in a wide variety of speaking situations that include ones that may be anticipated to be stressful.

The notion that stutterering is associated with or is caused by laryngeal spasm has an old history. Appelt (1929, Chap. 1) reviews this history and cites theorists and practitioners who held this view as long ago as the 1830s. Appelt notes that spasms of the laryngeal apparatus do occur in stammering (stuttering) and observes, "In severe cases of stammering the expiratory spasm is induced by the intention to speak and sets up at the first intention to open the mouth" (p. 79). However, Appelt is certain that the "spasms are, beyond all doubt, induced by psychic obstacles" (p. 80). Among his recommendations for treatment Appelt includes individual psychotherapy to help the stammerer deal with his neurotic needs.

Operant Conditioning and Behavior Modification

An approach that has come into increasing use by clinicians working with confirmed stutterers is operant conditioning. Stuttering is viewed as behavior that is subject to modification (conditioning or reconditioning). The underlying principle of operant conditioning is stated succinctly by Shames and Egolf (1976, p. 3).

"Specifically, it refers to a process of reinforcement whereby the frequency of a particular class of behaviors can be increased or decreased or maintained at a designated level by presenting or withdrawing certain stimuli immediately after a designated response has been emitted."

The use of operant procedures may be applied directly to the speech behavior of stutterers or to an aspect of behavior associated with stuttering. Wolpe (1969a and 1969b) assumes that when dealing with stuttering of long duration, regardless of the causes for the onset of stuttering, the stutterer eventually develops a neurotic anxiety about his speech. This anxiety maintains stuttering, and thus must be treated. Specific techniques for the modification of anxiety include encouraging the patients to talk about their feelings, and so reduce their strength. Relaxation based on Jacobson's *Progressive Relaxation*[8] is taught to stutterers and they are "trained" to assume the posture and recognize the feelings of relaxation. When the stutterer shows evidence of tension associated with anxiety, he/she is trained to relax voluntarily, so that relaxation replaces the tension state. In effect, the awareness of tension cues a state of relaxation. The stutterer is asked to list anxiety-producing (stuttering-producing) situations in order of severity (hierarchies). Each state is then a subject of therapy.

> When relaxation has become adequate and when the hierarchies are ready, one begins the central procedure, which is to present the weakest scene from a hierarchy to the *imagination* of the deeply relaxed patient for a few seconds, repeating presentations until the imagined item no longer evokes any anxiety at all. At each presentation the weak anxiety evoked by the scene is to some extent inhibited by the relaxation so that at the next presentation its evocation is weaker still, until it is eventually zero. The therapist then proceeds to the next scene, and so on, until the whole anxiety has been dealt with (Wolpe, 1969a, p. 19).

Wolpe observes that almost always there is complete transfer of the anxiety from the imagined situation to the corresponding real-life situation as reported by the patient.

Various behavior therapy techniques are based on these general approaches. Several of these techniques are presented in the monograph by Gray and England (1969). Another behavior therapy approach, more elaborate than the one that we have described, is presented in detail by Brutten and Shoemaker (1967) and by Shames and Egolf (1976). Most behavior therapists report success in the modification of stuttering symptoms after relatively few sessions as compared with other approaches. Perhaps the success is related to the readiness of the stutterers to do whatever they need to do to put an end to or at least to reduce the overt symptoms of stuttering.

The techniques of prolongation, easy articulation, negative practice, etc., described earlier are, of course, behavior modification approaches intended to change (modify) the oral (speech) practices of stutterers and to replace them with acceptable if not normal fluency patterns. Operant procedures, in a strict sense, are limited to the application of techniques according to schedules of contingent rein-

---

[8] The technique of *progressive relaxation* is described by E. Jacabson in his book *You Must Relax* (New York, McGraw-Hill Book Company, 1944.

A recent adaptation of the relaxation technique is included in H. Benson, *The Relaxation Response* (New York, Morrow, 1975).

forcements to strengthen selected desired behaviors and contingent "punishment" to weaken others not considered desirable.

Ultimate Objectives for the Stutterer

We would like to be able to recommend as a legitimate, ultimate objective for every confirmed stutterer the establishment of normal speech and a well-adjusted personality. Such an objective, however, cannot be recommended in the light of our experience with many stutterers. Perhaps a more reasonable and more moderate objective may be speech that is relatively free of the more severe characteristics of stuttering, and a relatively normal adjustment. We should not expect stutterers, not even those who are having psychotherapy, to become better adjusted than most of their peers because most of their peers have some traits that can stand improvement.

Many stutterers are able to free themselves of their significant aberrant speech symptoms. Some, however, continue to have excessive disfluencies under conditions of fatigue, ill health, or stress. For some, also, it is possible that disfluencies are likely to persist on a constitutional basis. For these, the acceptance of disfluency without accompanying apprehension and struggle behavior may be all that can be achieved. If this attitude can be established, the characteristics of stuttering generated by anxiety and apprehension are removed and the overall occurrence of abnormal disfluencies is, therefore, reduced.

The Role of the Classroom Teacher

The task of helping the confirmed stutterers toward better speech and the improvement of their associated adjustment problems are, as we have indicated, primarily for the speech clinician and not for the classroom teacher. There are, however, a number of ways the classroom teacher can be of appreciable help to the stutterer in his improvement program.

The teacher should make note of the class situations that appear to be conducive to stuttering. Unless the child volunteers, he/she should not be called upon to speak in these situations. If he/she does speak, the stutterer should not be stopped regardless of the severity of difficulty. If at all possible, however, the stutterer should be called upon for short replies rather than for ones that require lengthy communications.

If many children are to be called on during a recitation period, the teacher should call upon the stutterer early. Waiting induces anxiety and anxiety induces an increase in stuttering. The stutterer should

Pros and Cons of Stuttering Modification and Fluency Shaping Therapies with regard to: (A) Client, (B) Clinician, and (C) Training Program[1]

Stuttering Modification Therapy		*Fluency Shaping Therapy*	
A. CLIENT		**A. CLIENT**	
PRO	CON	PRO	CON
1. Does not require speaking in abnormal pattern.	1. Needs to confront and perform fear producing tasks.	1. Less need to confront and perform fear producing tasks.	1. May require speaking in abnormal pattern for a period of time.
B. CLINICIAN		**B. CLINICIAN**	
PRO	CON	PRO	CON
1. Therapy tends to be more spontaneous and enjoyable.	1. Therapy is nonstructured, more difficult decisions need to be made.	1. More structured programs available. Thus, less planning needed.	1. Therapy can be boring.
	2. Less data kept for measuring progress for IEP, etc.	2. More data kept for measuring progress for IEP, etc.	2. More charting of data needed.
C. TRAINING PROGRAM		**C. TRAINING PROGRAM**	
PRO	CON	PRO	CON
	1. More difficult to teach to clinicians.	1. Easier to teach to clinicians. There are fewer individual differences, clearer defined decisions based on observed behavior.	

[1] Source: Guitar, B., and T. J. Peters, *Stuttering: An Integration of Contemporary Therapies,* Memphis, Tenn.: Speech Foundation of America, 1980. Reproduced by permission of the publisher. (See footnote, p. 406.)

know that participation is expected, but that he/she will not have an indefinite period of anxious waiting for the moment of active participation.

The teacher should also note the conditions or situations when the stutterer is likely to have least difficulty with speaking and invite active participation when these situations are present. For example, if a stutterer can recite memorized poetry without difficulty, he/she should be given an opportunity to recite. If the child can read aloud much better than recite impromptu, he/she should be called upon to read aloud.

The teacher can get considerable information from the stutterer as to both easy and difficult speech situations. In most instances, an understanding can be reached with the stutterer as to participation in class recitations. We recommend a basic principle to be followed in regard to oral recitations: If the stutterer is exempt from any oral activity, he/she must compensate by some other form of activity. This may call for additional written work done at home, or for board work done in class. Exemption without compensation gives stuttering a positive value that may be difficult to surrender. The teacher should not become a partner to the creation of gains to be derived from stuttering; neither, of course, should the teacher become part of any classroom attitude that inflicts punishment on the stutterer because of the stuttering.

The teacher should try to reward the stutterer for fluent speech, but to do so without readily apparent fuss. "Very good, Johnny" is much better than a lengthy response of praise because Johnny has been fluent. If the teacher looks pleased, Johnny is likely to get the idea even without a verbalization of the pleasure. There is a very real danger that a remark intended as a verbal reward may actually backfire and become an implied penalty. For example "You spoke very well, Johnny" may be interpreted to mean that in most instances Johnny does not speak well, hence the need to point out the occasions when speech is good. As a general procedure, the teacher should try to avoid directing undue attention to good speech as well as to poor speech. The nature and form of the reward should depend upon the intellectual and emotional maturity of the child. Rewards should be given for good speech as for any other worthwhile performance. They should come quickly and inconspicuously.

The teacher should help to create a classroom atmosphere that will encourage the stutterer to talk. Such an atmosphere exists when any child, whether he/she stutters, has no defect in speech, or has some form of defective speech other than stuttering, feels free to volunteer to speak without fear of penalty or criticism. It may help to explain to the stutterer's classmates, *at a time when the stutterer is out of the classroom,* how they can be of help. Nothing said to the classmates should suggest that the stutterer is in need of pity or excessive sympathy. Instead, the teacher should emphasize that what the stutterer needs is to be given opportunities to talk and a group of patient listeners when he/she talks. If the stutterer is excused from any recitations, the classmates should be informed that the child is doing other work to make up for it. In this way the classmates will not feel resentful that the stutterer is a privileged member of the group. Rather they will feel that the stutterer is a member of their group who has a problem that all are helping to solve by their understanding.

Luper and Mulder (1964, Chap. 8) sum up approaches for the treatment of the stuttering child in a school setting, with special emphasis on the interrelated roles of the speech clinician and the classroom teacher.

CLUTTERING

Cluttering is usually included among disorders of rhythm and fluency. By some authorities (Weiss 1964), it is considered a forerunner of stuttering. Yet were cluttering to be designated as an articulatory disorder, or as a language disorder, it would be so labeled based upon verifiable observation. A description of cluttering should indicate why all of these designations might well be correct and why, therefore, it deserves its own classification. We are discussing cluttering at this point in our considerations because of its superficial resemblance to stuttering, from which, nevertheless, it needs to be differentially identified.

Superficially, cluttered speech suggests a torrent of words, poorly or partially articulated, with repetitions of monosyllabic words and first syllables of longer words. It is a "hot potato in the mouth" speech, with morphemes falling where they may. Cluttered speech spurts rather than flows, then stops and spurts again. Behind the speech is the clutterer who, unlike the stutterer at any stage, seems unaware of his perpetrations. Objectively, we may characterize cluttering as repetitious, poorly articulated utterance produced at a rate incompatible with the speaker's ability to speak intelligibly. Part of the lack of intelligibility is the clutterer's loose and poorly organized phrase and sentence structure. These last features make it difficult for a listener to anticipate and so comprehend or guess what the speaker is trying to say. Weiss (1964, p. 24) believes that clutterers may well be at a loss for the words to express their thoughts. "Because the clutterer is inept

Summary of Similarities and Differences Between Clutterers and Stutterers[1]

	Clutterers	*Stutterers*
Family history	May be present, especially on the male side	May be present, much more often in the males than females
Onset of speech	Often delayed	May occasionally be delayed, but not as often or as long as for clutterers
Likelihood of awareness	Usually unaware	Often aware to level of anxiety
Feeling about own speech	Indifferent	Fearful, anxious
Likely result of		
(a) speaking after instruction to be careful	Improves	Increase of stuttering symptoms
(b) Interruption and reminder to slow down	Improves	Worsens; anxious, tense, blocked speech
Speaking with awareness of importance of situation	Usually improves	Usually worsens
Speaking when relaxed, at ease	Worse	Improves
Reading new material aloud	Better at outset	Worse
Reading familiar material aloud	Worse	Improves

[1] This summary table is adapted from D. A. Weiss (1964, p. 69).

at finding the necessary words to express his ideas, his speech is studded with clichés and repetitions of words and phrases." We accept this position, with emphasis on the notion that the clutterer does not really have more than a vague idea of what he/she wants to say, along with an apparent compulsion to say it.

When the clutterer slows down, both articulation and intelligibility improve. Perhaps when a clutterer speaks slowly, at a rate compatible with his/her neuromuscular system when it operates efficiently, the clutterer also gives himself time to think and to formulate the utterance.

The table above summarizes similarities between clutterers and stutterers and how different situations affect their speech and language productions.

Background History of Clutterers

Clutterers often present a history suggestive of minimal brain disfunction and minimal brain damage (see Chapter 16). Weiss (1964, p. 51) reports a familial history of speech disorders other than but also including cluttering, especially on the paternal side. He views it, as do we, as a *central language imbalance (disorder)* that includes such features as delayed language onset, retarded language development, delayed articulatory proficiency, and vocal monotony. We would add to these characteristics slow development of vocabulary and syntax. As they grow older, clutterers are likely to have reading and writing difficulties, the latter both for legibility and sentence structure. Behaviorally and motorically, the clutterer is likely to show impulsiveness, late laterality development, and ambinondexterity. The clutterer gives the impression of a loosely assembled person, who is awkward and imprecise.

Differential Diagnosis: Stuttering and Cluttering

Most stutterers tend to speak better when they are relaxed and when they give minimal attention to their articulation. In contrast, clutterers tend to improve when they direct conscious attention to their utterance. Stutterers, especially in later stages, show apprehension and anxiety about their speech, and tend to have difficulties that are directly related to their apprehensions. Clutterers, as indicated, show a benign unawareness about their speech. With awareness, they tend to improve. Finally, the marked difficulties of clutterers in all language functions, written as well as spoken, distinguish them from most stutterers. Thus, though there is some evidence that stuttering has a familial, constitutional basis, the evidence of such etiology for the clutterer is clear and strong.

Cluttering as a Transitional Stage to Stuttering

Whether cluttering is a transitional stage, an early stage in the progression toward stuttering, is a moot point. It is possible that when some clutterers are directed to attend to their speech, they may develop anxieties and frustrations growing out of the awarenesses, and begin to speak like stutterers. Van Riper (1978, p. 59) observes: "Some clutterers become stutterers as well; most do not." Thus, though some stutterers may begin as clutterers, most do not show the early characteristics that we have described. However, we have known families that included both stuttering and cluttering siblings and a cluttering father. We have also known individuals who shifted periodically between cluttering and stuttering.

Therapy

The treatment for clutterers is implied in the differential diagnosis. Clutterers do tend to improve when they slow down and "mind their speech." They also tend to improve by being urged to formulate, to think through in words, before they begin to speak. Unfortunately, in conversation give-and-take we cannot ordinarily preformulate our utterances. Most of us have to learn to talk as we think. The best we can do for clutterers is to remind them to slow down, and cue them when their speech begins to accelerate, and so becomes unintelligible. These external controls must, with practice, become habitual. Clutters must, therefore, be taught to observe their listeners for indications that they may be talking too rapidly and are failing to make themselves understood. Rewards in the form of verbal and facial approval by the teacher, the clinician, and the family members when the clutterers do mind their speech should reinforce such behavior. Practice in making short announcements before the class and in therapy sessions with the speech/language/clinician are of help. Finally, we wish to re-emphasize that the clutterer's primary problem is with language. Each clutterer needs help in verbal expression, both oral and written. Clutterers need, to begin with, to learn to make simple statements simply. They need to learn to become slow and considered speakers. Most clutterers, we believe, will enjoy such a reputation if it can be achieved.

Problems

1. Define stuttering. Distinguish between early and confirmed stuttering.
2. What is meant by normal hesitation phenomena (NHP)? What is the relationship of NHP to disfluency? To stuttering?
3. Observe two or three speakers in a conversation. Note evidence of normal hesitation phenomena. How does this differ from stuttering?
4. What is the difference between a nonstutterer's "Well, well . . ." and a stutterer's postponement devices? What are your postponement devices?
5. Briefly describe Bloodstein's phases of stuttering and Van Riper's devel-

opmental sequence of stuttering. How are they the same? How are they different?

6. Talk to two or three stutterers about their feared word or speaking situations. Are there any common factors? Do they resemble yours?

7. Outline your own theory about the onset of stuttering.

8. Read J. Sheehan's essay on stuttering in J. Eisenson, Ed., *Stuttering: A Second Symposium*. Why does Sheehan regard stuttering as a learned form of behavior? What does Sheehan mean by his observation that stuttering is essentially an expression of an approach-avoidance conflict?

9. What is the evidence to support the position that stuttering is a manifestation of constitutional predisposition? What is a predisposition?

10. What is the evidence that the prediposition to stuttering may be inherited?

11. Read W. Johnson's position on stuttering in *Speech-Handicapped School Children*. How does Johnson explain the evidence of the heredity of stuttering on a nongenetic basis? Do you agree? Do you agree with Williams (1978) position?

12. Which of the positions on stuttering presented in this text best reconciles the therapeutic approaches with the onset causes? Which the poorest?

13. Suppose a four- or five-year-old child is sent to you by a parent with the complaint that the youngster is a stutterer. How would you go about determining whether the child has "normal disfluencies" or is *normally expressing* normal hesitations and repetitions? What would you tell the parent?

14. Why do most stutterers have less difficulty in reciting memorized material than in explaining or paraphrasing it? What are the easiest conditions for stutterers? The most difficult?

15. What is meant by "secondary gain?" What are some possible secondary gains, other than those mentioned in this chapter, that stutterers may entertain? How would you deal with them?

16. What is conditioning? What is deconditioning? How do they relate to therapy for stutterers? What is behavior modification?

17. What is meant by "desensitization" for stutterers? Can you give any examples of how you or a friend were desensitized against an anxiety or fear-producing situation? How were you initially sensititized to it?

18. Why should the treatment of an early-stage stutterer be directed toward the parent? Outline such treatment. What is the role of the classroom teacher?

19. What is meant by "negative practice?" How does this relate to stuttering therapy?

20. Distinguish between cluttering and stuttering.

21. How is the treatment of a young clutterer different from that of a primary stutterer? Of an adult clutterer and a confirmed stutterer?

22. Check the literature on delayed auditory feedback (DAF). How are the effects of DAF in most stutterers different from what they are for most non-stutterers? How is DAF used in therapy?

References and Suggested Readings

Andrews, S. G., and M. Harris, "Stammering," in *The Child Who Does Not Talk*, C. Renfrew, and K. Murphy, eds. The Spastics Society Medical Education Association, London: W. Heinemann Medical Books, 1964.

Appelt, A., *Stammering and Its Permanent Cure*. New York: E. P. Dutton & Co., Inc., 1929. (The author, who was a stutterer during his youth and early manhood, critically reviews the literature on theories and therapies of stuttering. Appelt regards psychotherapy as essential to deal with the neurotic attitudes of stutterers.)

Berry, M. F., "Twinning in Stuttering Families," *Human Biology*, **9,** 3 (1939), pp. 329–346.

Bloodstein, O., *Speech Pathology: An Introduction*. Boston: Houghton Mifflin Company, 1979, Chap. 4. (A good review of the development of stuttering and current treatment approaches to the problem.)

———— a, *Handbook on Stuttering*. Chicago: National Easter Seal Society for Crippled Children, 1975.

———— b, in J. Eisenson, Ed., "Stuttering as Tension and Fragmentation." In *Stuttering: A Second Symposium*. New York: Harper & Row, Publishers, Inc., 1975, pp. 1–95.

Bluemel, C. S., *The Riddle of Stuttering*. Danville, Ill.: Interstate Publishing Company, 1957. (A psychiatrist's exposition about the nature of stuttering as an underlying language disorder.)

Brown, S. F., "The Loci of Stuttering in the Speech Sequence." *Journal of Speech Disorders*, **10** (May 1945), 181–192.

Brutten G. J., and D. J. Shoemaker, *The Modification of Stuttering*. Englewood Cliffs, N.J.: Prentice-Hall, Inc. 1967.

————, in J. Eisenson, Ed., "Stuttering: Topography Assessment and Behavior Changing Strategies." In *Stuttering: A Second Symposium*. New York: Harper & Row, Publishers, Inc., 1975, pp. 199–262.

Coriat, I. H., "The Psychoanalytic Concept of Stammering." *The Nervous Child*, **2** (1943), 167–171.

Curry, F. K. W., and H. H. Gregory, "The Performance of Stutterers on Dichotic Listening Tasks Thought to Reflect Cerebral Dominance." *Journal of Speech and Hearing Research*, **12** (March 1969), 73–82.

Dell, C. W., *Treating the School Age Stutterer: A Guide for Clinicians*. Memphis, Tenn.: Speech Foundation of America, 1981. (The author describes programs and procedures that he has found to be effective with school age children.)

Eisenson, J. Ed., *Stuttering: A Second Symposium*. New York: Harper & Row, Publishers, Inc., 1975. (Six points of view are presented on the nature of stuttering with suggested therapies for stuttering consistent with the theoretic position. Van Riper provides a separate essay on "The Stutterer's Clinician." The contributors are O. Bloodstein, G. J. Brutten, J. Eisenson, R. J. Ingham, G. H. Shames, E. J. Brutten, and C. Van Riper.

————, In J. Eisenson, Ed., "Stuttering as Perseverative Behavior," in *Stutter-*

ing: A Second Symposium, New York: Harper & Row, Publishers, Inc., 1975.

———, *Aphasia in Children*. New York: Harper & Row, Publishers, Inc., 1973.

———, "Observations of the Incidence of Stuttering in a Special Culture." *ASHA*, **8** (1966), 391–394.

———, and E. Horowitz, "The Influence of Propositionality on Stuttering." *Journal of Speech Disorders*, **10** (March 1945), 193–198.

Emrick, C., "Language Performance of Stuttering and Nonstuttering Children." Doctoral Dissertation, University of Iowa, 1971. (Reported in *Dissertation Abstracts*, March, 1972, 5509–5510.)

Goldman-Eisler, F., "The Distribution of Pause Durations in Speech." *Language and Speech*, **4** (1961), 232–237.

Goldman-Eisler, F., "Hesitation, Information, and Levels of Speech Production." In A. V. DeReuck and M. O'Connor, Eds., *Disorders of Language*, Ciba Foundation, 1964.

Gray, B. B., and G. England, eds., *Stuttering and the Conditioning Therapies*. Monterey, Calif.: The Monterey Institute for Speech and Hearing, 1969.

Gregory, H. H., *Learning Theory and Stuttering Therapy*. Evanston, Ill.: Northwestern University Press, 1968.

Guitar, B., and T. J. Peters, *Stuttering: An Integration of Contemporary Theories*. Memphis, Tenn.: Speech Foundation of America, 1980. (The authors indicate how it is possible to teach stutterers how to modify their manner of utterance so that "they can be gradually shaped to normal sounding speech in all situations.")

Howie, P. M., "The Role of Genetic Factors in Stuttering." Address to American Speech and Hearing Association, 1976.

Hull, F. M. and R. J. Timmons, "The National Speech and Hearing Surveys; Preliminary Results." *ASHA*, **13** (1971), 501–509.

Ingham, R. J., "Operant Methodology in Stuttering Therapy." In Eisenson, J., Ed., *Stuttering: A Second Symposium*. New York: Harper & Row, 1975.

———, "A Comparison of Covert and Overt Assessment Procedures in Stuttering Therapy Outcome Evaluation." *Journal of Speech and Hearing Research*, **18** (June 1975), 346–354.

Johnson, W., in W. Johnson et al., *Speech Handicapped School Children*, 3rd ed. New York: Harper & Row, Publishers, Inc., 1967.

———, *Stuttering and What You Can Do About It*. Minneapolis, Minn.: University of Minnesota Press, 1961.

Jonas, G., *Stuttering: The Disorder of Many Theories*. New York: Farrar, Straus & Giroux, 1977. (A personal point of view about the nature of stuttering; the author, a journalist, reviews theories and therapies and tells what was effective for him.)

Kidd, K. K., T. Reich, and S. Kessler. Abstract of paper presented to the 12th International Congress of Genetics, *Genetics*, **74**, 2 (1973), p. 137.

Kimura, D., "Functional Asymmetry of the Brain in Dichotic Listening." *Cortex*, **3** (1967), 163–178.

Lanyon, R. I., "Speech: Relation of Nonfluency to Information Value." *Science*, **164** (April 3, 1969), 451–452.

Leske, M. C., "Speech Prevalence Estimates of Communicative Disorders in the U.S., Speech Disorders," *ASHA*, 23 (1981), 217–225.

Luper, H. L. and S. C. Ford, "Disorders of Fluency." In R. J. Van Hattum, Ed., *Communication Disorders*. New York: Macmillan Publishing Co., Inc., 1980, Chap. 7.

Luper, H. L., and R. L. Mulder, *Stuttering Therapy for Children*. Englewood Cliffs, N.J.: Prentice-Hall, Inc., 1964. (Addressed to public school speech clinicians and emphasizes therapeutic approaches for stuttering children that the authors have found to be practical, operational, and effective.)

McClay, H. and C. E. Osgood. "Hesitation Phenomena in Spontaneous Speech," *Word*, **15** (1959), 19–44.

McDearmon, J. R., "Primary Stuttering at the Onset of Stuttering: A Re-examination of Data." *Journal of Speech and Hearing Research*, **11** (September 1968), 631–637.

Muma, J. "Syntax of Preschool Fluent and Dysfluent Speech," *Journal of Speech and Hearing Research*, **14** (1971), 428–441.

Murphy, A. T., and R. M. FitzSimons, *Stuttering and Personality Dynamics*. New York: The Ronald Press Company, 1960.

Nelson, W. E., "The Role of Heredity in Stuttering." *Journal of Pediatrics*, **14** (1939), 642–654.

Orton, S., *Reading, Writing and Speech Problems*. New York: W. W. Norton & Company, Inc., 1937. (A pioneer but still highly relevant consideration of organic factors underlying language disorders.)

Perrin, K., *An Examination of Ear Preference for Speech and Non-Speech in a Stuttering Population*. Ph.D. dissertation, Stanford University, 1969.

Pratt, J. *Comparisons of Linguistic Perception and Production in Preschool Stutterers and Nonstutterers*, Doctoral Dissertation, University of Illinois (Urbana), 1972.

Records, M. A., K. K. Kidd, and J. K. Kidd. "Stuttering Among Relatives of Stutterers." Address to the American Speech and Hearing Association, 1976.

Sander, E., "Untangling Stuttering: A Tour Through the Theory Thicket, *ASHA*, **17** (1975), 256–262.

Schwartz, M. F., *Stuttering Solved*. New York, McGraw-Hill Book Company, 1977.

Shames, G. H., and D. B. Egolf, *Operant Conditioning and the Management of Stuttering*. Englewood Cliffs, N.J.: Prentice-Hall, Inc., 1976. (Intended for clinicians; describes how operant procedures can be used in the treatment of stutterers, including young ones.)

——, and C. E. Sherrick, "A Discussion of Non-Fluency and Stuttering as Operant Behavior." *Journal of Speech and Hearing Disorders*, **28** (February 1963), 3–18.

Sheehan, J. G., *Stuttering: Research and Therapy*. New York: Harper & Row, Publishers, Inc., 1970.

————, "Conflict Theory and Avoidance-Reduction Therapy," in J. Eisenson, ed., *Stuttering: A Second Symposium.* New York: Harper & Row, Publishers, Inc., 1975.

Slorach, N., and B. Noehr, "Dichotic Listening in Stuttering and Dyslalic Children." *Cortex,* **9** (1973), 295–300.

Sommers, R. K., W. A. Brady, and W. H. Moore, "Dichotic Ear Preferences of Stuttering Children and Adults." *Perceptual and Motor Skills,* **41** (1975), 931–938.

Stemach, G., Unpublished pilot study employing language sampling with stuttering children. Institute for Childhood Aphasia, San Francisco State University, 1977.

Travis, L. E., "The Unspeakable Feelings of People with Special Reference to Stuttering." in L. E. Travis, ed., *Handbook of Speech Pathology and Audiology,* New York: Appleton-Century-Crofts, 1971, pp. 1009–1033.

Van Riper, C., *Speech Correction,* 6th ed. Englewood Cliffs, N.J.: Prentice-Hall, Inc., 1978. (Chapter 8 presents Van Riper's revised and practical considerations of the nature and treatment of stuttering. The treatment is both objective and sympathetic, strongly recommended for teachers and clinicians.)

————, *The Nature of Stuttering.* Englewood Cliffs, N.J.: Prentice-Hall, Inc., 1971. (A major contribution in the area of stuttering. Van Riper reviews the literature on stuttering to provide a comprehensive view of the disorder. A monumental work!)

————, and J. V. Irwin, *Voice and Articulation.* Englewood Cliffs, N.J.: Prentice-Hall, Inc., 1958, chaps. 7–13.

Weiss, D. A., "Therapy for Cluttering." *Folia Phoniatrica,* **12** (1960), 216–228.

————, *Cluttering,* Englewood Cliffs, N.J.: Prentice-Hall, Inc., 1964.

Williams, D., "Stuttering." In J. F. Curtis, Ed., *Processes and Disorders of Communication.* New York: Harper & Row, Publishers, Inc., 1978, Chap. 8.

Wingate, M. E., "Evaluation and Stuttering, Part I: Speech Characteristics for Young Children." *Journal of Speech and Hearing Disorders,* **26** (May 1962) 106–115.

Wolpe, J., "Behavior Therapy of Stuttering: Deconditioning the Emotional Factor." In B. G. Gray, and G. England, *Stuttering and the Conditioning Therapies.* Monterey, Calif.: The Monterey Institute for Speech and Hearing, 1969 (a).

————, *The Practice of Behavior Therapy.* New York: Pergamon Press 1969(b).

Wyatt, G., *Language Learning and Communication Disorders in Children.* New York: The Free Press, 1969.

14

Impaired Hearing:
Implications for
Speech and Language

Most of us—parents, clinicians or teachers—have had experience with children who earnestly look as if they are listening and may in fact be listening hard and intently, yet on occasion fail to understand much of what is said to them. Many of these children may be impaired in hearing. Usually they are not so impaired as to give up trying to understand spoken language. Sometimes they succeed if the spoken words are accompanied by gestures, or if the speaker speaks "loud and clear." But there are other occasions when the task of comprehension is beyond them. A head cold or an allergic involvement of the upper respiratory system makes the effort of listening a frustrating one. We are describing children who may have a mild to moderate hearing loss, as well as some of the circumstances that enhance hearing and others that may aggravate difficulties in hearing and listening.

Any teacher who has taught 100 or more different children is likely to have at least one with some degree of impaired hearing. In some instances the child's articulation was also defective, and perhaps so was the extent of the child's vocabulary and competence for producing conventional syntactical sentences. Generally, the degree of the hearing impairment will be related to the presence and severity of the speech/language problems. A child may produce a voice that is either lacking in adequate loudness or, less frequently, overloud. Conductive losses, which are discussed later, are often associated with inadequate loudness. In contrast, a nerve (sensorineural) loss is associated with an overloud voice. We expand later on the types of speech problems associated with impaired hearing. First, however, we consider briefly some aspects of sound and the reception and perception of speech sound by the hearing mechanism.

SOUND AND THE SPEECH RANGE

Sound for our purposes may be considered the result of energy so applied to a body capable of vibration that it produces waves (disturbances of air) at a rate and in a manner that makes them perceptible to the human ear. Normal, young persons can hear sounds between 20 and 20,000 Hz (cycles per second or cps). Adults, after age 30 or 40, tend to lose hearing in the upper ranges, above 8,000 or 10,000 Hz. However, since most of the sounds of speech lie within the range 250–4,000 Hz, adults of "middle age" suffer no impairment of hearing for speech. Older adults frequently do, however.

The decibel or dB is the unit of intensity of sound. Very simply stated, intensity varies directly as the amount of energy applied to the body capable of vibration. However, sounds of different pitch are discernible to us at different intensity levels. This, we believe, is related to the differences in the sensitivity of the endings of the auditory nerve in the cochlea of the inner ear. Thus, we may hear sounds within one part of our pitch range at a relatively low intensity, as compared with sounds within a different part of the pitch range that may be perceived (heard) only at higher intensity levels.

THE HEARING MECHANISM

The External and Middle Ear

The external ear, or pinna, is part of the auditory mechanism that most of us refer to as the ear. Its function, to a limited degree, is to help us to "gather in" sound. This function may be enhanced by using a hand to cup over the ear. The pinna includes a skin-lined canal leading to the eardrum or tympanic membrane (see Figure 14).

The middle ear is a small cavity on the inner side of the eardrum. The middle ear includes three tiny bones, or ossicles: the malleus (hammer), the incus (anvil), and the stapes (stirrup). The named designations correspond to their resemblance to the objects (see Figure 15). The malleus is directly attached to the eardrum. The incus constitutes a connection or bridge between the malleus and the stapes. These os-

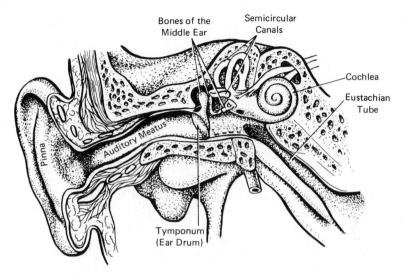

FIGURE 14. A sectional view of the ear.

sicles are connected but normally *not rigidly fixed* to positions within the middle ear by attachments of ligament and tiny muscles. Thus, the ossicles are able to move whenever the eardrum moves, as it does whenever it is stimulated by sound waves (air vibrations). The movements of the ossicles transmit the vibrations of the eardrum from the middle ear to the inner ear.

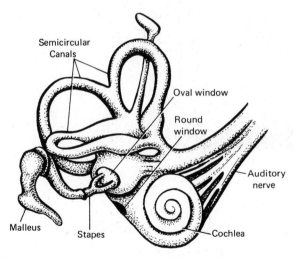

FIGURE 15. Enlarged representation of the middle and inner ear: the ossicles, cochlea, and semicircular canals.

The Inner Ear

The inner ear includes (1) the semicircular canals, (2) the cochlea, a snail-shaped structure that contains tiny hairlike structures of varying length, which are in fact the sensitive endings of the auditory nerve, and (3) the vestibule, a connecting area between the semicircular canals and the cochlea.

When air vibrations cause movements of the eardrum, the impulses are transmitted to the stapes, which in turn produces movements of the fluid that fills the vestibule. These vestibular-fluid movements stimulate the nerve endings in the cochlea. The stimulations received from the auditory nerve endings are carried by way of the auditory (eighth cranial) nerve to the temporal area of the brain cortex, producing the experience we refer to as sound perception or hearing.[1]

HEARING IMPAIRMENT

Classification

Although "functional" definitions of hearing loss are presented in this section, it is essential to appreciate that the effect of hearing loss is variable. For some persons, what may be regarded as a relatively small amount of hearing loss may be associated with greater impairment of hearing in particular and adjustment in general than a measurably greater amount of hearing loss for other persons. Even among persons born with severe hearing loss, some are able to make considerably better use of a small amount of residual hearing than others. With these reservations in mind, "practical" definitions are offered.

The *deaf* are those for whom the sense of hearing is so impaired as to have precluded normal acquisition of language. Somewhat more broadly, the deaf are those for whom the capacity to hear is so limited as to be considered nonfunctioning for the ordinary purposes of life. Children who are deaf either (1) are not able to learn speech through the avenue of hearing or (2), if their hearing impairment was acquired shortly after "natural" speech was learned, have lost their speaking ability or have become severely impaired in it.

The deaf may be divided into two subgroups according to onset of impairment. The *congenitally deaf* are those who are born without hearing. The *adventitiously deaf* are those who were born with hear-

---

[1] See the discussion of the speech mechanism in Chapter 5 for the function of the left temporal cortex in the analysis of speech sounds.

ing sufficient for the acquisition of speech but later, as a result of illness or accident, suffered severe hearing impairment.

The *hard of hearing* are those for whom the sense of hearing, although defective, is functional with or without a hearing aid. Hard-of-hearing children, although frequently with considerable defects, learn to speak essentially through the avenue of hearing.

Newby (1979, p. 393) classifies hearing loss into six groups that are associated with common descriptive terms as follows:

Hearing Loss*	Degree of Impairment
20–30 decibels	slight
30–45 decibels	mild
45–60 decibels	moderate
60–75 decibels	severe
75–90 decibels	profound
90–110 decibels	extreme

* Listener has difficulty hearing at intensity levels (decibels) below (less than) those indicated.

Northern and Downs (1978, p. 44), observe that the effects of hearing loss vary considerably according to whether it is unilateral or bilateral.

> The child with a totally dead ear on one side but with a normal ear on the other side may function quite well in most situations. . . . This youngster's auditory abilities will be lacking in circumstances where sound localization is needed or in instances when noise exists to compete with the signal of interest.

The practical and fundamental criterion for the distinction between the deaf and the hard-of-hearing is *in the manner in which* the child acquires an oral/aural language system. The deaf then include those who require specialized instruction to learn to talk, or to acquire a substitute (visual) system for the normal oral/aural system. The hard-of-hearing are those who learned to speak essentially in the normal developmental manner of hearing children.

Children with hearing impairments are educated in a variety of settings. Those who are deaf are most likely to be educated in special schools or in special classes in "regular" schools. Some deaf children continue to be educated in residential schools. Most hard-of-hearing children attend classes with normal-hearing peers.

For educational placement, Moores (1978) broke down levels of hearing loss into these categories according to loss in decibels (dB):

1. Level I, 35–54 dB. Individuals in this category seldom require special class/school placement; the children do require special speech and hearing assistance.
2. Level II, 55–69 dB. Only occasionally do children with this range of hearing loss require special class/school placement; they do require and generally benefit from special speech, hearing, and language assistance.
3. Level III, 70–89dB. In this category of deafness most children require special class/school placement; they also require special speech, hearing, language, and educational assistance.
4. Level IV, 90 dB and beyond. Children with hearing loss in this range almost always require special class/school placement; In addition they also require special speech, hearing, language, and educational assistance.

Incidence

It is difficult to arrive at "hard" figures for the incidence of hearing loss even in the school-age population on whom figures are relatively easy to gather. Silverman (1971, pp. 402–403) notes that on the basis of mass-testing surveys among schoolchildren, reported percentages of findings of hearing loss range from 2 to 21 per cent. "This great variability in reports of hearing impairment is undoubtedly due to differences in definitions of hearing impairments, in techniques, apparatus and conditions of testing, and in the socioeconomic status and climate of the communities in which the surveys were carried out." Silverman accepts that about 5 per cent of school-age children have hearing levels at least in one ear that are outside of the normal range.

The 1969 report of the Subcommittee on Human Communication and Its Disorders to the National Institute of Neurological Diseases and Stroke (1969, p. 15) includes an estimate of hearing loss in the United States. According to the report, about 250,000 children of school age have hearing losses of sufficient severity to impair their communication ability and their social efficiency. Approximately 40,000 children are deaf.

On the basis of recent available data, Davis and Hardick (1981, p. 141) believe that there are at least 20 times as many children who have mild to moderate hearing losses compared to those with severe to profound losses. They report several studies that indicate that children with mild to moderate losses have reduced language skills and some may be at risk for academic achievement when compared with children with less than 15 dB loss. Davis and Hardick conclude that "If all of these children are included in the incidence figures, there are probably more than two million of them in the public schools."

TYPES OF HEARING LOSS AND RELATED SPEECH AND LANGUAGE IMPAIRMENTS

Conductive Loss

Conductive loss is associated with external or middle ear abnormalities that impede the transmission of energy (vibratory energy producing sound) to the middle ear. Abnormalities may include an accumulation of hardened wax (cerumen), the presence of a foreign body, and structural malformations, such as an incomplete canal or an exceedingly narrow ear canal. The external ear may be inflamed by disease processes that may affect other skin surfaces. Except for the structural abnormalities, the resultant hearing loss is likely to be temporary, that is, lasting only as long as the abnormal condition persists.

Middle-ear involvements include conditions that impair the vibratory-transmassive functions of the ossicles, infections of the middle ear, which are often associated with upper respiratory disease (the common cold), allergies, or excessive fluid, often associated with inflammation in the middle ear, and enlarged adenoidal tissue growth in the area of the nasopharnyx.

Because conductive losses are usually the result of temporary pathologies, most children with such impairments are likely to have normal speech. Chronic involvements may be associated with an inadequately loud voice. This, as suggested earlier, may be the result of the child's hearing his/her own voice louder than he/she is able to hear the voices of other speakers. The child assumes, therefore, that he/she is speaking loudly enough to be heard, even though he/she may be barely audible to others. This interesting phenomenon takes place because the child with conductive loss hears himself/herself through the vibrations produced by his/her vocalization by way of the bones of the head. If the inner ear is normal, the nerve endings will respond to these vibrations. However, the child's self-hearing is not modified by the vibrations that normally would also come to him/her through air vibration by way of the external and middle ears. The child with conductive loss also hears the voices of others as less loud than they sound to normal ears.

Denasality is also likely to characterize the voice and the nasal consonant sound production of the child with respiratory infections or with enlarged adenoids. Speech, as far as articulation in general is concerned, is likely to be unaffected in children with mild conductive loss of hearing. Chronic conductive hearing impairment, if more than of mild degree, is likely to be associated with distortion and omissions of speech sounds.

Sensorineural Hearing Loss

Sensorineural hearing loss results from involvements of the inner ear or those of the eighth (auditory) nerve. Reception and perception (discrimination) of sound are impaired. Such losses, especially if they are congenital or had their onset before speech was acquired, are associated with vocal, articulatory, and linguistic defects. Children with severe degrees of nerve involvement may make little or no sense out of the speech to which they are exposed because they will have difficulty in the analysis of the complex sounds that constitute spoken language. Usually, high-pitched sounds, including those that comprise most of the consonants of speech, are within the range of impaired hearing. Voiced and vowel sounds, if produced with sufficient loudness, are usually heard and perceived. Some children may speak excessively loudly in order to hear themselves. They may produce vowels acceptably but have difficulty with consonants, especially the high-frequency sibilants and the velar stops, which are not readily visible. They may confuse voiced and voiceless cognate sounds. With severe impairment, children cannot readily hear functor words (prepositions, conjunctions, articles)—which normally are not given much emphasis in running speech—or grammatical markers (plurals, tense endings). Their verbal productions may also be characterized as ungrammatical or agrammatical. They will, therefore, be linguistically deficient.

Some bright children who are skilled in visual speech (lip) reading, which they may learn without direct teaching, may have good comprehension of speech and may themselves have fairly good articulation. Children who are not skilled in visual reading may have severe difficulty in comprehending speech. With the usual reservation for the exceptional child, the severity of speech and language impairment is generally related directly to the severity of the sensorineural loss. Usually the age at which the hearing loss, if progressive, became severe is another factor affecting the quality of speech. As a rule, the later the age after speech onset, the better is the overall speech quality.

Mixed Hearing Loss

Mixed hearing loss combines the impairments of conductive and nerve loss. The cause is the existence of both conductive (transmissive) and sensorineural pathology. In effect, the child with such combined pathology will have difficulty in receiving sound signals as well as difficulty in analyzing (perceiving) those signals that—however weakly—are received. Unless the conductive condition is chronic, the speech characteristics of the child will be related to the factors associated with sensorineural loss.

Central Auditory Impairment

Some children, fortunately few in number but complex in the severity of their impairments, may be able to respond to nonspeech auditory signals as most children do, but are still unable to make sense out of speech sounds. These children hear spoken language but have severe difficulty in interpreting what they hear. We consider these children—tentatively diagnosed as aphasic—in Chapter 16.

MEASUREMENT OF HEARING LOSS

Hearing loss is objectively measured in terms of decibels. From our point of view, we may consider a decibel the minimum unit of intensity necessary for us to appreciate a difference between the loudness of sounds.

The pure-tone audiometer, which is widely used as an objective instrument for measuring possible hearing loss, is an electrical instrument designed to produce a number of tones of discrete or individual frequencies at intensity levels that can be controlled. Most modern pure-tone audiometers cover the frequency range between approximately 125 and 12,000 Hz (cycles) per second. Many audiologists in their examinations, however, do not consider it necessary to go beyond 8,000 Hz. On a pure-tone audiometer the weakest sound that can normally be heard is considered as zero decibels.

Losses are measured in terms of the normal threshold of hearing for tones at specified pitch levels and are stated in decibels. The following tables suggest how we would evaluate the results of a pure-tone audiometric examination. We should always bear in mind, however, that many factors other than the "objective" amount of hearing loss enter into the effect of the loss for the given individual.

We strongly recommend Newby's (1972, p. 114) observation as to the need for assessing functional hearing as well as the results of pure-tone audiometry. Says Newby:

> Although the audiogram yields important information concerning the rehabilitative needs of patients, it is most valuable when the information it conveys is combined with the results of clinical speech audiometric tests, which measured directly a patient's ability to hear and understand speech. After all, the measure of the handicap of a hearing loss is how one's communicative ability is affected. Whereas predictions of how communication is affected can be made from the pure-tone audiogram with some certainty, actual measures of the communicative ability can be derived through speech audiometry.

See Table (Classes of Hearing Handicaps), p. 433.

Identification Audiometry

Identification audiometry signifies the application of appropriate hearing test procedures leading to an initial discovery of a hearing loss.[2] In the ordinary school situations, a screening test rather than a complete audiometric examination is likely to be given as the first step in the evaluation of a child's hearing. An early and still widely used screening device is the fading-numbers test. A recorded voice is played back and listened to through earphones, either by a single child or by a group of children.

The usual recording is of a sequence of numbers, which fade out at the end of the sequence. The results provide information *under the conditions of testing* about the intensity levels at or above which a selected speech sample—a sequence of numbers—can be heard. Unfortunately, as Newby (1979, pp. 296–297) points out, a fading-numbers test is not an accurate indicator of a child's ability to hear normal running speech. The test does have merit as a rough screening device that permits relatively quick assessment of the hearing of many children. Unhappily, as the *ASHA* Guidelines point out, the fading-numbers test often passed children with hearing losses in the range above 500 Hz.; actually, with losses as high as 50 decibels in the range of 1,000–2,000 Hz. Figure 16 is of a frequently used Audiogram Form. Figure 17 indicates the frequency range of modern telephones.

Other Hearing Tests

THE MASSACHUSETTS HEARING TEST. Another technique that permits screening of children on a group basis is the Massachusetts

[2] See ASHA Committee on Audiometric Evaluation, "Guidelines for Identification Audiometry," *ASHA* (February 1975), pp. 94–99.

Classes of Hearing Handicap

DB	CLASS	DEGREE OF HANDICAP	*Average Hearing Threshold Level for 500, 1,000 and 2,000 in the Better Ear**		ABILITY TO UNDERSTAND SPEECH
			MORE THAN	NOT MORE THAN	
	A	Not signi-ficant		25 dB (ISO)	No significant difficulty with faint speech.
25					
	B	Slight handicap	25 dB (ISO)	40 dB	Difficulty only with faint speech.
40					
	C	Mild handicap	40 dB	55 dB	Frequent diffi-culty with normal speech.
55					
	D	Marked handicap	55 dB	70 dB	Frequent diffi-culty even for loud speech.
70					
	E	Severe handicap	70 dB	90 dB	Can under-stand only shouted or amplified speech.
90					
	F	Extreme handicap	90 dB		Usually cannot understand even ampli-fied speech.

* Whenever the average for the poorer ear is 25 dB or more greater than that of the better ear in this frequency range, 5 dB are added to the average for the better ear. This adjusted average determines the degree and class of handicap. For example, if a person's average hearing threshold level for 500, 1000, and 2000 Hz/s is 37 dB in one ear and 62 dB or more in the other, his adjusted average hearing threshold level is 42 dB and his handi-cap is Class C instead of Class B. Source: Davis, 1978, p. 271.

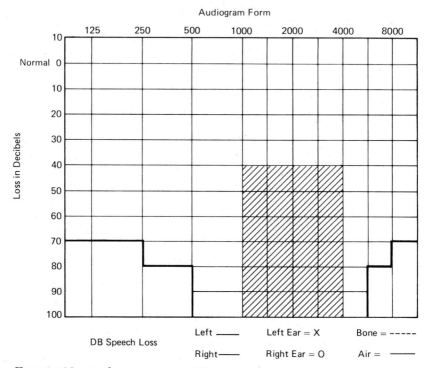

FIGURE 16. Audiogram Form. The shaded area indicates the hearing range most critical for the reception of speech.

Hearing Test.[3] This is a pure-tone rather than a speech-hearing test which was devised to permit screening testing of as many as 40 children at one time at three critical frequencies within the range of normal speech. The usual frequencies tested are 500, 4,000, and 6,000 Hz. Each of these frequencies is presented at sensation (loudness) levels of 20, 25, and 30 decibels, respectively. Responses are ordinarily entered on a prepared test blank and consist of a "Yes" or "No" to indicate whether the child who is being examined does or does not hear the spurt of pure-tone sound produced by the test instrument. An audiometrist signals the individual child or children when the response to the sound is expected. According to a prearranged plan, the audiometrist may not always present a tone and signal for a

[3] This and other testing techniques specially suitable in the school situation are described in some detail in Chapter 8 of H. Newby's *Audiology* (New York: Prentice-Hall, Inc., 1979). See also J. Northern and M. P. Downs, *Hearing in Children* (Baltimore: The Williams & Wilkins Co., 1978), Chap. 5 for an in-depth discussion of the purposes and types of identification audiometry for children beginning in early infancy.

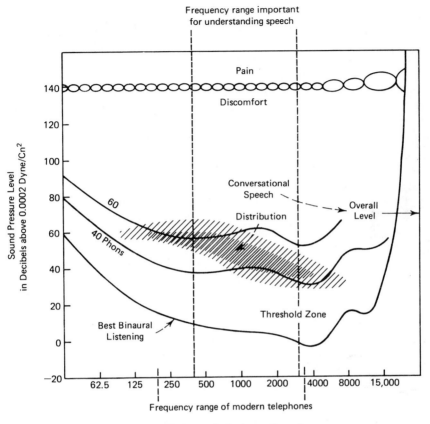

FIGURE 17. The Speech Area. Speech is a mixture of complex tones, wide band noise, and transients. Both the intensities and the frequencies of speech sounds change continually and rapidly. It is difficult to measure them and logically impossible to plot them precisely in terms of sound pressure levels.

response. Throughout this procedure, some "No" responses are expected, and such entries should appear on each test blank.

THE SWEEP TEST. Another approach for screening employing pure-tone audiometry is the sweep test. This testing is done with a pure-tone audiometer, and results are obtained in a very few minutes. In sweep testing the dial is set at a critical point, with allowances made for the room and the "free-floating" noise in the surroundings. The most usual setting is 15 decibels. The examiner then "sweeps" through the frequency range. The child is instructed to signal whether or not the tone produced is heard at each frequency.

A NEW TEST. A recent addition to screening tests utilizing standard audiometric equipment (pure-tone audiometry) and headsets is described by Hollien, Wepman, and Thompson (1969). Up to 40 children at a time can be screen-tested in about 15 minutes. This test can be administered by a classroom teacher, a school nurse, or any trained adult. The frequencies employed are 500, 1,000, and 4,000 Hz; the hearing levels used are 35, 25, and 20 decibels. ASA standards are used.

As the name suggests, the purpose of screening tests is to single out individuals who may have significant losses of hearing at the time of the testing. Final evaluations should include more thorough individual pure-tone testing as well as speech testing through speech audiometry. In addition, of course, an otological examination should be routine. For a review of individual and group hearing screening procedures, see Anderson (1978).

Hearing Conservation in the Schools

In many public schools, the responsibility for discovering hearing loss among the children has become an integral part of the overall health conservation program. The development of this aspect of the detection and treatment of children's health needs has received considerable impetus from the availability of instruments and techniques for assessing hearing loss that can easily be used in school settings.

School hearing conservation programs have two fundamental purposes. The first is the earliest possible detection of hearing loss so that children, whenever possible, may be referred for medical treatment in the hope that in many instances permanent hearing impairment may be prevented. The second purpose is to provide for the special needs —educational, speech, language and audiological—of children whose hearing may not be directly subject to improvement but who can be helped to conserve and make maximum use of their hearing capacities.

Responsibility for the actual assessment of hearing loss varies considerably among school systems. Many large school districts conduct their own hearing testing and conservation programs. Some smaller school districts may contract for hearing services with professional agencies or audiology clinics associated with colleges or universities. In some school districts, audiologists or audiometrists are engaged whose responsibilities include the assessment of the children's hearing throughout the grades.

The concentration, as Newby (1979, p. 293) points out, should be in the primary grades. Children in these grades are likely to have a higher percentage of upper respiratory ailments and other conditions associated with temporary hearing loss that may become chronic if untreated. Fortunately, most of these conditions respond favorably to medical treatment. As a result, the discovery of treatable conditions that produce hearing loss will appreciably reduce the incidence of hearing impairment and associated educational and social problems in the upper school grades.

In many schools, including those that provide organized audiological services, the detection of possible hearing loss continues to be the responsibility of the classroom teacher or the school nurse. The nurse may note a child's difficulty in hearing in her routine examination of the children. The classroom teacher, however, has a daily opportunity to detect whether a child, habitually or occasionally, seems to have difficulty in hearing. Children who frequently misunderstand directions, or who ask that questions be repeated, or who look blankly at the teacher talking or at classmates should be checked for possible hearing loss. The teacher should also watch for the child who seems to hear only when spoken to from one side of the room but fails to hear what is said when spoken to from the opposite side. Some children unconsciously turn their heads to favor the better ear. If these habits and manifestations are associated with poor articulation and with voice production that is inappropriate in quality and loudness, hearing loss should be suspected. Additional significant signs of hearing loss include poor coordination, poor balance, occasional dizziness, and complaints of earaches and of running ears. A child suspected of hearing loss should be referred to the school physician for further examination. If the school has no physician, the possibility of the child's hearing loss should be discussed with the principal and, of course, with the parents, and then referred to a physician for medical evaluation and whatever other referral may be needed.

THERAPY FOR THE CHILD WITH A HEARING IMPAIRMENT

Hearing Aids

Many children whose hearing losses range from moderate to severe are able to get considerable help from a properly fitted hearing aid. The decision whether a hearing aid is needed should be made by the otologist, a medical specialist. The actual fitting of the hearing aid may be done either by the otologist or an accredited professional audiologist.[4] Although many individual factors enter into the usefulness of hearing aids, experience indicates that hearing aids are usually indicated for children when the hearing loss is between 35 and 70 decibels in the pitch range most important for speech. This range is roughly between 200 and 4,000 Hz (ASA standard). For children with more severe hearing losses, exceeding 70 decibels in the pitch range, the help to be derived from a hearing aid is limited. In some instances, only the awareness that there is noise and activity about is made available to the user. This may be important, however, in preventing the child from feeling isolated by inner silence if a hearing aid is not used. To be able to anticipate that someone is about to enter a house because the ringing of a doorbell is heard is often considerably better than to be caught by surprise, or to fail to answer a doorbell because it is not heard.

If a hearing aid is indicated, training in its care and proper use is in order.[5] Such training may be provided by the otologist or by the audiologist associated with a medical center, college, or university speech and hearing clinic, or in private practice.

It is imporant to appreciate that a hearing aid does not serve to give the user normal hearing in the same sense that properly fitted eyeglasses give most users essentially the equivalent of normal vision. The hearing instrument, as its name suggests, is only an aid. It helps the wearers make more complete use of the hearing they have. If the hearing loss is moderate rather than severe, and an individual learns how to employ the aid effectively, hearing that is functionally close to normal may be achieved. If, in addition, the individual learns speech reading (lip reading), comprehension close to normal may be achieved. For the severely impaired, speech reading is of greater importance than for those with moderate hearing loss. The hearing aid has more limited application and value for the deaf, but together with speech reading, it can be of significant help.

Speech reading implies the use of all visual cues in interpreting (decoding) what a speaker says. Speech reading entails more than the

---

[4] Many college and university clinics, as well as medical centers, provide services for the selection of hearing aids. Professionally accredited audiologists may also engage in private practice.

[5] Criteria for determining the need for a hearing aid are considered by H. A. Newby, *Audiology*, 4th ed. (New York: Prentice-Hall, 1979), pp. 187–188 and by J. Northern and M. P. Downs, *Hearing in Children* (Baltimore: The Williams & Wilkins Co., 1978), pp. 227–252. Both of these sources emphasize the need for flexibility and the responses of the individual child rather than fixed audiometrically determined level of hearing loss.

See also Ross in Katz, J., *Handbook of Clinical Audiology*, Baltimore: Williams and Wilkins, 1978, Chap. 43.

reading of lips. It requires that the listener be attentive to all of the visible movements of the speaker that are involved in the communication of a message.

Speech and Hearing Therapy

Proper medical attention may help many children as well as adults to conserve whatever hearing they have. Proper speech and listening training should help them make the maximum use of their hearing and conserve the quality and intelligibility of their speech.

The hearing therapist helps the child to make maximal use of his/her residual hearing as well as effective use of the hearing aid, if one is used. In addition, the child is made aware of all the aspects of sound production so that tactile as well as auditory and visible cues are recognized and utilized. In this way, the child not only becomes more completely responsive to how other persons speak but also responds to his/her own speech with greater awareness. The result is better articulation, better voice, and improved intelligibility. In working with the schoolchild, specific instruction is correlated with academic subject matter. The vocabulary of a new subject is introduced and becomes the core of the speech and hearing instruction.

Newby (1979, pp. 431–433) summarizes the goals of an auditory training program along the following lines:

1. Persuade the child to accept the hearing aid.
2. Teach the child to operate the hearing aid so effectively that he/she will not want to do without it.
3. It may be desirable in the early stages of training to prevent the child from observing visual cues so that concentration and attention may be given to auditory signals. However, the long-range objective is to help in the development of the child's overall communicative abilities to their fullest extent. "Therefore, auditory training should usually be combined with speech reading, and while the comprehension of speech is being taught emphasis must also be placed on helping the child to improve his own speech."

THE ROLE OF THE CLASSROOM TEACHER WITH THE HARD OF HEARING

The classroom teacher shares social and educational responsibilities with the speech/language clinician in the interests of the hard-of-hearing child that are like those for other children in the classroom, but just more so. The teacher can help the child to obtain a sense of social competence and to function normally in a school setting. Hard-of-hearing children are inclined to withdraw and isolate themselves from others, especially when the going is rough. The teacher must be on the alert for such signs and behaviors, and attract the child to group activities. Through the assignment of regular as well as inspiration-of-the-moment responsibilities, the teacher can help the hard-of-hearing child to feel and be accepted as a fully participating member of the group.

Perhaps more than anything else, the teacher should encourage oral language through recitation activities in class as well as in less formal discussion and conversation. Reading is of especial importance for the hard-of-hearing child. Through reading, grammatical markers, functor words, and syntactic structures may become more readily apparent than in heard speech.

The physical placement of the hard-of-hearing child in the classroom is particularly important. The following suggestions will enhance the likelihood that the child will have full awareness of what is going on in the classroom:

1. Make certain that the child is seated where speakers are best seen and heard.
2. Seat the child where there is the least amount of interfering noise. A seat up front in the aisle farthest from the window should accomplish this objective. However, the child should be permitted to move as freely as space permits if the teacher needs to move to another part of the classroom.
3. Make certain that there is no light glare in the child's eyes.
4. When addressing the hard-of-hearing child, speak naturally but somewhat more loudly and slowly than otherwise might be necessary.
5. Use appropriate gestures freely but without exaggeration, especially if the word or idea is new.
6. Emphasize the use of prepared visual materials. Use the blackboard for writing words, phrases, and sentences associated with the essential material of the oral presentation.
7. Remember to observe the child for signs of lack of comprehension or confusion. If material is repeated, it should as closely as possible be an exact repetition. If rephrasing is in order, provide cues that you are indeed rephrasing and not repeating. Something such as, "I will say it another way." should do. The "other way" should be in clear syntactic structures.
8. If the child is using a hearing aid, make certain that it is operational, batteries are on and working, and ear piece is properly fixed.

EDUCATION OF THE HEARING IMPAIRED: THE DEAF

Silverman, Lane, and Calvert (in Davis and Silverman, 1978, Chap. 17) review the educational problems of preschool and elementary-school-age deaf children and emphasize the need for their early education. Silverman et al. are aware that the deaf tend to lag behind their hearing age peers in educational achievement at all levels of schooling. They note:

> The deaf child generally does not learn at the same rate as the hearing child. With the need to master new vocabulary and language, it takes about two or more years to achieve second-grade level and an additional one and a half to two years to complete third grade. This plateau in learning may be discouraging, but it is not the fault of the child or teacher. It can be attributed to the time necessary to build a foundation for future progress.

With important individual exceptions, the deaf have difficulty in acquiring syntactic (grammatical) systems on a level with the hearing. These difficulties become readily apparent in their writing. Quigley and Power (1977) report on investigations on the development of syntax in deaf children. They note errors in verb tense, in the use of auxiliaries, and in constructions involving relative clauses. To a lesser degree, deaf children have difficulties with question constructions, negation, and conjunctions. Silverman et al. (p. 470) are not certain whether the differences in syntactic proficiency are products of instructional methods or are in some way the result of learning difficulties imposed by deafness.

Furth (1973, pp. 92–93) sums up his view of the underlying educational problem of the deaf in no uncertain terms. Says Furth:

> Here in a nutshell is the problem of the education for deaf children. The one educational objective to which nearly all energies are turned is language. The colossal reading failure . . . reflects a deficiency in the knowledge of language and not, as would be the case with hearing children, a reading disability.

Furth also notes that

> A person who has been profoundly deaf from birth and who can read at Grade 5 or better is invariably an exception.

Apparently there are exceptions to the delayed and impaired language acquisitions and the retarded educational achievements of the deaf. Some deaf children and adults are educated in settings for the hearing and are able to make progress comparable with that of their hearing peers. It would help considerably to know what makes these

exceptional deaf different from others with, at least by objective measurements, an equal amount of hearing loss. Why can't many more, if
not most, of the deaf be educated in classes along with the hearing?
These questions, to which we have no answers, suggest the nature of
the controversy between those who are still advocates of the oral
method of instruction and those who believe that the "natural" approach for teaching deaf children is through a manual (sign) system.

The Oralists, the Manualists, and Total Communication

Oralism

The proponents of *pure oralism (auditory stimulation)* recommend
that from the beginning—when a child is identified as deaf—the
child should be exposed to environmental sounds and spoken language at all possible opportunities. If possible and as early as possible, they feel, the deaf child should be fitted with a hearing aid. Northern and Downs (1978, pp. 263–267) explain the aural/oral approach
and present the arguments, pro and con, for this method of establishing language and teaching for the deaf. Furth (1973, Chap. 4), we
think with considerably less objectivity than Northern and Downs,
presents his arguments against oralism. Furth considers oralism in its
extreme form as "nothing less than the denial of deafness" and so considers it to be psychologically wrong. Furth strongly recommends the
total approach (signing accompanied by speaking on the part of the
parent or instructor).

The oral method, as developed and practiced in the Clarke School
for the Deaf in the United States, discourages the use of all signing.
Lip reading (speech reading) is emphasized, progressing from the recognition and imitative production of isolated phonemic elements,
sound combinations, words, and finally speech utterances.

As of 1970, Silverman and Lane report that 85 per cent of deaf children who were enrolled in schools for the deaf were, at least in their
early schooling, instructed by the oral method. The basic argument of
the proponents of the oral method is that every deaf child deserves
and should be afforded an opportunity to learn to communicate by
speech. Proponents of the oral method also argue that an early use of
signing will create a dependence on this (manual) approach and the
deaf child will not readily or willingly accept the more strenuous demands of the oral/aural approach. Consequently deaf children will be
limited in their social world and in vocational situations as compared
to the nonoral deaf. In effect, they will be socially and vocationally
isolated from the hearing world.

The opponents of pure oralism point to the low language and educational achievement of most deaf children as an argument against the method. Further, they argue that it is simply not natural for a deaf child to learn an oral/aural system of language. They point out that most deaf children, when left to themselves and presumably unobserved by their teachers, resort to signing because it is a natural mode for them. Other arguments to which we are sympathetic are that the oral method is a slow one and tends to retard language comprehension and production in the critical early years of life when such acquisition is readily and easily established. Specifically in regard to English, lip reading as a mode of speech reception must contend with too many "invisible" sounds and others that are so closely alike in manner of production as to cause confusion. At best, few persons become sufficiently skilled in lip reading to be at ease in conversation. Even those who do become skilled in lip reading need ideal environmental situations of light and distance, and a speaker who articulates carefully.

The Manual Method

A fundamental question in regard to the manual method (signing) is whether sign language is, in fact, a natural language or a limited and artificial one, comparable to pidgin.[6] The answer, at least since the late 1960s, as signing has been developing in the United States, is that whatever sign systems may once have been, some sign systems now incorporate many of the essential features and functions of a natural language. Perhaps the most widely used of the sign languages in the United States is the *American Sign Language* or *Ameslan*. A variant of *American Sign Language* is *SEE* (*Seeing Essential English*). The *SEE* system employs morphemes, English word order, and syntax. Still another system based on *Ameslan* is *SEE 2* (*Signing Exact English*). Mayberry (in Davis and Silverman, Chap. 15) describes the features of most of the sign systems now used in the United States.

It should be apparent that critics of the oral method recognized the limitations of older manual methods. The newer sign systems are attempts to provide a natural language system for the deaf that will permit communication more nearly comparable to the oral/aural systems of hearing persons.

Total Communication

The total approach to language education for the deaf combines manual, auditory, and oral methods. Children who are identified as deaf are exposed to this total approach as early as possible in their own

---

[6] Pidgin, by definition, is a simplified language used for special purposes and situations by speakers who are primarily speakers of different languages.

homes. Hearing parents of deaf children are themselves encouraged to learn signing and finger spelling and to use these visible methods along with oral speech.

The Total Communication approach is now being used experimentally in classes for the deaf in public schools. We earnestly hope that investigation can be carried on that will provide objective evidence of the values of all of these approaches and what kind of deaf child can best be taught by each one of the approaches. It is also possible that an issue we may need to assess is *when* one approach may be more effective than another.

Problems

1. Why is it not advisable to assess the effects of hearing loss solely in terms of the percentage of loss below normal hearing? What is normal hearing?
2. Distinguish between the deaf and the hard-of-hearing.
3. What are the most frequently used nonobjective techniques for detecting the presence of hearing loss?
4. Define or explain each of the following: (a) cps or Hz, (b) decibel, (c) pure tone, (d) audiometer, (e) audiogram, (f) sweep test, (g) hearing aid, (h) residual hearing.
5. Does a hearing aid give the same assistance to its user as properly fitted glasses do for most persons with visual impairment? Justify your answer.
6. What does *identification audiometry* mean? Describe three techniques commonly used in identification audiometry.
7. Why does Newby (1979) recommend testing for functional hearing, as well as pure-tone audiometry, in the assessment of hearing loss?
8. What specifically can the classroom teacher do for the child known to have a hearing loss? What can a hearing parent of a deaf child do?
9. What is the implication of age and acquisition of oral language in relation to an acquired hearing loss?
10. What are the characteristic voice and articulatory defects of a child with sensorineural hearing impairment?
11. How are children with hearing loss educated in your school district?
12. What are the objectives of an auditory training program?
13. What are the basic philosophical and methodological differences between oralists and manualists? In effect, can there be any *pure oralists*?
14. Describe some recent advances in sign languages. Which sign language meets the criteria of a natural language?
15. Why was a sign language (The American Sign Language) chosen to train chimpanzees in the use of a linguistic system? Why wasn't an oral/aural system selected?
16. Furth (1973) argues that too much attention is paid to teaching "correct" English to the deaf. Furth also believes that our priorities for the deaf are faulty. What priorities does he recommend? Indicate whether and why you either agree or disagree with him.

References and Suggested Readings

Anderson, C. V., "Hearing Screening for Children," in Katz, J. *Handbook of Clinical Audiology*, 2nd ed., Baltimore: Williams and Wilkins Company, 1978, Chap. 5.

ASHA Committee on Audiometric Evaluation, "Guidelines for Identification Audiometry." *ASHA*, **17**, 2 (1975), 94–99.

Davis, H., and S. R. Silverman, *Hearing and Deafness*, 4th ed. New York: Holt, Rinehart and Winston, Inc., 1978. (A lucidly written survey of research, including some of their own investigations, on problems of hearing.)

Davis, J. M. and E. J. Hardick, *Rehabilitative Audiology for Children and Adults*, New York: John Wiley and Sons, 1981.

Eagles, E. L., W. G. Hardy, and F. Catlin, *Human Communications*, Washington, D.C.: U.S. Dept. of Health, Education, and Welfare, 1968.

Furth, H. G., *Deafness and Learning*, Belmont, California: Wadsworth Publishing Co., Inc., 1973.

Hollien, H., J. M. Wepman, and C. L. Thompson, "A Group Screening Test of Auditory Acuity," *Journal of School Health*, **39**, 8 (1969), 583–588.

Moores, D., *Educating the Deaf: Psychology, Principles and Practices.* Boston, Massachusetts: Houghton Mifflin Company, 1978.

Newby, H., *Audiology*, 4th ed. Englewood Cliffs, N.J.: Prentice-Hall, Inc., 1979.

————, 3rd ed. New York: Appleton-Century-Crofts, 1972.

Northern, J. and M. P. Downs, *Hearing in Children*. Baltimore: Williams and Wilkins, 1978.

Northcott, W. H., *The Hearing Impaired Child in a Regular Classroom: Preschool, Elementary and Secondary Years.* Washington, D.C.: The Alexander Graham Bell Association for the Deaf, 1973. (Emphasizes the kind of planning needed by teachers, audiologists, speech pathologists, social workers, psychologists, and administrators in planning for the teaching of hearing-impaired children in integrated school programs.)

Quigley, S. P. and D. J. Power, "The Language Structure of Deaf Children." *Volta Review*, **79** (1977), 85–92.

Ross, M. "Hearing And Evaluation," In Katz, J., ed., *Handbook of Clinical Audiology*, Baltimore: Williams and Wilkins, 1978.

Sanders, D. A., "Psychological Implications of Hearing Impairment." In W. M. Cruickshank, *Psychology of Exceptional Children and Youth.* Englewood Cliffs, N.J.: Prentice Hall, 1980.

Silverman, S. R. "The Education of Deaf Children." In L. E. Travis, Ed., *Handbook of Speech Pathology and Audiology*, New York: Appleton-Century-Crofts, 1971, 399–430.

Silverman, S. R. and H. S. Lane, "Deaf Children." In Davis, H. and S. R. Silverman, *Hearing and Deafness*, New York: Holt, Rinehart, and Winston, 1970.

————, H. S. Lane, and D. R. Calvert, "Early and Elementary Education." In H. Davis and S. R. Silverman, *Hearing and Deafness*. New York: Holt, Rinehart and Winston, 1978.

Subcommittee on Human Communication and Its Disorders, *Human Communication and Its Disorders: An Overview.* Washington, D.C.: National Institute of Neurological Diseases and Stroke, U.S. Dept. of Health, Education and Welfare, 1969.

Van Riper, C., *Speech Correction,* 6th ed. Englewood Cliffs, N.J.: Prentice-Hall, Inc., 1978, Chap. 10.

Additional Recommended Readings

Culatta, B., and D. Horn. "Systematic Modification of Parental Input to Train Language Symbols." *Language, Speech, and Hearing Services in Schools,* **12,** 1 (1981), 4–12. (This article describes how teaching parents to teach their children specific language symbols at home enhanced the functional language output of four hearing-impaired children.)

Dee, A. D., "Meeting the Needs of Hearing Parents of Deaf Infants: A Comprehensive Parent Education Program." *Language, Speech, and Hearing Services in Schools,* **12,** 1, (1981), 13–19. (The author found that a "Structured parent-education program that focuses on the parent's psychological and cognitive needs results in impressive gains for both parent behavior and child behavior.")

Fisher, C. G. and K. Brooks. "Teachers' Stereotypes of Children Who Wear Hearing Aids." *Language, Speech, and Hearing Services in Schools,* **12,** (1981) 139–144. (The authors found that many classroom teachers have negative stereotypes about children who wear hearing aids.)

Leske, M. C., "Prevalence Estimates of Communicative Disorders in the United States: Language, Hearing and Vestibular Disorders," *ASHA,* **23,** 3, (1981), 229–237. (The author reviews the causes and prevalence of hearing impairments in the United States and associated problems of speech and language. The author notes that one in 1,000 newborns has a congenital hearing impairment. "Prevalence rises gradually with age and increases steeply over the age of 60 years. More than 60,000 children are enrolled in programs for the hearing impaired.")

The author notes that national studies to determine impaired hearing in the United States have used different criteria and definitions; these factors must be considered in discussing the implications of findings.)

Schmaman, F. D., and G. Straker, "Counseling Parents of the Hearing-Impaired Child During the Post-Diagnostic Period." *Language, Speech, and Hearing Services in Schools,* **11** (October 1980), 251–259. (Shows how professionals dealing with the hearing-impaired child can provide supportive counseling to parents following the diagnosis of a hearing impairment. Deals with parents' feelings, the source of their feelings, and ways in which the professional can deal with these feelings.)

15

Facial Clefts:
Cleft Lip and
Cleft Palate

A facial cleft is any opening in the oral cavity, lips, or nasal cavity that may be caused either by prenatal developmental failure or by accident or disease at or following birth. The vast majority of facial clefts are developmental failures. That is, during the embryonic state of the fetus, parts of the facial area failed to fuse and develop normally. Facial clefts may involve the palate as a whole, or be limited to parts of the hard or soft palate. Clefts may also involve the upper gum ridge (alveolar process), the upper lip, and one or both of the nares (the passageways from the nostril to the nasal cavity). Extensive clefts may involve any two or more of the parts of the oral cavity or upper lip. An insufficient palate, though not technically an oral cleft, is believed to be associated with the anomaly. An insufficient palate is one that does not have a normal amount of soft palate. The uvula may be missing or be shortened, and part of the soft palate anterior to the uvula may be smaller than is normal. We shall use the term *facial cleft* to comprise what is frequently included in the terms *cleft lip* and *cleft palate*.

Although the specific cause of congenital facial cleft is not known, there is little doubt that heredity plays an important role in its etiology. Other factors that may be associated with congenital facial clefts are believed to be the diet and health of the mother and intrauterine pressure on the developing fetus.

447

INCIDENCE

The incidence of facial cleft varies somewhat according to geographic distribution. Surveys record ranges from one in about 600 to one in 1,000 in the population. Probably a moderate estimate is that one child in 600 is born with some form of facial cleft that will require special care and training. Morris (1978, p. 158) also notes that "Although there is some lack of consistency in the research findings concerning the incidence of the various cleft types, a reasonable, approximate generalization is that one-fourth of the total number of

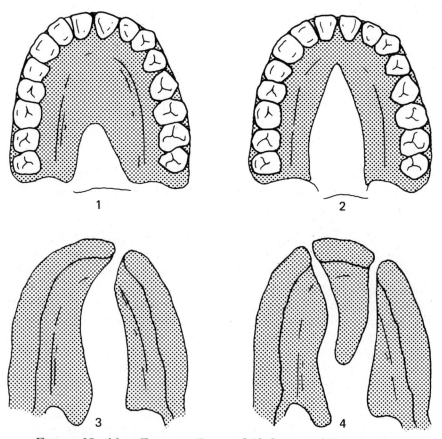

FIGURE 18. Most Frequent Types of Cleft Lip and Palate.

1. Incomplete palate (partial cleft of the velum or soft palate).
2. Cleft of most of the hard and all of the soft palate.
3. Unilateral, complete cleft (alveolar ridge, hard and soft palate).
4. Bilateral clefts of the alveolar ridge, hard and soft palate.

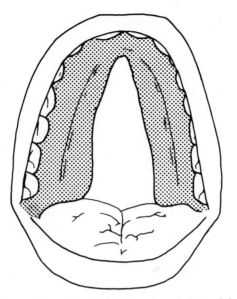

FIGURE 19. View of mouth of child with a bilateral but incomplete cleft; the alveolar (gum) ridge is not involved.

individuals born with clefts have cleft lip only, one-half have cleft lip and palate, and one-fourth have cleft palate only." Figures 18 and 19 are representations of the most frequent types of palatal clefts.

Voice and Articulation Characteristics

From the description of the inadequacy of the mechanism, the speech difficulties are readily discernible. In the speech of the child with a palatal cleft, all sounds pass directly into the nasal cavity where normal oral reinforcement is not possible. Therefore, all the vowel sounds are nasalized and most of the consonants have nasal characteristics. For example, /b/, /d/, and /g/ take on the characteristics of /m/, /n/, and /ŋ/. Other articulatory difficulties are obvious. The stop sounds /p/, /b/, /t/, /d/, /k/, and /g/ are defective because they are emitted nasally rather than orally. The fricatives /f/, /v/, /s/, /z/, /ʃ/, /ʒ/, /θ/, and /ð/ are also defective, because the air stream coming through the mouth cannot be controlled adequately. Because *s* and *z* require the direction of an air stream down a narrow channel, they are likely to be the most seriously affected of the fricative sounds. Other distinctive traits include frequent inhalation and considerable use of the glottal stop, particularly before vowels. The resulting speech of a child with a severe cleft-palate condition may be a series of snorting sounds.

Westlake and Rutherford (1966, p. 30) make an interesting observation in regard to the sound substitutions made by young cleft-palate children. They point out that normal children tend to substitute [w], /f/, /t/, /d/, /b/, /θ/, /ð/ (th), and /tʃ/ for the sounds they are unable to make. In each instance, the sound substituted is one that requires articulatory adjustments similar to the appropriate sound. Thus, we may say that normal sound substitution is close to the required sound and the articulation, and the child with "infantile" speech is moving toward his target. In contrast, cleft-palate children produce substitutes that are quite different from the correct ones. "More than half of their substitutions are glottal stops and pharyngeal fricatives. These sounds, in addition to the [m], [n], and [ŋ], and nasal emissions, account for three fourths of cleft-palate substitutions." Thus, the cleft-palate children are far from the target sounds in their defective articulation.

Related Problems

Certain facial mannerisms are frequently associated with cleft palate. Some children seem to engage in nasal twitching; others look as if they are habitually sniffing. The alae, the winglike structures of the nose, constrict; this constriction compensates for the failure of the nasal port to close.

The child with a facial cleft faces a variety of problems. One of the first likely to be encountered is difficulty in feeding, with some possible consequences of poor nutrition. As the child grows older, there are frequently dental conditions that require orthodontia. Teeth may fail to erupt, or they may grow in an irregular alignment. The child tends to suffer from the effects of colds, with chronic infection of the nasal areas and of the Eustachian tubes. These may produce conductive hearing loss. Pannbacker (1969) found that about two-thirds of a population of 103 cases of cleft lip and cleft palate (60 males and 43 females) had hearing losses of 15 decibels or more on audiometric assessment. However, cases with cleft lip alone, and those with congenital palatal insufficiency, did not have "socially significant audiological defects." Based on their review of the literature, Westlake and Rutherford (1966, p. 18) state: "All researchers agree that there is a high incidence of hearing loss in the cleft-palate population." Morris (1978, p. 163) observes: "With rare exception the hearing loss . . . is for air conduction only; it may be unilateral or bilateral; it rarely exceeds levels of 30 to 40 dB; and although it may be relatively chronic until about the age of 6 years, it usually shows marked fluctuation, depending on the middle ear/Eustachian tube function."

Linguistic Competence

Although we are inclined to think of the cleft-palate child as one whose primary difficulties are with voice and articulation, recent evidence suggests that language competence as a whole may be delayed or improficient in many such children. Morris (1978, pp. 165–166) sugests that a combination of factors may explain the delay and differences in language proficiency, especially among the younger children. These factors include hearing deficit, the amount of dental and surgical treatments required, and the time spent in hospitals rather than in preschool and primary school settings. "By the age of five or six, however, the child with a cleft will probably have acquired normal language patterns."

Earlier reports on the language proficiency of cleft-palate children are less optimistic. For example, Smith and McWilliams (1968) assessed the linguistic abilities of 136 cleft-palate children ranging in age from 3.0 to 8.11. The population included 86 males and 50 females. Of these, 71 had both cleft lip and cleft palate, 46 had cleft palates without cleft lip, and 19 had cleft lip alone. Smith and McWilliams used the Illinois Test of Psycholinguistic Abilities (ITPA) as their investigative instrument. They compared the standard age scores for the nine subtests of the ITPA with the scores for their experimental population. "The data revealed that cleft-palate subjects manifest a general language depression with particular weakness in vocal expression, gestural output, and visual memory. Moreover, in the samples studied, there was a tendency for language weaknesses to become more marked as age increased." Both male and female subjects with cleft lip alone showed relative weaknesses in motor expression and visual memory, and generally similar linguistic profiles to the children with cleft palate.

Moll (1968, p. 110) after reviewing the literature concludes:

> it appears that individuals with cleft lips and cleft palates are retarded in some degree in language development. This retardation seems to exist on almost every dimension measured in the various studies: these children exhibit less verbal output and a more simple language structure than children without clefts.
>
> . . . it must be emphasized that the conclusions about retarded language development refer to cleft palate subjects on the average; obviously not all children exhibit retardation in language skills.

Intelligence

Another factor deserving study and consideration in determining the therapeutic needs of the cleft-palate child is his/her intellectual development. A carefully conducted control study by Goodstein (1961), in which the Wechsler Intelligence Scale for Children was used to assess the intellectual status of cleft-palate children and a matched group of children without cleft palate, indicates that there are significant differences in intelligence levels between the two groups. An appreciably larger percentage of the cleft-palate children fell in the categories of dull normal, borderline, and mentally defective intellectual classifications than did the control children. The latter group of children tended to distribute very much according to the expected intellectual classification levels. This study points to the need for the individual assessment of the intelligence of the cleft-palate child as well as the related need to adjust the therapeutic program so that the objective, materials, and rate of progress are realistically geared to the child's intellectual capacity.

Westlake and Rutherford (1966), after reviewing some of the literature on the intelligence of cleft-palate children, suggest that one of the reasons for the somewhat lower intelligence test scores may be in involvements such as hearing loss that are associated with, or etiologically related to, the clefts. They conclude (Ibid., p. 17) that "present information gives little reason for assuming that a person with a cleft is more likely to have a lower I.Q. than any other person." This observation is consistent with the general position taken by Westlake and Rutherford that cleft-palate persons vary individually as much as persons without cleft, and that generalizations are to be avoided in favor of intensive study of the individual who may have a facial cleft.

Based on his own study and a review of the literature, Goodstein (1968, pp. 209–212) concludes: "The findings . . . suggest a generally mild to moderate degree of intellectual impairment, with the distribution of I.Q. for the group of children with cleft palate displaced to the lower end of the distribution." The differences are generally more pronounced in the verbal than in the performance areas. Though the mean I.Q. of cleft-palate children ranged from 94 to 99, it needs to be reemphasized that a given child with cleft palate can be found anywhere on the intelligence range, including genius.

Medical Therapy: Surgical Repair

The first step, if possible, is the repair of the oral mechanism to the fullest extent that can be achieved for life processes and speech. The first step may in fact be a series of steps taken over a period of years, through infancy and childhood. The primary goal of surgery is to provide the cleft-palate child with the best possible functioning of the palate and the vocal mechanism as a whole. A secondary but exceedingly important goal is cosmetic; to do whatever can be done to make the child as good-looking and as normal in appearance as possible.

A variety of procedures is used to close the palate, to lengthen it if possible, and to provide an oral cavity that will serve both the functions of articulation and reinforcement (resonance). Often, as we have indicated, the teeth need to be arranged or rearranged, or dentures provided when this is not possible.

Usually the repair of extensive facial clefts requires a series of operations. Since surgical repair of facial clefts is a highly specialized area of oral surgery, most of the work is done in fairly large medical centers. Surgeons must not only make the oral cavity adequate for the present but must also predict how future growth will affect and be affected by the surgery.

Descriptions of some of the surgical procedures are presented in Westlake and Rutherford (1966, pp. 79–82), Perkins (1977, pp. 186–188), and Bloodstein (1979, pp. 354–360).

Prosthetic Appliances

In some cases, the surgeon may advise against or postpone an operation. It may be desirable for the child to be older or to be in better health before surgery. The surgeon may decide that the available tissue is insufficient for the purpose of "covering" the area of the cleft. In such instances the physician may recommend that the child be fitted with an obturator, a prosthetic device that substitutes or "supplements" the cleft palate according to need. Some prosthetic appliances are inserted into the hard palate, others are inserted into the soft palate area, and still others "cover" both the hard and soft palates. Soft palate appliances usually include a bulb for the area of the nasopharynx, which, if carefully fitted, may help considerably in reducing nasality. If the bulb is too large, denasality may result.

In some instances, prosthetic appliances are used temporarily, while the child is growing. These devices may need changing as the child grows. With maturity, if surgery is not indicated, "permanent" prosthetic appliances may be designed and fitted. Figure 20 is an illustration of a typical velo-pharyngeal prosthesis.

The Therapeutic Team

The congenital defects of cleft lip and/or cleft palate present problems that from the outset require the intervention of a variety of specialists as well as greater than usual involvement in the early and continued care of the child. The surgeon—orofacial and cosmetic—the ortho-

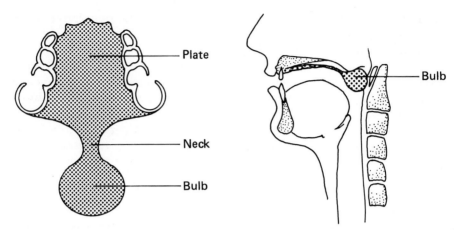

FIGURE 20. A. Typical Velo-Pharyngeal Prosthesis. B. Prosthesis in place.

dontist, the prosthodontist, the psychologist, and the speech/language clinician in cooperation with the parents and child constitute the therapeutic team. All, including the child as he/she grows older, must have an in-depth knowledge of the others' goals if not of their methods. When the child is of school age, the classroom teacher joins and for many years continues to be part of the team.

SPEECH REMEDIATION

Muscle Strengthening

The speech clinician must help the child to make maximum use of the oral cavity musculature as modified either by the surgeon or by the prosthodontist. Objectives should include making the oral musculatures stronger and more flexible so that they may be used more adequately for speech. Control of breath and the prevention or reduction of leakage of breath into the nasal cavities are the primary goals. This may be accomplished through nonenergetic "blowing exercises."[1] The gentle, sustained blowing of a feather, a Ping-Pong ball, a candle flame, or a paper butterfly helps to improve the child's ability to direct the breath stream outward toward the front of his mouth, and so to increase oral resonance when application is made to speech production. Swallowing, sucking through a straw, and yawning are also of some help in strengthening the soft palate and throat muscles. Young chil-

[1] Note that we use the term *nonenergetic blowing*. Energetic blowing that requires great tension is contraindicated. Further, at no time should the child be permitted or directed to constrict the nostrils to achieve blowing. Such constricted blowing efforts may produce a backing up of the nasal fluids and may result in middle-ear infection.

dren may enjoy the interesting noise effects of blowing through the teeth of a comb against which a piece of tissue paper is fixed. A more musical result may be obtained from playing a harmonica.

It must be emphasized, however, that all of these exercises are merely token indicators of what a child may be able to do in speech activities. A child may be able to achieve complete success in blowing exercises and yet not be able to control his velum in a manner and at a rate necessary to avoid nasality while speaking. In the final analysis, what matters is how a child with a repaired cleft, or one with an oral prosthesis, uses his mechanism for intelligible speech and, if possible, appropriate nasal reinforcement. Of the two, *intelligibility should be the primary objective.*

Realism should dictate the remedial speech efforts and objectives for the cleft-palate child. Along this line we accept the basic philosophy for speech therapy of Van Riper (1978):

"We make the person's speech better and we make him a happier person. . . . Within the limits of our time and energy and knowledge, and with an awareness of the limitations which the case also possesses, let us do our utmost and be content with that." So, with the clinician's direct help and the teacher's support, cleft-palate children should be taught to speak as well as they can. This means with as little abnormality as possible, and with major emphasis on intelligible communication.

Visualizing Palatal Movement

Actual movement of the palate and the oral mechanism as a whole can now be visualized by means of X-ray photography, taken while the patient is talking. Perhaps the best technique is that of X-ray motion pictures (cinefluorography), which is now available in many medical centers. Information derived from such films enables the clinician to know what needs to be done to improve palatal action and to counteract the tendencies of a person with repaired cleft to use inappropriate articulatory movements. It may be possible to see as well as hear the differences when the child speaks slowly and when the child speaks at what may be a normal rate of utterance, but not an optimum rate for this child. However, X-ray photography is not always available, so that other less sophisticated methods may need to be used. Simple devices include the use of long bits of light feather glued to the end of a tongue depressor or, perhaps better, an ice cream stick. Placed under the nostrils, the feather should respond to the emitted air. If the air is inappropriately emitted, the clinician and child have a visual cue for this misfunction. Westlake and Rutherford (1966, p. 91) also suggest the use of a small plastic rectangular box, fashioned so that an open space on one of the shorter ends fits against the upper lip so that the nose may extend into the area of the box. Air escaping from the nostrils will cause the feather or paper to move about in the box. Westlake and Rutherford (1966, p. 91) realistically observe that "all these methods are difficult to use with young children, many of whom seem diabolically driven to make the papers fly instead of trying to speak without moving them." We would suggest a counterdiabolic procedure by directing the child alternately to make things move and to talk without producing such movement. This is an application of the principle of negative practice in learning!

In some instances, a child may have a short palate, insufficient in length to close the nasal part. Excessive nasality is then almost inevitable. A physician can advise whether this is the situation and whether a prosthetic device is considered advisable as an adjunct to the soft palate. Occasionally we find a child who sounds like one with a cleft palate but who, upon cursory examination, appears to have a complete palate. In some instances, the palate does indeed have a cleft, but is covered by a thin layer of tissue (submucous cleft), which results in hypernasality as well as deviant articulation

Improving the Vocal Quality

Careful ear training and voice training often reduce the excessive nasality. We are not sure how excessive nasal resonance is produced, although we do know that it occurs when the opening of the nasal cavity is too large as compared with the opening of the mouth cavity. The clinician will strive for a satisfactory acoustic balance of nasal and oral resonance. Thus, if the child speaks with a "tight" (hypertensive) oral musculature and a small oral opening, effort should be directed to help the child change to the use of a more relaxed and larger mouth opening. It is often not possible to get rid of all hypernasality. Continued effort to achieve the not realistically achievable may frustrate both the clinician and the child.

For extended discussions and specific details for vocal therapy for cleft-palate children see Shelton *et al.* (1968), Van Riper (1978, pp. 366–372) and McWilliams (1980, 421–425).

Correcting Articulatory Defects

Although excessive and inappropriate nasality is a major problem of most cleft-palate children, constant attention should be paid to improving articulation. Investigations indicate that cleft-palate speakers with intelligible articulation are likely to be judged as having less nasality then do cleft speakers with poorer articulation (Moll, 1968, pp. 96–97).

The speech clinician must help the cleft-palate child to improve overall articulatory efforts. Exercises should be directed at increasing the child's mobility and control of jaw, lip, and tongue movements.

In some instances, a hearing loss may increase the difficulties of the cleft-palate child. Impaired hearing may account for the misarticulation of some of the sounds. If the hearing loss is moderate or severe, the use of a hearing aid may be indicated.

The clinician first teaches the sounds that are easiest for the child. For example, h is usually fairly easy to teach. Some of the later sounds to be established are k, g, s, and z. Since k and g involve the soft palate and since the stream of air for s and z needs very careful control, these four sounds are difficult for the child with a cleft palate. In many instances, there is a persistent tendency for sibilant sounds to be emited nasally. Considerable effort and time are needed to overcome this tendency.

Voice and speech therapy for the cleft-palate child require patience, sustained effort, and continued motivation. Because the results often seem small for the time and energy involved, both child and clinician may become discouraged. But most children can be helped a great deal if the objectives of intelligible communication are kept realistically in mind.

The Role of the Classroom Teacher

Classroom teachers must augment the efforts of the clinician. Teachers appreciate that the degree of normalcy of the child's speech will depend on the condition of the speech mechanism after its repair, as well as on speech training, motivation, intelligence, and hearing. At times a teacher is the liaison between the clinician and the home. The teacher and the clinician advise the parents that the training period for correcting the child's speech may be long and that the work will be hard. They explain to the parents how the parents can help the child. Such advice includes providing good speech models, recognizing and rewarding small increments of improvement, and not rejecting or punishing the child for deficiencies that are not the fault of the child.

The teacher helps the child to carry over the work from the correction session into everyday speech. The teacher promotes such activities as creative dramatics, in which the child may sell newspapers on the corner or popcorn at the ball park. This activity gives the child practice in the use of the acceptable speech.

Children with cleft palates must be helped to "accept" and adjust to their difficulties. Adjustment includes efforts to improve the child's voice and overall speech intelligibility. Beyond this, cleft-palate children must be helped to feel that they are worthwhile, adequate, and loved. In the classroom the teacher must help the cleft-palate child to such attitudes. It may also be necessary to modify the reactions of the classmates so that the child is neither ridiculed nor pitied. The teacher's attitude of acceptance will go a long way to influence the behavior of the classmates.

Parents often unconsciously and sometimes even consciously reject their child with a facial cleft. The rejection may be accompanied by feelings of shame and guilt. If these feelings become apparent to the teacher or to the clinician, recommendation for counseling is in order. In some instances, the teacher's attitude of acceptance may help the parents to modify their own attitudes.

Another result of rejection by parents may be overprotection. So some parents who, because of their concern about their cleft-palate child, overindulge the youngster and do more than they should if social, psychological, and intellectual development are to have a chance for normal potential. Oversolicitude may also be shown by the teacher. The child with a facial cleft must be encouraged to perform according to his/her potential. In the interests of the child, it should be made clear that classroom obligations are to be carried out, and the child's best performance effort is regularly to be expected. Allowances, when they are made, are based on knowledge of a given child's limitations, but these should not be flaunted. Allowance must, of course, be made on the basis of hazards to health. Here a physician's guidance is important.

Problems

1. What are the types of facial clefts? What are the chief causes of clefts?
2. What is meant by the term *cosmetic problem*? What can be done to avoid or minimize such a problem in cleft-palate children?
3. Contrast the positions of Westlake and Rutherford and Van Riper (see References) on the psychological and social implicatons of a facial cleft for a child or an adult. Compare those with Goodstein's findings.
4. What problems, other than speech, are often associated with cleft palate?
5. The voice of the cleft-palate child, even after repair, is often excessively nasal. Why? When may the voice become denasal?
6. Why is it especially important to ameliorate any hearing loss that may be associated with cleft palate? Why are the hearing losses usually conductive rather than sensorineural?
7. One of the new surgical procedures for reducing nasality is called the "surgical flap." Check the literature for a description of this operation and the circumstances that indicate when it is the procedure of choice.

8. Why is the strengthening of the oral musculature important in the thera-peutic program for a child with cleft palate?
9. What should be the primary objective in speech training for a cleft-palate child?
10. What are the most frequent articulatory errors made by young cleft-palate children? How are these errors different from those made by most young children? What are the implications of the differences?
11. Describe some techniques that may be used by clinicians to help them, and their cleft-palate children, to visualize excessive nasal emission?
12. What is a prosthetic appliance? When is its use indicated for a person with a cleft palate?
13. What are the findings relative to the intelligence of cleft-palate children?
14. Can you explain the bases for the findings that as a total "special" popula-tion, cleft-palate children are behind their age peers in early language de-velopment?
15. Read an article or a chapter in a book that deals with cleft palate published in the 1960s and one in the late 1970s or 1980s. Is there any change in point of view as to etiology or treatment.

References and Suggested Readings

Bloodstein, O., *Speech Pathology.* Boston: Houghton Mifflin Company, 1979, Chap. 9. (Includes good diagrams of types of cleft palate and surgical proce-dures; many recent references.)

Bzoch, K. R., *Communicative Disorders Related to Cleft Lip and Palate.* Bos-ton: Little Brown and Company, 1972.

Goodstein, L. D. "Intellectual Impairments in Cleft Palate," *Journal of Speech and Hearing Research,* 4, (1961), 287–294.

————, "Psychosocial Aspects of Cleft Palate." In D. C. Spriestersbach, and D. Sherman, eds., *Cleft Palate and Communication,* New York: Academic Press, 1968.

McWilliams, B. J. "Communication Problems Associated with Cleft Palate" in Van Hattum, R. J. ed. *Communication Disorders,* New York: Macmillan Company, 1980.

Moll, K. L., "Speech Characteristics of Individuals with Cleft Lip and Cleft Palate." In D. C. Spriestersbach, and D. Sherman, Eds., *Cleft Palate and Communicaton,* New York: Academic Press, 1968.

Morley, M. E., *Cleft Palate and Speech,* 7th ed. Baltimore: Williams and Wil-kins, 1970. (This book is a virtual classic on the treatment of the multifa-ceted problems of cleft palate.)

Morris, H. L., "Cleft Lip and Palate." In J. F. Curtis, Ed., *Processes and Disor-ders of Human Communication.* New York: Harper & Row, 1978, Chap. 7.

Pannbacker, M., "Hearing Loss and Cleft Palate." *Cleft Palate Journal,* **6** (Oc-tober 1969), 50–56.

Perkins, W. H., *Speech Pathology,* 2nd ed. St. Louis: C. V. Mosby Co., 1977, Chap. 8.

Powers, G. L., and C. D. Starr, "The Effects of Muscle Exercises on Velopharyngeal Gap and Nasality," *Cleft Palate Journal,* **11** (1974), 28–35.

Prather, W. F., and C. M. Kos, "Audiological and Otological Considerations." In D. C. Spriestersbach and D. Sherman, Eds., *Cleft Palate and Communication,* New York: Academic Press, 1968.

Shelton, R. L., E. Hahn, and H. L. Morris, "Diagnosis and Therapy," (Chap. 7). In D. C. Spriestersbach and D. Sherman, Eds., *Cleft Palate and Communication,* New York: Academic Press, 1968.

Shprintzen, R. J., G. N. McCall, and M. L. Skolnick, "A New Therapeutic Technique for the Treatment of Velopharyngeal Incompetence." *Journal of Speech and Hearing Disorders,* **40,** 1 (1975), 69–83.

Smith, R. M., and B. J. McWilliams, "Psycholinguistic Abilities of Children with Clefts." *Cleft Palate Journal,* **5** (April 1968), 238–249.

Spriestersbach, D. C., and D. Sherman, Eds., *Cleft Palate and Communication.* New York: Academic Press, 1968. (A high level scientific approach by ten contributors to the multiple aspects of cleft palate.)

Van Riper, C., *Speech Correction,* 6th ed. Englewood Cliffs, N.J.: Prentice-Hall, Inc., 1978, pp. 348–373. (Has excellent illustratons for types of cleft palate. Discusses the psychological and social problems of persons with cleft palate, which Van Riper believes are often as severe as for many stutterers.)

Wells, C., *Cleft Palate and its Associated Speech Disorders.* New York: McGraw-Hill Book Company, 1971. (The emphasis in this writing is on the assessment and therapeutic procedures for cleft palate.)

Westlake, H., and D. Rutherford, *Cleft Palate.* Englewood Cliffs, N.J.: Prentice-Hall, Inc., 1966. (A study guide for the understanding of the problems of persons with cleft palate. Emphasis is on the individual with cleft palate and the need to determine therapy based on his special problems.)

Yules, R. B., and R. A. Chase, "Pharyngeal Flap Surgery: A Review of the Literature." *Cleft Palate Journal,* **6** (1969), 303–308. (Indicates that there is a lack of available criteria for determining when the pharyngeal flap procedure should be used.)

16

Brain Damage,
Brain Difference,
Brain Dysfunction, and
Language and Learning
Disabilities

In this chapter we consider the implications for language acquisition
and related learning by children who are congenitally brain different,
or who, because of acquired brain damage, have become brain different. Essentially, we will be considering children who have either congenital or acquired causes for their learning disabilities, which are basically for language functions and for normal linguistic behavior. The
groups, whose symptoms often overlap, include the "minimally"
brain damaged (brain different), the congenitally aphasic, the cerebral
palsied (those with apparent neuromotor dysfunctions), and children
with acquired aphasia.

THE CONCEPT OF MINIMAL BRAIN DIFFERENCE AND
BRAIN DYSFUNCTION

During the 1960s and 1970s, but less so more recently, teachers and
clinicians have been confronted with the terms *minimal brain damage* and *minimal brain dysfunction*. The second term assumes the
presence of the first, but not on the basis of the "hard signs"—the
physiological and structural alterations that many neurologists require
as evidence of brain damage. In brief, children with minimal brain
dysfunction are not frankly (obviously) cerebral-palsied. They do not
have clear and unquestioned indications of sensory and motor impairments, or of aberrant reflexes, that are the "hard-sign" indications of
brain damage. Neurologists, psychologists, and teachers who do ac-

461

cept the concept of minimal brain dysfunction do so on the assumption that there are relationships between brain functioning and dysfunctioning, and behavior. So, they agree:

> we must accept certain categories of deviant behavior, developmental dyscrasias, learning disabilities, and visual motor perceptual irregularities as valid indices of brain dysfunctioning. They represent neurologic signs of a most meaningful kind, and reflect disorganized central nervous system functioning at the highest level. To consider learning and behavior as distinct and separate from other neurologic functions echoes a limited concept of the nervous system and of its various levels of influence and integration (Clements, 1966, pp. 6–7).

THE SYNDROME OF MINIMAL BRAIN DIFFERENCE AND DYSFUNCTION (MBD)[1]

The term *minimal brain dysfunction* (MBD) refers to a combination of manifestations (syndrome) present in children who are of near-average, average, or above-average intelligence. These manifestations, all of which are not necessarily present for any given child, include problems of attention and memory, impulsivity, mild motor disabilities (awkwardness, delayed laterality), perception, conceptualization, and speech and language development. These children are *perceptually* and *intellectually inefficient,* so that they do not meet the expectations for educational achievement based on their intelligence test scores, especially for those scores derived from "nonlanguage" or performance inventories. Often, in fact, they present problems in learning during the school years, and become so identified. They are often among the "underachievers," especially in the language subjects—reading, spelling, and often arithmetic as well. Their thinking tends to be concrete and ego-oriented and they may have difficulty with abstract conceptualization and abstract language. Occasionally, however, some children show surprising flashes of insight as well as an ability to appreciate the abstract. Thus, they may be inconsistent and puzzling performers who show wide day-to-day variations in their accomplishments. For a detailed testing of the symptomatology of the child with minimal brain dysfunction, see Clements (1966,

---

[1] We prefer the use of the term *minimally brain different* to the term *minimally brain damaged.* The notion of a "different" brain, even one that may be "minimally" different, has implications for deviant functioning. The term *damage,* even though it is presumed to be minimal, is often difficult to establish. Moreover, the term *damage* has semantic implications that may be excessive and discouraging.

pp. 11–12) and Kenny and Clemmens (1975, pp. 48–57) and McGrady, (1980).

Kenny and Clemmens (1975, p. 48) point out that we have no clearly defined clinical prototype of minimal brain dysfunction. Usually the child is identified between the ages of six and nine because of behavior and learning problems. Other behavioral "symptoms" include awkwardness, difficulty in fine motor coordination, hyperactivity, distractability and associated behaviors, tendency to act impulsively (acting out), low frustration tolerance, and perseveration.

In general, the term *minimal brain dysfunction* is employed to describe a group of children who have determined deficiencies in learning and/or motor functioning. However, the children's intellectual level is usually well above the range for the mentally retarded. The concept of minimal brain dysfunction implies that there are brain abnormalities that underlie and contribute directly to the aberrations observed (Kenny and Clemmens, p. 48).

The *learning problems* of these MBD children are especially apparent in their language. Often they are delayed in language acquisition and present a variety of speech problems that suggest articulation defects, but may in reality be problems of morphology and/or syntax (such as failure to understand plural and tense endings). Writing problems include both legibility and those that parallel difficulties in oral language development. Despite these characteristics, most MBD children come well within the normal range on nonverbal tests of intelligence. Their potential for learning must, therefore, be presumed to be adequate.

We agree with Kenny and Clemmens (p. 50) that "It is obvious that the current state of our knowledge about minimal brain dysfunction is far from complete and acceptance is far from universal." These children, insofar as they can be identified, constitute problems and challenge for classroom teachers and speech and language clinicians. Fortunately, their intellectual potential provides a basis for an optimistic outlook for most MBD children. We believe that many MBD children are probably congenitally aphasic (dyslogic). We discuss this problem in the succeeding pages. In the meantime we direct your attention to the use of the term *learning disabilities* for children who have central auditory processing problems. Says Sanders (1977, p. 185):

> The term *learning disabled* has replaced the far more misleading label of *minimal brain damage*. This term was developed to soften the even more negative aspects of the broader label *brain damage*. The term *minimal brain damaged* was initially used to identify children who evidenced problems in processing information despite normal sensory end-organs and intact mental and motor function. The label was clearly in-

tended to imply the presence of a dysfunction of the brain arising from deficit or damage insufficiently severe to manifest gross neurological symptoms.

DEVELOPMENTAL APHASIA AND BRAIN DIFFERENCE

In a literal sense, *aphasia* means "without language" or "without speech." However, the terms *aphasia* and *aphasic* are used by professional persons concerned with problems of language related to brain damage as designations for language impairments that were acquired at a stage after language was established. These problems include impairments in the comprehension and production of spoken as well as written language. The terms may also be used for a child who incurs damage and language impairment following accident or disease of the brain (encephalopathies). Fortunately, the young child, up to the age of early adolescence (12 to 14 or so) has such great plasticity of the brain and such great reorganizational and recuperative capacity that usually almost full recovery and resumption of language functioning may ordinarily be expected. Exceptions are found, however, among children who incur bilateral or profuse damage of the cerebrum. Residual deficits in acquired aphasia will be considered later.

In our earlier discussion of minimal brain damage and minimal brain dysfunction, we anticipated our consideration of children whose impairments are so severe as to make them essentially nonverbal. We use the terms *developmental aphasia*, and *congenital aphasia* synonymously to designate such severely linguistically delayed and impaired children.

The Child with Developmental Aphasia and Brain Dysfunction

Children who are born with brain damage because of a prenatal condition, or who have incurred brain damage as a result of a birth injury or a cerebral pathology before the age at which speech usually begins, are frequently severely retarded in their speech onset and development. Often, even after these children begin to speak, their articulation, voice, and vocabulary development are impaired. In very severe cases, usually associated with damage to both hemispheres of the brain, even the comprehension of language may be severely and sometimes completely impaired. It is likely that most of these children who are bilaterally brain damaged also suffer from an appreciable degree of mental impairment, and others suffer from hearing loss with or without mental deficiency. Our own experience with brain-damaged children leads us to believe that, where hearing loss and mental deficiency are not complicating factors, language learning may be delayed but is usually established by age four or five. In most cases where hearing and intelligence are relatively normal, language is acquired and speech, however defective, is usually established by the time the child has reached school age.

There are, however, a small group of children with slow maturation of the central nervous system, or who, because of minimal brain damage and considerably more than minimal brain dysfunction, do not "spontaneously" acquire speech. *These children must be taught directly what most children acquire naturally—by listening, identifying, and finally by imitating and then creating on their own an infinite number of utterances they could not possibly have learned through imitation.* These children who do not acquire language "naturally" are *developmentally* or *congenitally aphasic* (without language). The following are some critical differences that distinguish such children from their speaking as well as nonspeaking age peers.

1. The developmentally aphasic child has *perceptual difficulties* related to one or more sensory modalities, but primarily for the perception of those auditory events that constitute the sounds of speech. [See Eisenson (1972, Chap. 4) for an exposition of this point.]

   Recent research indicates that the essential problem with aphasic children appears to be difficulty in processing (discriminating and keeping in mind a sequence of sounds) rapidly changing features that are inherent in an aural/oral language system. Based on the results of a series of studies by Tallal and coinvestigators, Tallal and Piercy (1978, p. 75) conclude:

   > These findings suggest that the speech production deficits of these dysphasic children mirror their defects of speech perception. Those speech sounds incorporating rapid spectral changes critical for their perception are most difficult for dysphasic children to perceive and are also most often inaccurately produced. These results add further support to the hypothesis that developmental dysphasia[2] can be accounted for, at least in part, by a failure to develop an auditory perceptual process necessary for the perception of speech.

2. The aphasic child is often *slow in developing laterality*. At the age of five or even later he/she may not have established a preferred hand or foot or an eye or an ear. Often associated with this developmental lag is confusion in directional and spatial orientation.

---

[2] The term *dysphasia* implies a less severe degree of impairment than *aphasia*. If we take the implied meanings of the terms literally, we would assume that a developmentally (congenitally) aphasic child's difficulties with language and learning are generally more extreme than those of a child designated as dysphasic.

3. *Inconsistency of response* is almost a universal characteristic of the aphasic child. A response made to a situation on one occasion may not be made on a succeeding occasion. A response that may be completely appropriate when first made may simply fail to be made on successive occasions.

4. *Morbidity of attention* is associated with inconsistency of response. Occasionally the aphasic child may become so completely absorbed with the situation to which he/she is attending that he/she cannot shift attention to new situations, despite the intensity of a new stimulus. Thus, loud noises may be ignored, or at least are not immediately able to compete for attention with what is already concerning the child. In contrast with this compulsive and persistent manner of attending to a situation, the aphasic child may sometimes have such fleeting attention as to seem to be reacting to everything, and adequately to nothing.

5. Associated with inconsistency of response and morbidity of attention is *lability* (instability) *of general behavior.* The aphasic child may behave excessively and exhibit uncontrolled emotionality because of seemingly trivial disturbances. If the child is disturbed at all, he/she is disturbed a great deal. Along with emotional lability there may be accompanying hyperactivity. The child may suddenly change from being relatively docile to being active beyond easy control.

6. A characteristic feature of the language development of the aphasic child, aside from the initial retardation, is *unevenness of ability.* Even after this child begins to use language, he/she does not show the expected increments or the "ordered" pattern by which most children increase their linguistic abilities for day-to-day communication. Many aphasic children learn to say a few words at intervals far apart, but during these periods may have a normal or better than normal increase in their comprehension vocabularies. Later, they may show parallel disparities in learning to read and write. The result may be that even after the children are in the midprimary grades, their educational achievements are so uneven as to cause considerable concern to their teachers, their parents, and to themselves. They are often painfully slow in achieving an integrated pattern of development with those features that go together and that are ordinarily found together.[3]

The features we have reviewed of developmentally aphasic children may be understood in terms of the impaired efficiency of their

[3] For example, most children begin to combine words into rudimentary two-word utterances when they have a base vocabulary of about 50–75 words. Aphasic children usually do not begin to produce two-word utterances until they have a base vocabulary of from 250 to 500 words.

neurological mechanisms. The overall effects of the cerebral differences in this brain-different child aggravate any sensory impairments they may have—some have slight to moderate degrees of hearing loss —and reduce their perceptual and intellectual potentials. Functionally, these children do not hear as well as audiometric results would suggest they should be able to hear. Otherwise stated, they do not hear (in reality, listen) as proficiently as non-brain-damaged or brain-different children do with the same amount of "objectively measured" hearing. Similarly, and more generally, they often function considerably below the upper limits of their mental potential. They disturb easily and have very good cause for such reactions.

Clinical Assessment

Severely linguistically retarded children who are suspected of being aphasic should be evaluated by highly competent specialists. These children are often not easy to diagnose into clear-cut categories. They often respond, or fail to respond, in the manner of deaf children. Sometimes they seem to respond with the slowness and limited understanding of severely mentally retarded children. Often they behave as if they were emotionally disturbed. It is essential, therefore, that a team of clinicians, including a physician and, if possible, a neurologist, an audiologist, a psychologist, and a speech/language clinician make the assessment. It may well be that a given child may actually have brain damage and hearing loss, and the general lability may be a reaction to his/her own impairments. Even when language learning is proceeding, the child, as well as the teachers and parents, may be responding to the child's uneven abilities with repeated frustration.

The most severely developmentally aphasic children do not have enough language when they reach school age to enter and perform competently in regular classes. In some school districts they may be accepted in special classes for aphasic or neurologically handicapped, or severely orally linguistically handicapped (impaired) children. Usually they need prior training to be prepared for such classes. Such training is now offered in clinics or in medical or educational centers here and abroad. Approaches that have been found useful emphasize speech-sound discrimination, visual stimulation in association with oral language, sequencing of visual materials and of oral language presented more slowly and in smaller units than in normal speech utterance, and the direct teaching of syntax. We have found that many preschool developmentally aphasic children do well by an almost exclusively visual approach that introduces arrangements of pictures to tell something (visual semantic sequencing), which later becomes associated with oral language. Essentially, the child learns that utterances, whether visual or audible, have "law and order," or rules out of which sense and meanings are derived. By approaching the child primarily through the visual and less impaired modality, which incidentally and importantly permits looking as long and as often as necessary to derive meaning from the input, the notion of representation and symbolization becomes established. Thus, some children begin to be able to read on a primer level before they are able to do much talking.

Programs for congenitally aphasic children have been developed at the Institute for Childhood Aphasia at San Francisco State University (Eisenson, 1972). Programs with a different emphasis and orientation have been published by Barry (1961), McGinnis (1963), and Gray and Ryan (1973).

Therapeutic Approaches

Approaches to improve the speech and language impairments of the school-age aphasic child should be shared by the language clinician and the classroom teacher. Many aphasic children continue to need specialized help—either ancillary to regular class teaching or, as we have indicated, in special classes—throughout the primary grades, and some even beyond this level. If the child has made sufficient progress to be attending grade school, he/she still requires the additional therapy that is a product of understanding and patience. The classroom teacher may help the child to work to maximum level of ability by motivation that is timed to the child's periods of best effort. Aphasic and post-aphasic children, more than most children, need encouragement because they are never quite certain what they may expect of themselves. In the absence of severe sensory or motor disability, many, if not most, may be helped to achieve at least a normal level of overall proficiency. Care must be exercised that they are not pushed too hard, or urged too soon, as they begin to acquire language and learn how to behave in a world of linguistic symbols. With good timing, and with an educational schedule geared to awareness of their labile inclinations and their intellectual and cognitive limitations, the teacher and clinicians can balance their demands to the children's manifest abilities so that proficiencies may develop despite early unevenness in developmental patterns.

ACQUIRED APHASIA IN CHILDREN

Children can become aphasic, can suffer from impairments in previously established language functions, from the same causes as adults. That is, they can incur damage to the brain, specifically and usually to the language centers of the left hemisphere, as a result of head wounds, blood vessel obstructions, hemorrhages, or pathologies that invade the cerebral system. From a functional point of view, no child should be considered to have *acquired aphasic involvements* who had not previously established language behavior as a practical, communicative system.

Unless the child suffers bilateral brain damage, the outlook for recovery is generally good. This is so because young persons seem to be able to have the hemisphere that is normally subordinate for language functions—usually the right—take over linguistic processes that are ordinarily served by the left. Up to the 1960s neurologists and speech pathologists were generally optimistic that the "switch" from the left to the right hemisphere for language decoding and encoding could take place without significant loss or reduction in proficiency. This position was especially held for children below age twelve. More recent evidence indicates that this is not necessarily so. Long term follow-up studies by investigators including Alajouanine and Lhermitte (1965) and Hécaen (1976) indicate that there may be residual impairments in language functioning. These include difficulties in word finding, reading, spelling, writing, and to a lesser degree, in arithmetic.

Prognosis

The important implications of these findings is that we should not take it for granted that children with acquired aphasia are all likely to recover either spontaneously or completely without therapeutic intervention. With the combination of considerable spontaneous recovery and language remediation, the prospect improves. Therapeutic approaches may include encouraging the child to self-correct, reviewing reading, spelling and writing, and possibly "regressing" the child and "reteaching" until he/she catches up. Fatigue, anxiety, physical illness may temporarily reduce proficiency. It often helps to have the child know that when these negative factors are reduced, language proficiency increases. The encouragement and patient understanding of the teacher and clinician go a long way to helping the child with acquired aphasia to re-establish language functioning.

NEUROMOTOR DYSFUNCTIONS (THE CEREBRAL PALSIED)

Definition and Problems

In a narrow and literal sense the term *cerebral palsy* refers to motor involvement (palsy or paralysis) on the basis of brain damage. The motor involvement may vary in type or degree and may include obvious severe paralysis, motor weakness, and/or motor incoordination. It is usually possible to relate the nature of the motor disability with localized pathology in the brain. However, in some instances, pathology and manifest impairment are not easily associated.[4]

In a broader sense, cerebral palsy refers to several conditions that are associated with the cerebral pathology, but not necessarily specific to the motor impairments. Perhaps it would be more accurate to say that many cerebral-palsied individuals have such impairments as hearing loss, visual difficulties, and other sensory difficulties such as the integration of sensory stimuli, perceptual and intellectual decrement, and related behavioral problems. These involvements, which all too often occur multiply among the cerebral-palsied, underlie general learning disabilities and specific difficulties in the comprehending of speech and in acquiring and developing language proficiency, both oral and written. We should note and emphasize that many individuals who are known to have congenital brain damage and who have manifest motor involvements are essentially free of any other associated impairments. Thus, we cannot stress the point too strongly that for any child, regardless of whether motor or sensory involvements are evident, a complete assessment of potential abilities as well as limitations is in order. High-level intelligence and high-level potential achievement are definitely represented among the population of the frankly cerebral-palsied.

Prevalence

Figures as to the prevalence of cerebral palsy vary considerably according to criteria. Prevalence would be high if the collector of the data assumes that the existence of any of the conditions mentioned previously is presumptive evidence of cerebral palsy, or if the condition cannot be attributed to some other specific cause. Behavioral disturbances, especially of the "acting out" variety, are perhaps all to frequently considered to be associated with brain damage. The figure is likely to be considerably lower if the investigator demands clear-cut positive evidence of brain damage, such as would satisfy a pediatric neurologist who might be concerned with "hard-sign" indications of neuropathology. Psychologists, and neurologists as well, who view

---

[4] Cruickshank (1976, p. 2) provides a *practical definition* of cerebral palsy. "From such a point of view cerebral palsy is seen as one component of a broader brain-damage syndrome comprised of neuromotor dysfunction, psychological dysfunction, convulsions, or behavior disorders of organic origin. In some cerebral palsied individuals only a single factor may appear; other individuals may be characterized by any combination of the factors mentioned."

the assessment of perceptual and cognitive functioning as an extension of a neurological examination, would stress the significance of findings of perceptual impairment (the failure to derive meanings from sensory input) and impairment of intersensory integration as evidence of brain damage, even when motor disabilities are minimal. Investigations along this line are reviewed in monographs by Birch (1964) and Allen and Jefferson (1962). A conservative estimate of the prevalence of cerebral palsy is about 1.7 per 1,000 of population (Wilson, 1973, p. 466). Interestingly, this prevalence may have been somewhat higher in the 1960s than in previous decades because many children who survived the conditions that make them cerebral-palsied would have died in the first half of the century. We may hope, however, that immunization against measles and rubella may continue to reduce this number sharply in future years.

The Causes of Cerebral Palsy

The causes of cerebral palsy are, unfortunately, both numerous and varied. By definition, whatever the specific cause, it must be one that damages or retards or impairs the development of one of the centers of the brain that is involved in the production and control of motor activity. There is also a high incidence of sensory defects, predominantly hearing and vision, as well as mental retardation. These impairments are associated with pathologies of the cerebrum, cortical and subcortical, in the cerebral palsied.

The major causes of congenital cerebral palsy include developmental maturational failure beginning in the embryonic stage. In many instances, such failure is associated with illness incurred by the mother during the early months of pregnancy. Rubella, or German measles, is high among such illnesses. Trauma affecting the brain, associated with the mother's prolonged labor or precipitous labor, is also one of the more frequent causes. Any condition that cuts off or sharply reduces the oxygen supply to the child's brain and that occurs immediately before, during, or after the child is born may cause cerebral palsy. Such conditions include maternal hemorrhaging, a tightened umbilical cord around the child's neck, an injury that occasionally, but fortunately rarely, may result from forceps delivery, or cerebral hemorrhaging of the child from unknown causes. Prematurity (babies born before full term and weighing less than five pounds) is high among the conditions associated with cerebral palsy. Even after the child has survived the first hazardous journey through the mother's birth canal, damage to the brain may be incurred from head trauma or from some infectious involvement that produces brain damage.

Although all causes of brain damage cannot be specifically related to the type of cerebral palsy a child may have, certain etiological correlates are recognized. External trauma to the brain (head injury that affects the brain) is likely to produce spastic cerebral palsy. Anoxia (a cutting off or sharp reduction in the supply of oxygen to the brain) tends to be associated with athetoid (tremerous) cerebral palsy. In the embryonic state, the stage of the development of the child's central nervous system may be affected by the illnesses of the mother.[5]

Disturbances Related to Cerebral Palsy

As we have indicated, many cerebral-palsied children have multiple handicaps usually associated with the basic brain damage. On the physical side these handicaps include epilepsy and impairments of hearing and vision. Many children also show considerable mental retardation even when allowances are made for the inadequacy of the test procedures. In addition, there are often subtle disturbances in perceptual ability, such as the ability to recognize and reproduce forms and appreciate spatial relationships. This impairment interferes with the children's learning potential and with their attempts at adjusting to their physical environment.[6]

Another area of difficulty is emotional stability. Many cerebral-palsied children are disturbed children. Some of the disturbances arise out of a reaction to their multiple handicaps. Other disturbances arise out of the reactions of the parents and siblings to the cerebral-palsied children, and theirs in turn to their parents and siblings. Perhaps an even greater cause of emotional disturbance may be attributed to the frequent failures in attempts at communication, which may have the unfortunate result of allowing quick and chronic frustration to become an established mode of behavior.

Intelligence and Educability

Intelligence

Until very recently, testing instruments used for estimating the intelligence of cerebral-palsied children have had severe limitations.

---

[5] E. T. McDonald and B. Chance, *Cerebral Palsy* (Englewood Cliffs, N.J.: Prentice-Hall, Inc., 1964), chap. 2 present an excellent brief review of the neurophysiology and etiology of cerebral palsy.

W. H. Perkins, *Speech Pathology* (St. Louis: The C. V. Mosby Co., 1977), pp. 134–143 discusses the types of cerebral palsy, their neuropathologies, and related disorders of speech (language, voice, and articulation).

[6] See the discussion of the multiple-handicapped child by Lewandowski and Cruickshank in *Psychology of Exceptional Children and Youth*, 4th ed., (Englewood Cliffs, N.J.: Prentice-Hall, Inc., 1980) pp. 345–354, for an explanation of these factors.

Most tests used were initially standardized on populations that did not include a significant number of children with motor handicaps or the other handicaps often associated with cerebral palsy. Tested by such instruments, the cerebral-palsied population showed a large incidence of mental retardation. Fortunately, several instruments are now available that require little or no verbalization and call instead for relatively gross motor actions in the test situations. Such tests enable us to make a more adequate estimate of the intelligence of the cerebral-palsied. These tests include the Ammons Full Range Picture Vocabulary Test, the Revised Peabody Vocabulary Test, the Revised Columbia Mental Maturity Scale, and Raven's Progressive Matrices. The results obtained from surveys employing these tests suggest that there is probably less mental retardation among the cerebral-palsied than was earlier reported. There is little question, however, that the prevalence of mental retardation is considerably greater among the cerebral-palsied than among the population at large. Estimates as to the amount of mental retardation among the cerebral-palsied range from 25 per cent to more than 50 per cent.

While becoming aware of the intellectual limitations of many of the cerebral-palsied, we should not overlook the important fact that intellectual genius is also present in this physically handicapped group. Taken as a whole, all levels of intellectual capacity are represented among the cerebral-palsied, as they are among the population at large.[7]

Perhaps the most realistic as well as the fairest way to deal with the results of psychological (intelligence) testing is to accept the scores as minimal indicators of a child's intellectual potential. They provide a baseline, a place from where to begin and to plan education and other treatment programs. The test results should not be regarded as the ceiling of a child's intellectual capacity.

Educability

Because many cerebral-palsied children have multiple handicaps, including mental retardation, a large percentage of the children have been classified as uneducable. Many are "trained" in resident institutions rather than in schools; others are educated in day schools. Of late, increasing numbers of cerebral-palsied children are being educated in special classes in regular public schools. Private schools spe-

---

[7] R. M. Allen and T. W. Jefferson, in their manual on the *Psychological Evaluation of the Cerebral-Palsied Person* (Springfield, Ill.: Charles C Thomas, Publisher, 1962) describe tests and suggestions for the modification of procedures needed in the assessment of the cerebral-palsied. See also T. E. Newland, in Cruickshank, W. M., ed., *Psychology of Exceptional Children and Youth*, 4th ed., (Englewood Cliffs, N.J.: Prentice-Hall, 1980), pp. 100–105.

cializing in the treatment of the handicapped are also accepting the cerebral-palsied and giving them the benefit of improved understanding and teaching techniques. A majority of cerebral-palsied children have sufficient intellectual capacity for education along with the non-handicapped in the normal classroom situation. Many of these children, however, will require special attention from the speech clinician as well as understanding from the classroom teacher.

THERAPY FOR THE CEREBRAL PALSIED

The Cerebral Palsy Team

For children with more than minimum or residual cerebral palsy, a program of training calls for the cooperation of a team of professional specialists. Included in the team are the physician, the psychologist, the social worker, the physical therapist, the occupational therapist, the teacher, and the speech/language clinician.

The physician or physicians must estimate to what extent the child's neurological involvements may affect his/her learning. Frequently, an orthopedic surgeon is called upon for recommendations as to how classroom equipment or home furnishings are to be constructed or adapted to the child's needs. The orthopedic surgeon's advice is also needed in matters relating to the improvement of motor abilities and the prevention of physical disabilities.

The physical therapist, working with the physician, strives to improve the child's performance in coordination and motor activity. Specific therapeutic measures may be employed that may help the child to learn how to control speech musculature so that a proper degree of relaxation and synergy of movement is achieved. Such therapy prepares the cerebral-palsied child for the work of the speech/language clinician.

The occupational therapist functions as an observer of the child's motor activity and trains the child specifically in "occupational" skills. Essentially, the occupational therapist supplements the work of the physical therapist.

The psychologist, through testing and observation, makes an appraisal of the intellectual capacities and the present and potential abilities as well as the disabilities and limitations of the cerebral-palsied child. Recommendations as to the child's educability and type of education are made by the psychologist. Periodic reappraisals are made so that objectives and goals may be changed according to the manner and rate of the child's development.

The social worker investigates the home situation of the cerebral-palsied child. This specialist obtains information about the child's home and the attitudes of the parents and other key members in the household. In addition, the social worker helps to adjust the members of the family to their problem in relationship to the child and in the interest of the child.

The speech/language clinician evaluates the child's speech and language problems and trains him/her to improve communicative skills. Speech disabilities are found in 50 to 75 per cent of cerebral-palsied children. Some of the disabilities can be considerably improved; others can be modified only slightly. Realistic goals must be established that are consistent with the child's sensory and motor abilities and intellectual capacity. Progress, it must be recognized, is often slow and amounts of improvement are not likely to be discerned on a day-to-day basis.

SPEECH THERAPY FOR THE CEREBRAL-PALSIED CHILD

We cannot overemphasize the point that the establishment of some functional language system should be the first and immediate objective for the communicatively impaired cerebral-palsied child. If the communicative system to be established is the aural-oral one, then reasonable intelligibility and not refined and precise articulation is the goal. We should also expect that many cerebral-palsied children will be severely delayed in their acquisition of language. Procedures for delayed language children are, therefore, indicated. Such procedures include establishing a base vocabulary of at least 100 words (it may be as many as 300–500) before expecting the child to produce two-word utterances. Language teaching should include providing models of syntactic structures that incorporate features of grammar that approximate the order of a normal child's language acquisition. A program based on their principle is provided in *Aphasia in Children* (Eisenson, 1972). In using this syntactic-semantic approach we should also provide the child with the opportunity to enjoy and express all the functions of language considered in Chapter 1.

At the risk of being simplistic, we emphasize that except for the most severely mentally retarded, no syntactic construction is taught merely by rote as a conditioned response. For all educable cerebral-palsied children the clinician and/or teacher should make certain that the child understands the content—the contextual meaning—of any given language construction. It follows that both the meaning and the construction should be functionally useful for the child and so can be practiced in the non-school environments in which the child lives.

The suggestions that follow pertain primarily to the motor aspects of speech. They include procedures for enhancing intelligibility and so communication. At all levels, realism should determine expectations.

Specific speech therapy for the cerebral-palsied child with speech disabilities must be adapted to the child in terms of specific involvements. If a child has a hearing loss, speech signals must be intensified. This can be accomplished through the use of a hearing aid or through the use of amplification and headset earphones. For many cerebral-palsied children, an overall program would include the following:

1. *Relaxation and voluntary control of the speech musculature.* Often much of this work has been accomplished through the training given by the physiotherapist.
2. *The establishment of breathing control* for vocalization and articulation. Many cerebral-palsied children breathe too deeply or too shallowly for purposes of speech. Frequently children attempt to speak on inhaled breath. For most cerebral-palsied children, a normal length of phrase is not to be expected. Short, uninterrupted phrasing is a more modest and more possible achievement. Devices such as blowing through a straw, "bending" a candle flame, and moving ping-pong balls on flat surfaces and up inclined planes are helpful in establishing breath control. Application to speech must follow if the technique is to be more than a game.
3. *Control of the organs of articulation.* Considerable exericse is needed to establish directed and independent action of the tongue and to overcome the frequently present tendency of cerebral-palsied children to move the jaw as they attempt to move the tongue. Children enjoy such exercises as licking honey from their lips, or reaching for a bit of honey or peanut butter placed on the upper gum ridge. A lollipop held outside the mouth for licking provides a sweet objective for the tip of the tongue. The child should be shown what he or she does by observing himself or herself and the speech clinician in a mirror.
4. *Work on individual speech sounds.* The sounds most frequently defective are those that require precise tip-of-the tongue action. These include *t, d, l, n, r, s,* and *z.* Intense auditory stimulation, even if the child has no significant hearing loss, often helps to create awareness of what the child is expected to produce. Sound play, calling for repetition of sounds the child can produce, may give him or her a feeling of accomplishment in the early stages of speech

training. For many children, normal proficiency of articulation may not be expected. The production of "reasonable facsimiles" of sounds so that speech, though defective, is intelligible is frequently all that we have a right to expect.

5. *Incorporation of sounds in words and phrases.* Many cerebral-palsied children have considerable difficulty in making the transition from the production of individual sounds to connected speech. Abrupt stops are frequent, especially when words include stop plosive sounds or others that call for rapid articulatory action. The child should be encouraged to keep the sounds moving, to keep the articulators in action, even if there is a resultant lack of precision in the effort as a whole. Articulation must, of course, be coordinated with breathing and vocalization.

Van Riper (1978, pp. 393–395) describes an approach to speech therapy that coordinates with the Bobath system of physical therapy for cerebral-palsied children. A more detailed explanation of this and other procedures is provided by McDonald and Chance (1964, pp. 63–75).

Non-speech (Non-articulated) Communication

Some cerebral-palsied children are unable to control their articulatory mechanisms well enough to make oral speech at almost any level of proficiency a realistic expectation. For such children, and for adults as well, non-speech (non-articulated) functional communication may still be possible. Systems that bypass the vocal-articulatory mode include:

- *Communication Boards.* These are displays of pictures with or without printed words that permit the user to point to one or more (a sequence) of pictures to encode and communicate a message.
- *Blissymbolics.* This system is based on Chinese ideographs. It consists of about one hundred pictorial (ideographic) symbols and printed words on communication boards.
- *Premack-Type Plastic Word Symbols.* This is the basic system by which Premack taught a chimpanzee to "read." It is ideographic but not pictographic; each symbol is a geometric form that has been assigned a meaning—a specific word or a concept (idea).

These and other non-speech communication systems, including some that are electronically generated, have been used with varying degrees of success with the cerebral palsied. The systems are described and evaluated by Silverman in his book *Communication for the Speechless* (Prentice-Hall, Inc., 1980).

The Classroom Teacher's Responsibility for Cerebral-palsied Children

Because the cerebral-palsied child may look different, because frequently the child is unable to participate in many of the activities of other children, because the family may have been oversolicitous or may have unconsciously rejected the child, the cerebral-palsied is likely to have difficulty in adjusting to a group. When the teacher accepts this situation, appears to be casual about it, but still demands performance that is within reach and is compatible with the child's capabilities, the teacher is doing the child a real service. If the teacher does not let his/her sympathy show but accepts the child in a friendly fashion with cheerful affection, the child's adjustment is made easier. As far as possible, the teacher should consider the cerebral-palsied child as just another member of the group who enjoys and likes living with the classmates, and should provide new experiences that give adequate scope for individual abilities and energies.

Cerebral-palsied children speak better when they are relaxed. They do better when they have confidence in themselves and in their abilities. When they are anxious or frustrated, cerebral-palsied children have more difficulty with their speech. When the teacher can help a child to feel that he or she is making a contribution to group living, and that he or she is accepting and carrying through responsibilities for successful group activity, a feeling of "belongingness" with the classmates and a feeling of security in this particular environment may be established. The teacher must provide the cerebral-palsied child with frequent opportunities to relax. At times, the teacher or children may make things easy for the cerebral-palsied child physically; for example, the child's seat may be moved to a particular spot that is more readily accessible for the current activity. Whatever is done should be done in as casual a manner as possible so that no attention is attracted to the activity and the cerebral-palsied child will be able to feel comfortable rather than self-conscious.

Problems

1. Children now referred to as being cerebral-palsied were once generally referred to as spastics. Why is the term *cerebral-palsied* more appropriate than *spastic*? What is your response to the term *neuromotor disability?*
2. What are the characteristics of the chief types of cerebral-palsy conditions?
3. Why are many cerebral-palsied children multiply handicapped? What are the most frequent types of handicaps?
4. Why is it difficult to be certain about the intellectual assessments of cerebral-palsied children?

5. Is it reasonable to believe that all cerebral-palsied children can achieve normal speech? Justify your answer.
6. Can a cerebral-palsy condition be acquired by an adult? Justify your answer.
7. What is meant by *minimal brain dysfunction?* What are the arguments for and against this concept? Why might *minimal brain difference* be a better term?
8. What does the term *perceptual dysfunction* imply?
9. Compare an obviously (frankly) cerebral-palsied person with one designated as having minimal brain dysfunction and so presumably minimally brain damaged. What are some similarities? What are some essential differences?
10. What does the term *emotional lability* signify when applied to the brain-damaged child?
11. What is developmental aphasia? In what respects does the developmentally aphasic child resemble the one with minimal brain damage?
12. Why may it be said that a developmentally aphasic child often shows maximal brain dysfunction and minimal brain damage?
13. What is the rationale for approaching the developmentally aphasic child through the visual modality?
14. Why is the developmentally aphasic child described as one who is perceptually and intellectually inefficient?
15. What is the difference between hearing impairment and auditory perceptual dysfunction?
16. How would you go about establishing a differential diagnosis for the developmentally aphasic child and one who may be either mentally retarded or severely impaired in hearing?
17. Compare the approaches of Barry and McGinnis (see References) for the developmentally aphasic child. What are the chief similarities? The chief differences?
18. Compare the approaches of Gray and Ryan to those of Eisenson (see References). What is the basic rationale of each of the approaches?
19. Why do we emphasize the need for intelligibility rather than "standard" articulation for cerebral-palsied children?
20. Check the literature for some writers who have reservations about the use of the term *aphasic* for children. What is the nature of the reservations or objections? What is your position?
21. Describe some non-speech communicative systems. What is the evidence that they can be effective?
22. What are the causes of acquired aphasia in children? Are they any different from those for congenital aphasia? From acquired aphasia in adults?
23. Why is the recovery outlook for children with acquired aphasia better than it is for most adults?

References and Suggested Readings

Alajouanine, T., and F. Lhermitte, "Acquired Aphasia in Children." *Brain*, **88**, 4 (1965), 653–662.

Allen, R. M., and T. W. Jefferson, *Psychological Evaluation of the Cerebral-Palsied Person.* Springfield, Ill.: Charles C. Thomas, Publisher, 1962.

Barry, H., *The Young Aphasic Child.* Washington, D.C.: Alexander Graham Bell Association for the Deaf, 1961.

Birch, H. G., Ed., *Brain Damage in Children.* Baltimore: The Williams & Wilkins Company, 1964. (Includes a selective annotated bibliography on brain-damaged children.)

Brown, S. F., "Cleft Palate; Cerebral Palsy." In W. Johnson et al., *Speech-Handicapped School Children.* New York: Harper & Row, Publishers, Inc., 1967.

Clements, S. D., *Minimal Brain Dysfunction in Children.* NINDB Monograph 3, Washington, D.C.: U.S. Department of Health, Education, and Welfare, 1966.

Crothers, B., and R. S. Paine, *The Natural History of Cerebral Palsy.* Cambridge, Mass.: Harvard University Press, 1959. (An authoritative medical presentation of cerebral palsy, based on a review of 1,800 cases.)

Cruickshank, W. M., Ed., *Psychology of Exceptional Children and Youth,* 4th ed. Englewood Cliffs, N.J.: Prentice-Hall, Inc., 1980.

———, Ed., *Cerebral Palsy: A Developmental Disability,* 3rd ed. Syracuse: Syracuse University Press, 1976. (A multi-authored book that considers the various aspects and problems of cerebral palsied persons.)

Eisenson, J., *Aphasia in Children.* New York: Harper & Row, Publishers, Inc., 1972. (Considers the nature, assessment, and treatment of children with congenital or developmental aphasia).

———, "Developmental Aphasia: A Speculative View with Therapeutic Implications." *Journal of Speech and Hearing Disorders,* **30,** 1 (February 1968), 3–13.

———, "Perceptual Disturbances in Children with Central Nervous System Disfunctions and Implications for Language Development." *British Journal of Disorders of Communication,* **1,** 1 (1966), 21–32.

Gray, B., and B. Ryan, *A Language Program for the Non Language Child.* Champaign, Ill.: Research Press, 1973.

Hécaen, H., "Acquired Aphasia in Children and the Ontogenesis of Hemispheric Functional Specialization." *Brain and Language,* **3** (1976), 113–134.

Kenny, T. J., and R. L. Clemmens, *Behavioral Pediatrics and Child Development.* Baltimore: The Williams & Wilkins Co., 1975.

Lewandowski, L. J. and W. M. Cruickshank, Eds., *Psychology of Exceptional Children and Youth,* 4th ed. Englewood Cliffs, N.J.: Prentice-Hall, Inc., 1980.

McDonald, E. T., and B. Chance, *Cerebral Palsy.* Englewood Cliffs, N.J.: Prentice-Hall, Inc., 1964.

McGinnis, M., *Aphasic Children.* Washington, D.C.: Alexander Graham Bell Association for the Deaf, 1963.

McGrady, H. J., "Communication Disorders and Specific Learning Disabilities" in Van Hattum, R. J., ed. *Communication Disorders,* New York: Macmillan Company, 1980, Chap. 13.

Myklebust, H. R., "Childhood Aphasia: An Evolving Concept," and "Childhood Aphasia: Identification, Diagnosis, Remediation." In L. E. Travis, ed., *Handbook of Speech Pathology and Audiology,* New York: Appleton-Century-Crofts, 1971, pp. 1181–1217. (Traces the concept of childhood aphasia and differentiates it from other disorders that are associated with severe language delay. Emphasizes the underlying problems in auditory perception and verbal sequencing, and stresses the need for identifying the aphasic child early, and developing special education programs that should begin at the preschool level.)

Newland, T. E., "Psychological Assessment of Exceptional Children and Youth." In W. M. Cruickshank, Ed., *Psychology of Exceptional Children and Youth,* 4th ed. Englewood Cliffs, N.J.: Prentice-Hall, Inc., 1980, Chap. 3.

Perkins, W. H., *Speech Pathology.* 2nd ed. St. Louis: The C. V. Mosby Co., 1977, 134–140.

Perlstein, M., *Cerebral Palsy.* National Society for Crippled Children and Adults, Chicago: December 1961. (A booklet in the *Parent Series,* in which a medical authority on cerebral palsy provides answers to questions parents might ask about their cerebral-palsied child.)

Sanders, D. A., *Auditory Perception of Speech.* Englewood Cliffs, N.J.: Prentice-Hall, Inc., 1977.

Silverman, F. H., Communication for the Speechless. Englewood Cliffs, N.J.: Prentice-Hall, Inc., 1980.

Tallal, P., and M. Piercy, "Defects of Auditory Perception in Children with Developmental Dysphasia." In Wyke, M. A., Ed., *Developmental Dysphasia,* New York: Academic Press, 1978, 63–84.

Trombly, T., "Linguistic Concepts and the Cerebral-Palsied Child." *Cerebral Palsy Journal,* **29** (1965), 7–8. (A realistic approach to the basic language needs for cerebral-palsied children.)

Van Riper, C., *Speech Correction,* 6th ed. Englewood Cliffs, N.J.: Prentice-Hall, Inc., 1978, 389–398.

Wender, P., *Minimal Brain Dysfunction in Children.* New York: John Wiley & Sons, Inc., Interscience, 1971.

Westlake, H., and D. Rutherford, *Speech Therapy for the Cerebral Palsied.* Chicago: National Society for Crippled Children and Adults, 1961.

Wilson, M. I., "Children with Crippling and Health Disabilities." In L. Dunn, Ed., *Exceptional Children in the Schools,* 2nd ed. New York: Holt, Rinehart and Winston, Inc., 1973.

APPENDIX I

Articulation Exercises

We have arranged the following exercises for articulatory remediation. The first section includes short stories with emphasis on a particular sound. The second section shows how the teaching of a particular sound can be accomplished within a framework where language learning is taking place. You may select those concepts appropriate for the age level and for the kind of language program in the school in which you are working. These few examples merely show the kind of training that may take place. They are not meant to be inclusive in terms of syntactic structures, of language functions, or of the context of a particular sound.

SECTION 1. Exercises Emphasizing a Particular Sound—Grades 1–4

/t/—A TRIP IN THE WINTER

Two little boys, Tom and John, wanted to take a trip in the winter. One day a snowstorm came and their big sister, Mary, told them she would take them out down the street. After they put on their snowsuits, they went out into the storm. The trees, houses, and even the streets were covered with snow. The wet snow came down so fast and it was so cold they decided not to go any farther but to turn and go back home. When they got home, they wrote a note to their aunt to tell her about their cold, cold trip in the wet, wet snow.

Answer the following questions:

1. Who went on a trip?
2. What kind of weather did they have?
3. Why did they not go very far?
4. When did you go on your last trip?
5. What did you take with you on your trip?

/d/—NINE DREAMS

One day nine little children were deciding what they would like to have if some kind lady or man would make their dreams come true. Jim would like real live Indians to play with. Dan wanted peace in the world. Dick wished for good food for everybody. Mary wanted a sandpile in her own backyard. Tom would like to have a window full of colored glass. Elizabeth wanted to be able to dance like her mother. Arthur wished for a dog. They knew they would not find the kind lady or man who would give them what they wanted but liked telling each other about their dreams.

1. Which one of these dreams do you like best?
2. If you could have anything in the world, what would it be?

/k/—THE SICK PRINCE

The King, Queen, and the Prince lived high on a hill in a castle. The King was a funny man who loved to laugh and laugh. The Queen was a kind, sweet lady who loved to smile and smile. The Prince was a happy little fellow who loved to play and play. But one day the little fellow became very, very sick. The funny King didn't laugh any more. The kind, sweet Queen had a hard time smiling. The little Prince didn't play and play.

The King called all kinds of Doctors to Court. But they could not find out what was wrong with the Prince. The King began to sigh. The Queen began to cry. The little Prince just stayed in bed.

One day a new doctor, called Doctor John, came to Court. He said to take the sick little prince to the lake, put him in the water twice while music played, and then give him a big glass of milk. The King and Queen took the little Prince to the lake, put him in twice while music played, and gave him some milk. Quickly the Prince became well.

The funny King again laughed and laughed. The kind, sweet Queen smiled and smiled. The Prince played and played, and they all had a happy time.

1. What happened when the Prince got sick?
2. How did Doctor John cure the Prince?

/g/—RAIN

No rain, no rain, no rain!
I'm sad, sad, sad,

For the brown, brown grass
Will die, die, die.
Rain, rain, rain!
I'm glad, glad, glad
For the green, green grass
Will grow, grow, grow.

1. What happened when the rain came?

/f/—THE FIVE WISHES

One day I met a man who looked like a fish. He told me that I could have any five wishes I wanted if I found a real red fruit. One afternoon I found a real red apple. When I showed it to the man who looked like a fish, he asked me to decide what five wishes I wanted. Finally, I decided on these five:

I want to fly and follow the birds.
I want to live a long, long life.
I want never to be afraid.
I want to become famous.
I want to grow millions and millions of flowers.

Now life is fun! I'm never afraid when I fly like a bird. I grow flowers by the million. And just imagine! I'll live a long, long famous life. Just imagine!

1. What other animals can men look like?
2. What would be your five wishes?

/v/—TRAVELING TO THE WONDERFUL VILLAGES

One day I discovered that travel can be a wonderful adventure. I was wandering down the valley by the river, and decided I'd take my boat and visit a village along the river. The first village was all silver. The houses were silver. The stores were silver. The churches were silver. The streets were silver. It was good to see everything shining.

Because the visit was such a wonderful adventure, I decided to visit one more village. In the next village, I heard voices of children. I found seven of them around a corner playing King, Queen, and Royal Court. They voted for me for King. I loved being King. We all had a good time. My visit over, I wandered back up the valley, up the river home.

1. What was the village near?
2. What color was it?

/s/—MARY LIKES SUMMERTIME

Mary likes the summer time because she plays outside almost every day. John, Mary's friend, and Mary play hospital; and they take care of all the sick children. John is the doctor and Mary is the nurse. On very sunny days Mary's sister takes her to the sea to swim and to play in the sand. Some days she builds a very special house in the sand with shells for windows. Once in a while her sister takes her sailing over the sea. Mary likes summer better than fall, winter, or spring. She likes summer best of all.

1. Where does Mary's sister take her on sunny days?
2. What season does Mary like best?
3. What season do you like best? Why?

/ʃ/—THE SAD SHIP

The ship went sailing over the ocean.
The ship was in a very sad condition.
She dashed and dashed and dashed some more
Then rushed and rushed and rushed ashore.

1. What happened to this sad ship?

/l/—NIGHT

The silvery night rolls along.
The trees and flowers sing a song.
The stars and moon play a tune.
The dawn comes gently and too soon.

AUTOMOBILES

Millions of automobiles travel along,
Dashing and rushing and racing around,
Covering millions and millions of miles of ground
Powerful, wonderful, and very, very, very strong.

1. Tell me something else about night. What happens at night?
2. Where have you seen the most automobiles? Tell me about it.

/r/—MARY'S REPORT

Mary gave a report on the American people and the British people. She explained to the class how the British have a queen and how the Americans have a president. She brought pictures to show the class. She told the children how the British live near Europe, across the sea from the Americans, and that the Americans and British are good friends. The children enjoyed hearing her report.

1. What report did Mary give?
2. Who rules Britain and who rules America?

/dʒ/—JOHN AND HIS CLUB

John joined a club of little soldiers. Jim, his big brother, suggested the idea to him when John reached the age of eight. John was soon chosen to be the general. Because he did a good job as general, he enjoyed being general. He led his soldiers on long marches where they met many dangers. When he left the village to go to a new town, he left his club of little soldiers behind him.

SECTION 2. Exercises that Help to Build Language Concepts and that Concurrently Contain Sound Drill

/r/—Early Grades

You can help the child make nouns from verbs such as *farm, write, school, pitch*. For example, the speech clinician might say, "This is the picture of a _____. Tell me, who runs this farm?" "This man pitches the baseball. What is he called?" "This man is writing a book; he is a _____?" "Tell me, if you were a writer, what would you like to write about?"

You can help with the organizing processes of language. The following are examples:

1. I write with a pencil. I type with a _____.
2. (*Using pictures of roller skates and of a rolling pin*) How do you use this? This?
3. Tell me all you can about a rat. What other animal is he like?
4. Put in the missing sound:
   a. _inging a bell.
   b. Bo_owing a book.
   c. Fa_ away.
   d. Catching a t_ain.
   e. Absolutely _ight.
5. The meaning of *right* and *wrong* and the distinction between the two meanings of *right* can be taught through a discussion of America's and England's driving rules, followed by these questions:
   In America driving on the right side is _____.
   In England driving on the right side is _____.
   In America driving on the left side is _____.
   In England driving on the right side is _____.

/r/—Upper Grades

Teaching of /r/ clusters can be accomplished while teaching irregular verb forms. The following examples illustrate this principle: (Each answer would result from discussion.)

1. /br/ Johnny brings me mangoes each day. Yesterday he _____ me some.
   Did Brian break the window? Yes, he _____ the window yesterday. How's the window now? It's _____.
   /dr/ My Siamese cat drinks water. Yesterday he did what?
   /kr/ This baby is learning to creep. Yesterday all day she _____.

Other examples of furthering language acquisition are the following:

1. You may talk about names of places. For instance you might explain how the towns Virgil and Cicero in New York State got their names. You then would ask the boys and girls what strange names of places they know.
2. You may have the children use *never* in sentences. For instance, "What would you never want to be?"
Answer: "I would never want to be a teacher," or "I would never want to be a policeman." The children could then tell why. You can also use "Where would you never want to go?"

/l/—*Primary Grades*
In the following you can use either a flannel board or a blackboard drawing stick figures:

1. This is a short line. This is a long line. This is a longer line. This is the longest line.
2. This is a short man. This is a tall man. This man is taller. This man is the tallest.
3. These men are lining up for the bus. This man is first. This man is last.

You collect a variety of articles that include the sound /l/, such as wool, a ball, a clothespin, a lock, a block, a pencil, and a small flower pot. The children look at each article and discuss its use. You then place the articles in a large paper bag. The children are blindfolded, pick out an article, and then tell all they know about it without seeing it.

/l/—*Upper Grades*
You may make use of the parlor game in which you act out activities in the manner of the adverb. For example, the children may shake hands *gladly,* open the door *slowly,* throw a pencil *angrily,* or read a book *thoughtfully.*
You can teach the masculine, feminine, and offspring terms for:

Common Term	Masculine	Feminine	Offspring
horse	stallion	mare	foal
cow	bull	cow	calf
sheep	ram	ewe	lamb
dog	dog	bitch	puppy

Children can categorize the following foods into main dish or entrée, vegetable, dessert, and drink: *ladyfingers, lamb, lasagna, lemonade, lettuce, lima beans, liver, lobster, lyonnaise potatoes.*

They can compare a *lemon* with an *orange,* a *leopard* with a *lizard, lovely* with *delicious.* Or they can contrast *love* and *hate, light* and *dark, leap* and *stroll.*

/s/—Lower Grades

Have the children combine these nouns (*scarf, skirt, sweater, socks, stockings, slip,* and *slippers*) with a choice of these adjectives (*silk, soft, thin, heavy, nylon, woolen*). As a child combines *woolen skirt,* the clinician may ask, "Who has a woolen skirt?" A child may answer, "She has a woolen skirt."

Teach the difference between *some of* and *most of.* Using blue and red pencils, teach *Some of these pencils are red; most of them are blue.* You then can go on to *Some of the boys in my class wear red sweaters. Most of the girls in my class are brunettes.*

Ask for an explanation of this situation:

Sam's brother came into Sam's bedroom while Sam was there. His brother took Sam's favorite game, his roller skates, and his wallet. Why didn't Sam say something?
An answer such as *Sam must have been sleeping* can be expected. The other children in the group who hear this explanation will benefit.

/s/—Upper Grades

Ask the children to reduce the following sentence to five words: *Atlanta is a city in the South.* Ask them to make one word from *sun, shines; waste, basket; police, man.*

/f/ and /v/—Fifth Grade

Which of these ring? *Fire alarm, doorbell, telephone, firebell, village choir.* The following conversation may ensue:

CLINICIAN: Why does the fire alarm ring?
CHILD: It rings to ask the Fire Department to come.
CLINICIAN: After it has rung, what happens?
CHILD: After it has rung, the firemen arrive with all kinds of fire-fighting equipment.
CLINICIAN: What kind of fire-fighting equipment do the firemen bring?

The clinician may ask the children to read the conversation from *Bambi* between the fawn and the butterfly. The children could then act out the situation—with one child Bambi, the other the butterfly.

/ð/

Arrange small trucks quite near the child, and big trucks away from the child. "These trucks are _____. Those trucks are _____."

This truck is for _____ ; that truck is for _____ . Both of these trucks are dump trucks. They are used for _____ ."

During these exercises, children can be taught to evaluate each other's utterances. Each member of the group can take turns becoming the judge of a particular aspect. This can be accomplished directly or through a creative drama activity with children becoming the engineer who fixes the train, the judge who makes the decision, or the teacher who is helping the child.

As noted earlier, you use games judiciously. You make sure that the main goal is correcting the sound, not merely winning the game. Games do supply interest, however. For example, you may play a game similar to Bingo in which the children place beans on cards that contain ten or more pictures. The teacher, who has a duplicate set of pictures, shuffles them, holding up first one, then another picture. The child who has the picture of the object that the teacher holds up on his/her card says its name. Several children with particular sound difficulties can play this game, since the teacher gives them cards with pictures of words that contain their particular sound difficulties. The child who fills his/her card first calls out, "Word!" and wins the game.

A bus route that involves towns with sounds with which the children have difficulty can be arranged. The bus carries a driver who drives the bus and a hostess who explains the points of interest en route. A small toy bus travels over the route, which is drawn on the blackboard or on a large sheet of paper. The driver may either *chug, chug* [tʃʌg tʃʌg], or *bur, bur* [bɝ bɝ], or *si, si* [si si] along while the hostess takes care of the passenger. The driver stops, calls the towns, and assists the passengers on and off the bus. If the *chug, bur, bur,* or *si, si* is incorrect, the inspector sends the bus to the garage to be fixed. When the teacher drives, he/she occasionally says the sound incorrectly to train children in recognizing the incorrect sound.

Bibliography of Children's Books That Provide Practice Material for the Indicated Sounds

- /k/ 5, 9, 10, 13, 20, 27
- /g/ 5, 9, 10, 12
- /s/ 1, 3, 5, 9, 10, 12, 13, 18, 22
- /z/ 3, 10, 15, 17, 18, 32
- /ʃ/ 6, 18, 21, 23, 28
- /tʃ/ 4, 6, 18, 23
- /dʒ/ 4, 7, 12, 19
- /f/ 3, 18, 22, 30

- /v/ 7, 23, 31
- /θ/ 9, 15, 18, 20
- /ð/ 9, 15, 18, 20
- /l/ 1, 7, 13, 19, 28, 30
- /r/ 2, 3, 9, 10, 17, 20, 30, 31
- All sounds 3, 4, 8, 14, 17, 21, 24, 25, 26, 29

1. Aliki, *My Five Senses*. New York: Thomas Y. Crowell Company, 1962. (Each sensory organ and its function are presented as "I can see. I see with my eyes.")
2. Bright, R., *My Red Umbrella*. New York: William Morrow & Co., Inc., 1959. (The story of an umbrella that expands in the rain to cover a multitude of animals.)
3. Brown, M., *All Butterflies*. New York: Charles Scribner's Sons, 1974. (Alphabet book with phrases beginning with two sequential alphabet letters as "All butterflies; Cats dance; Elephants fly."
4. ———, *Peter Piper's Alphabet*. New York: Charles Scribner's Sons, 1959. (Tongue twisters that provoke mirth.)
5. Browner, R., *Everyone Has a Name*. New York: Henry C. Walck, 1961. (Clues to the names and characteristics of different animals.)
6. Breinburg, P., *Shawn Goes to School*. New York: Thomas Y. Crowell Company, 1974. (Shawn really wants to go to school but is frightened until the teacher calms him by getting him interested in other children and toys.)
7. Christopher, M., *Jinx Glove*. New York: Coward, McCann & Geoghegan, (Old baseball gloves are best.)
8. Crews, D., *We Read: A to Z*. New York: Harper & Row, Publishers, Inc., 1967. (Concepts that begin with letters; *a* is represented by *almost*.)
9. Dugan, W., *The Truck and Bus Book*. New York: Golden Press, Inc., 1966. (Short descriptions of various trucks and buses.)
10. Fassler, J., *Howie Helps Himself*. Racine, Wis.: Albert Whitman, 1975. (Howie can't run, skip, or ride a bike, for he has cerebral palsy. The story of Howie's going to a special school for the handicapped.)
11. Fife, D., *Adam's ABC*. New York: Coward, McCann & Geoghegan, 1971. (One day in the life of a black child in an urban setting.)
12. Fort, J., *June the Tiger*. Boston: Little, Brown and Company, 1975. (The story of a dog, his old mistress, and the enemy, a bear.)
13. Freeman, D., *The Seal and the Slick*. New York: The Viking Press, Inc., 1974. (Children clean the flippers of a seal who has been caught in an oil slick and who then returns to his family who move to another spot where there is no oil slick.)
14. Gag, W., *The ABC Bunny*. New York: Coward, McCann & Geoghegan, 1933. (The alphabet in rhyme centered around a bunny.)
15. ———, *Nothing at All*. New York: Coward, McCann & Geoghegan, 1941. (The story of three litle orphan dogs.)
16. Hoberman, M. A., *Nuts to You and Nuts to Me*. New York: Alfred A. Knopf, Inc., 1974. (An alphabet of poems. Fun.)

17. Holl, A., *The ABC's of Carts, Trucks, and Machines*. New York: American Heritage Press, 1970. (Rhymes about police cars, dump trucks, and the like.)
18. Joseph, S. M., ed., *The Me Nobody Knows*. New York: Avon Books, Inc., 1969. (Poems and essays written by black or Puerto Rican ghetto children. Includes four sections: (1) How I see Myself, (2) How I See My Neighborhood, (3) The World Outside, and (4) Things I Can't See or Touch.)
19. Klein, L., *How Old Is Old?* New York: Harvey House, Inc., Publishers, 1967. (The concept of age is presented using as a base the ages at which different animals are considered old. Ages of people vary, and *how old is old* depends on who is doing the evaluating.)
20. Kuskin, K., *Any Me I Want to Be*. New York: Harper & Row, Publishers, Inc., 1972. (What it would be like to be something other than you—like a bird, a sandwich, or a front door key.)
21. Lear, E., *A Was Once An Apple Pie: A Nonsense Alphabet*. New York: Scholastic Book Services, 1969. (An old favorite in paperback version with delightful illustrations.)
22. Lester, S. A., *Lost*. New York: Harcourt Brace Jovanovich, Inc., 1975. (A little boy gets lost at the zoo but finds another smaller boy who is also lost and whom he helps. Finally the boys are reunited with their families.)
23. Lobel, A., *The Man Who Took the Indoors Out*. New York: Harper & Row, Publishers, Inc., 1974. (Nonsense tale about a man who loved all the things in the house and felt they should have a taste of the outdoors. And so he took outside tables, chairs, dishes, a sink, and so on, which then refused to go back in the house.)
24. Matthiesen, T., *ABC: An Alphabet Book*. New York: Platt & Munk, 1966. (Letters based on everyday experiences.)
25. McGinley, P., *All Around the Town*. Philadelphia: J. B. Lippincott Co., 1948. (A tale of city sights beginning with *A* and ending with *Z*.)
26. Peppé, R., *The Alphabet Book*. New York: Four Winds Press, 1968. (Based on objects familiar to children.)
27. Prelutsky, J., *The Pack Rat's Day and Other Poems*. New York: Macmillan Publishing Co., Inc., 1974. (Fifteen poems about different animals. Fun verse.)
28. Rice, E., *New Blue Shoes*. New York: Macmillan Publishing Co., Inc., 1975. (Rebecca goes shopping for new shoes and really wants blue ones but is persuaded to get the sturdy kind.)
29. Dr. Seuss, *ABC*. New York: Random House, Inc., 1963. (An exciting ABC book.)
30. Simon, M., and H. Simon, *If You Were An Eel, How Would You Feel?* Chicago: Follett Publishing Company, 1963. (The eel, bear, tortoise, bat, cat, and seal are introduced with "If you were a—." Motivates oral communication.)
31. Sullivan, J., *Round Is a Pancake*. New York: Holt, Rinehart and Winston, Inc., 1963. (Shapes related to children's experiences.)
32. Udry, J., *A Tree is Nice*. New York: Harper & Row, Publishers, Inc., 1956. (Many concepts about trees are pictured.)

APPENDIX II

Influence of
Public Law 94-142
on Speech, Language and
Hearing Services

FUNDING

A state through its official educational agency and each of the local educational agencies may receive federal funds under Part B of the Education of the Handicapped Act as amended by Public Law 94-142. Part B provides formula grants to both state and local educational agencies to assist them in educating handicapped children. As a condition for receiving the funds, however, each state and local agency must comply with the provisions of P.L.94-142.

LEAST RESTRICTIVE EDUCATIONAL ENVIRONMENT

The law requires that the handicapped children be placed in the "least restrictive educational environment" (Sec. 504—Sec. 84.33(b)). Whenever possible, the child is to be educated in a regular classroom but with supporting services. When he cannot be educated in a regular classroom, he may be placed in a special class. The local education agency must then provide the necessary special class or resource room.

CARRYING OUT THE LAW

For the speech/language clinician the steps involved in carrying out the law are:

1. Identification of speech, hearing and language impaired.
2. Assessment of the suspected area of deficit by a team.
3. Placement by a team accompanied by appropriate services.
4. Planning an individual education program with parental approval.
5. Evaluation of the plan by a team including the parents. The parents have the right to a hearing if they believe that the intervention involved is inadequate.
6. Evaluation.

Identification of Speech and Language Impaired

Both the local and state educational agencies must conduct an annual program to identify, locate, and evaluate all handicapped children in their respective jurisdictions regardless of the severity of their handicaps. Obviously the identification of speech-, language-, and hearing-handicapped children is a necessary prerequisite to planning, programming, and appropriating funds for them to attend school.

Assessment of the Suspected Area of Deficit by a Team with Parent Participation

The speech/language clinician usually participates in the workings of the law under two conditions:

1. As a major coordinator. Since speech/language pathology and audiology are included under both *special education* and *related services*, when all the remediation the child needs is in the field of speech and/or language, the primary responsibility lies with the speech/language clinician. In this instance, the speech/language clinician provides the necessary special education.
2. As a member of the support team. When the child's primary disability is a handicap such as mental retardation, the major responsibility for special education lies with the Director of the Mentally Retarded or some similar professional. The speech/language clinican, however, is one of the team members who supplies support services.

The team for the assessment of a speech disorder may consist of the speech/language clinician and the child's regular classroom teacher.

For the assessment of a language disorder, the team may include, besides the classroom teacher, other school personnel such as a psychologist, audiologist, reading specialist, medical officer, and/or an educational examiner. Before the team begins its assessment, the parents must be notified and their consent obtained, When the parent does not respond, the school may either compel him through a due process hearing, start the assessment after giving notice, or retain the child in the present placement until the consent is obtained.

The team must include someone able to give the necessary diagnostic tests, and the placement must be based on more than one test. For example, for a child with an articulatory disability, the pathologist might well administer an articulation test, then tape and analyze a sample of his conversational speech—showing missing phonemes, error phonemes, and the distinctive features of the error phonemes.

Where necessary, the child is referred to other specialists, such as an otologist in the case of a hearing difficulty. When the medical service is needed for diagnostic purposes, it is provided at no cost to the parent. When the medical services are restorative in nature, they are not, however, funded under P.L.94-142. But if a hearing aid is an essential element of the child's special education to overcome his handicap so that the child can be part of a regular classroom, the aid is paid for under the law.

Turnbull and Turnbull (1978, p. 101) summarize the requirements for evaluation succinctly: P.L. 94-142 requires that the interpretation of evaluation results and the decision about the student's placement be made by a team of persons who are familiar with the student, the placement options, and the meaning of the evaluation results. The team must include at least one teacher or other specialist knowledgeable in the area of the suspected disability. The team must also include the child's regular teacher (or a regular teacher qualified to conduct the class he might be placed in), and a person qualified to conduct individual diagnostic examinations. Thus, a variety of educators within a school system must be competent in administering and interpreting evaluations.

The Individual Education Program

The term *indivualized educational program* (IEP) involves a written statement for each handicapped child. It must include:

1. A statement of the child's present levels of educational performance. This statement must be based on at least two assessment procedures.

2. A statement of annual goals, including short term instructional objectives.
3. A statement of the specific special education-related services to be provided to the child and the extent to which the child will be able to participate in regular educational programs.
4. The projected dates for initiation of services and the anticipated duration of the services.
5. Appropriate objective criteria for evaluation and evaluation procedures and schedules for determining, on at least an annual basis, whether the short-term instruction objectives are being achieved. These do not need to be elaborate; simple records of correct and incorrect responses, test scores, and check lists of behavior are ample.

The team for developing the IEP must include a representative of the public agency who is qualified to supervise, the child's special educator, the child's teacher, one or both of the child's parents, the student when appropriate, and other individuals at the discretion of the parents or agency. One member of the IEP team must have attended the previous assessment procedures so that he/she can interpret the results of the evaluation. The parents must be given advance notice of the meeting and when necessary an interpreter must be furnished (as when the parents cannot hear or cannot speak English). The meeting can only be held without the parents when the agency can document that it was impossible to get them to participate. The documentation must include detailed records of telephone calls, copies of letters sent and results of visits to the parents' home or places of work.

Evaluation

The evaluation process is not to be viewed as a tool for placement but rather as an aid in individual program planning. It is conducted at various points in the educational process, beginning with the initial assessment, which indicates the type of educational handicap, specifies the child's current level of performance, and gives continuous assessment of the short-term objectives specified in the student's individual education plan. Its purposes are to aid in developing the individual program, to give daily or weekly measurement of the child's progress, and to monitor progress in meeting the long-term objectives outlined in the IEP.

Parents have the right to obtain an independent evaluation at their own expense. When parents provide this information to the school team, the agency must take it into consideration as a basis for providing the child with an appropriate education. The person who does the independent evaluation, however, must be qualified in terms of certification, licensing, or registration.

Due Process

Since parental involvement is a goal in the development of the IEP, the parents must receive written notices indicating any proposal to assess a handicapped child, to confer about his/her IEP, or to initiate a change in the identification or educational placement of the child. Either or both parents may participate at an IEP conference and, consequently, they must be notified in ample time to make the necessary arrangements. The notice must include a description of actions proposed or refused by the agency, the options available, and the reasons why any of the options were rejected. The notice must further contain a description of each evaluation procedure, test, record, or report that serve as a basis for recommendations for placement and/or remediation. The parents must give consent to conducting a placement evaluation and to the initial placement of a handicapped child in need of special education services. They may revoke their consent as the program proceeds.

Parents have the opportunity to present complaints "with respect to any matter relating to the identification, evaluation or educational placement of the child or the provision of a free appropriate public education to such child." (Sec. 615(b)(1)(E) The complaint then takes place when the parents are dissatisfied. Section 615(b)(2) states:

> Whenever a complaint has been received, the parents or guardian shall have an opportunity for an impartial due process hearing which shall be conducted by the state educational agency or by the local educational agency or intermediate educational unit, as determined by state law by the state educational agency. No hearing conducted pursuant to the requirements of this paragraph shall be conducted by an employee of such agency or unit involved in the education or care of the child.

From the time when the complaint is received, the school district has 45 days in which to hold the hearing and to mail a final decision to the parties. Either party can request an extension of time.

At the early stages of disagreement, the school and the parents try to work together to agree on the IEP and to compromise on some of their differences and finally to come to mutually acceptable solutions. When the differences cannot be worked out, parents may call for a hearing, which is conducted by a person who does not have a professional or personal interest in the outcome. The purpose of the hearing officer is to assure procedural fairness during the meeting. All evidence to be used must be disclosed to the other party. Obviously, it is incumbent on the speech/language clinician to write the IEP carefully, to keep accurate records of therapy sessions, of evaluation, of test results—all the items that go into making the assessment, the IEP, and its management. The hearing officer then hears the witnesses on both sides, examines the written statements. Each side is cross-examined on its statements. The parties are both given a chance to make closing statements indicating why the evidence supports or does not support their positions. The parent has the right to be represented by counsel. Witnesses are examined on their strategies of therapy, their qualifications, their familiarity with the child, their experiences with children with similar handicaps. The reasons for the particular placement and for the IEP are examined. As noted earlier, no single test can justify a placement; the evaluation must be made by a team, must be administered in the child's language, and by trained personnel. When a child has impaired sensory, manual, or speaking skills, the test must accurately reflect the child's abilities rather than the child's impairment.

The hearing officer's decision must be based on the evidence and testing in the record. The officer can accept, reject, or modify the plan or can require the district to start a new plan. The officer must present a written document giving the reasons for the decision, which document is available to both parties. Decisions are final and both the parents and the school must accept them as such. The decision, however, can be appealed by filing a civil action in either a state court or a federal district court.

EXAMPLE OF A P.L.94-142 HEARING

Miller, Miller, and Madison (1980) report on a P.L.94-142 hearing that resulted from a dispute between a local school district (a large urban district) and the parents of an acoustically handicapped student. The hearing was the culmination of a series of unsuccessful meetings between the parents and school district officials regarding the student's Individualized Education Program for the 1977–78 school year. The subject was a 16-year-old eighth grader with a profound bilateral sensorineural hearing loss. He read at fourth-grade level and functioned below grade level in all academic areas except mathematics. The speech/language clinician determined that the boy had limited communication skills. Less than 10 per cent of his speech was intelligible. He used manual deaf signs as a primary means of communication but he was somewhat confused in the use of these for he had been exposed to a variety of manual sign systems.

The initial IEP conferences was attended by the boy's teacher, the clinician, the student advisor representing the school administration and the district Coordinator of Services for the Deaf and Hearing Impaired. The Initial IEP was formed and was changed several times during the year. Finally a hearing, requested by the parents under the due process of P.L.94-142, was held with a number of concerned personnel presenting evidence: the boy, his parents, the classroom teacher, three of the boy's former teachers, the local school district Supervisor of Special Education, the Coordinator of Services for the Deaf and Hearing Impaired, the Budget Director for the district, the President of the local Deaf Parent Teacher Organization, and the speech/language clinician.

The specific charges brought included:

1. The boy did not receive an appropriate education because the goals and objectives as specified in the IEP did not attempt to bring his levels of achievement, such as reading ability, up to the normal range for his age group.
2. The district did not provide the boy with an individualized program, because others in his class received the same number of hours of intervention by the speech/language clinician and the same number of hours of language arts instruction by the teacher.
3. The subject was not placed in the least restrictive environment, because he was not allowed to attend the school closest to his home. Instead, he was bused across the city to a school where the program for the acoustically handicapped was housed.
4. The district's compliance with P.L.94-142 consisted of the paperwork and IEP conferences rather than any substantive changes from previously existing programs for handicapped students.
(Miller, Miller & Madison 1980, page 78).

The parents asked that he be allowed to attend the high school nearest his home, which offered no special services for the deaf, that he be provided with the services of an interpreter assigned solely to him who would attend all his classes, and that he receive the services of a speech/language clinician for two hours of daily one-to-one instruction.

The clinician's role was important. She gave testimony in these areas:

1. Selection criteria of clients.
2. The clinician's case load. She was asked to produce data on how

many students she serviced per year, how many of these students were enrolled in her remediation program, and what progress she noted in those with whom she had worked. She was also asked about the number of hours of remediation provided for children with various categories of handicap severity.

3. Extent of services. The clinician was questioned about the number of hours provided for the boy on a weekly and yearly basis. She explained why she was unable to provide one hour of daily one-to-one intervention during 1977–78.

4. One-to-one instruction. She was asked if, in her professional opinion, one-to-one instruction in language would bring the boy up to grade level in reading and communication skills.

5. Extent of the boy's handicapping condition. She was asked to read her formal assessment of the boy's speech and language skills. In addition, the attorney for the plaintiff read paragraphs written by the boy and asked the clinician to comment on the subject's level of skill in written communication.

6. Parent contacts. The clinician testified regarding the parents' attitudes—their cooperation and their willingness to work with the clinician on a program of follow-up after intervention.
(Miller, Miller, and Madison, 1980, p. 80)

This hearing points first of all to the need for the clinician to keep careful records. The clinician needs to be aware of accountability procedures, to write formal assessments, and to pinpoint the deficiencies of handicapped students. Consequently the clinician keeps records on the numbers and names of students seen, students enrolled in the service program and the severity of their handicaps, the dates of contacts with parents including notes on exchanges between parents and clinician. He/she plans the schedule in September with enrollment dates and a rationale for scheduling children at specific times.

Secondly, it points to the need for explaining to parents what behavior changes are realistic. Probably the communication between parents and school should begin before the initial formal meeting. The IEP should be changed according to the needs and progress of the child. Every effort should be made to avoid the formal public hearings.

1982 SUPREME COURT HEARING

Dena Kleiman (New York Times, March 24, 1982, page B1) reports that the Supreme Court for the first time will clarify the meaning of "free appropriate public education" as applied to the handicapped in Public Law 94-142. The case involves the parents of a fourth grade deaf child in the academic upper half of her class and a New York State school district. So far the district has provided the deaf child with a wireless FM hearing aid, services of a speech/language clinician and a sign-language teacher, and such other help as a special teletype machine to allow the school personnel and the parents who are both deaf to communicate from the home to the school.

The lawyer for the parents is asking that a sign-language interpreter be assigned to the child so that the child can benefit more fully from classroom instruction through knowing what the teacher and the other children are communicating in the classroom at all times during the school day. On the other hand, the lawyer for the school district is challenging the jurisdiction of federal courts to determine the meaning of "appropriate public education;" the two lower federal courts have already decided in favor of the parents of the child. The decision of the Supreme Court will provide answers to such questions as: Does an appropriate education mean one that enables a child to become a "functioning member of society" or does it mean giving the child the kind of assistance that will provide an "opportunity to achieve his/her full potential?" The Supreme Court decided in favor of the school district.

Since the Federal Government is presently contemplating: 1) changes in the regulations of P.L. 94-142 and 2) legislation to amend P.L. 94-142, we recommend that you read S. Dublinske, "Action School Services," *Language, Speech, and Hearing Services in Schools*, 13 (April 1982), 134–136. We also suggest that you follow the Action School Services Reports in subsequent issues of *Language, Speech, and Hearing Services in Schools*.

References and Suggested Readings

Anderson, R. M., J. G. Greer and S. J. Odle, *Individualizing Educational Materials for Special Children in the Mainstream*. Baltimore: University Park Press, 1978. (Explains how to provide individualized institutional materials for handicapped students while they are being mainstreamed. Outlines the components of the Individual Educational Plan.)

Arena, J., *How to Write an IEP*. Novata, California: Academic Therapy Publications, 1978. (Explains P.L.94-142—mainstreaming, due process, and formulation of the IEP.)

Downey, M., "Due Process Hearings and P.L.94-142." *ASHA*, **22** (April 1980), 255–257. (Explains what may trigger a hearing and the nature of the due process hearing.)

———, "Conduct of the Due Process Hearing." *ASHA*, **22** (May 1980), 332–334. (Reveals the kind of information requested during a hearing.)

335–337. (Reveals summaries of decisions made in some appeal hearings that are relevant for speech/language clinicians and audiologists.)

———— and E. Sarnecky, "Evaluating P.L.94-142 Plans." *ASHA,* **22** (February 1980), 90–93. (Tells how to get involved in the review of the state's P.L.94-142 plan and indicates the many levels of involvement.)

LaVor, M. L., "History of Federal Legislation Dealing with Children with Specific Learning Disabilities." *ASHA,* **18** (August 1976), 485–490.

Gearhart, B. R., and M. W. Weishahn, *The Handicapped Child in the Regular Classroom.* St. Louis: C. W. Mosby Company, 1976.

Guralnick, M. J., Ed., *Early Intervention and the Integration of Handicapped and Nonhandicapped Children.* Baltimore: University Park Press, 1978. (Explores the possibilities of the handicapped child in the least restrictive environment.)

Miller, S. Q., J. K. Miller and D. L. Madison, "A Speech and Language Clinican's Involvement in a P.L.94-142 Public Hearing: A Case Study," *Language, Speech, and Hearing Services in Schools,* **11** (April 1980), 75–84. Reprinted by permission.

Sunderlin, S., Ed., *The Most Enabling Environment: Education for All Children.* Washington, D.C.: Childhood Education International, 1979. (Explains the implications of P.L.94-142—providing the least restrictive environment and the most enabling environment.)

Tolkoff, E. "Mainstreaming: A Promise Gone Awry." *New York Teacher,* **22** (January 18, 1981), 9–15.

Turnbull, H. R., and A. P. Turnbull, *Free Appropriate Public Education: Law and Implementation.* Denver, Colorado: Love Producing Company, 1978. (Explains clearly and very thoroughly all the implications of the law. An unusually good reference book on the law.)

Turnbull, A. P., B. B. Strickland and J. C. Brantley, *Developing and Implementing Individualized Educational Programs.* Columbus, Ohio: Charles E. Merrill, 1978. (Explains the essential elements of the individualzed educational plan as specified in P.L.94-142; describes the processes and procedures necessary in developing an IEP. Makes clear the need for an understanding of the responsibilities imposed upon teachers, administrators and parents by P.L. 94-142.)

Yater, V. V., *Mainstreaming of Children with a Hearing Loss.* Springfield, Ill: Charles C. Thomas, 1977. (Presents the legal, legislative, and education principles for the academic integration of hearing-impaired children.)

AUTHOR INDEX

SUBJECT INDEX